Midwifery Emergencies at a Glance

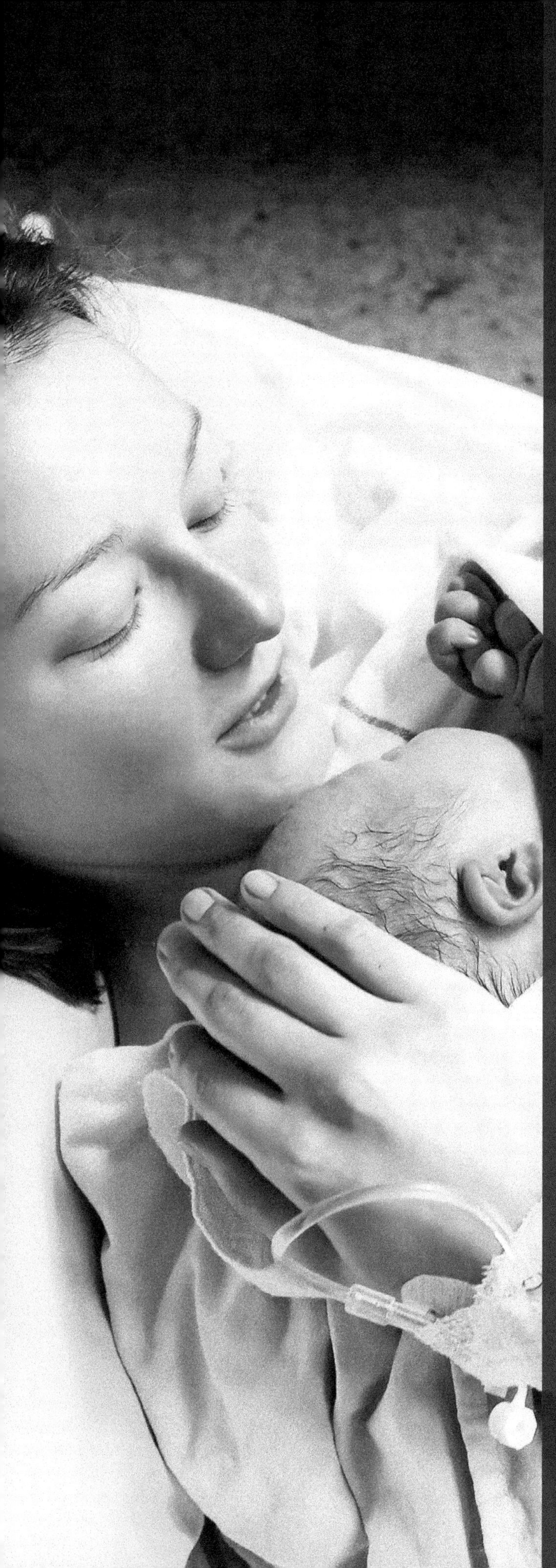

Midwifery Emergencies at a Glance

Denise (Dee) Campbell

MA, PgDip, BSc, RM, RN, FHEA
Principal Lecturer and Programme Tutor in Midwifery (*retired*)
University of Hertfordshire
Hatfield, UK

Susan M. Carr

MA, PgCert, BSc, RM, RN, FHEA
Principal Lecturer and Programme Leader in Midwifery
University of Hertfordshire
Hatfield, UK

Series editor:
Ian Peate OBE, FRCN

WILEY Blackwell

Registered Offices:
John Wiley & Sons, Inc., 111 River Street, Hoboken, NJ 07030, USA
John Wiley & Sons, Ltd., The Atrium, Southern Gate, Chichester, West Sussex, PO19 8SQ, UK

Editorial Office:
9600 Garsington Road, Oxford, OX4 2DQ, UK

For details of our global editorial offices, customer services, and more information about Wiley products visit us at www.wiley.com.

Wiley also publishes its books in a variety of electronic formats and by print-on-demand. Some content that appears in standard print versions of this book may not be available in other formats.

Library of Congress Cataloging-in-Publication Data
Names: Campbell, Denise, 1961– author. | Carr, Susan M. (Susan Mary), 1954– author.
Title: Midwifery emergencies at a glance / by Denise (Dee) Campbell, Susan M. Carr.
Description: Hoboken, NJ : John Wiley & Sons, Inc., 2018. | Series: At a glance series | Includes bibliographical references and index. |
Identifiers: LCCN 2018015376 (print) | LCCN 2018015920 (ebook) | ISBN 9781119138020 (pdf) | ISBN 9781119138044 (epub) | ISBN 9781119138013 (pbk.)
Subjects: | MESH: Obstetric Labor Complications | Midwifery | Emergency Treatment—methods | Handbooks
Classification: LCC RG571 (ebook) | LCC RG571 (print) | NLM WQ 165 | DDC 618.2/025—dc23
LC record available at https://lccn.loc.gov/2018015376

Cover image: © Natalia Deriabina/Getty Images
Cover design by Wiley

Set in 9.5/11.5pt Minion Pro by Aptara
Printed and bound by CPI Group (UK) Ltd, Croydon, CR0 4YY

10 9 8 7 6 5 4 3 2 1

Contents

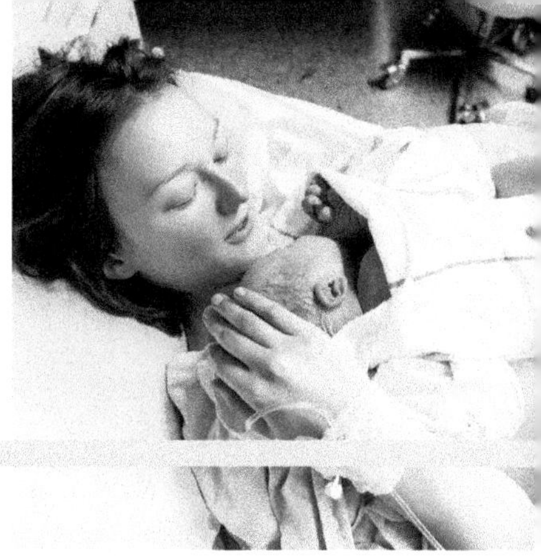

Preface viii
Abbreviations ix
About the companion website x

Part 1 **Professional issues 1**

Section 1 Professionalism
1 Professional standards 2
2 Communications during an emergency 4

Part 2 **Emergency skills 7**

Section 2 Resuscitation
3 Maternal resuscitation 8
4 Neonatal resuscitation 10

Section 3 Haemorrhage
5 Antepartum haemorrhage 14
6 Primary postpartum haemorrhage 16
7 Secondary postpartum haemorrhage 18

Section 4 Malpresentations and multiple pregnancy
8 Occipito posterior positions 20
9 Face and brow presentations 22
10 Breech presentations 24
11 Cord presentation and prolapse 26
12 Twins 28

Section 5 Dystocia
13 Shoulder dystocia 30
14 Uterine dystocia – failure to progress 32

Section 6 Placental separation problems
15 Manual removal of the placenta 34
16 Adhered or partially adhered placenta 36

Section 7 Uterine emergencies
17 Uterine inversion 38
18 Uterine rupture and scar dehiscence 40

Part 3 Medical and psychological emergencies 43

Section 8 Psychological disorders

19 Post-traumatic stress disorder 44
20 Postnatal depression (mood disorder) 46
21 Puerperal (postpartum) psychosis 48

Section 9 Hypertensive disorders of pregnancy

22 Pre-eclampsia 50
23 Eclampsia 52

Section 10 Embolic and coagulation disorders

24 Venous thromboembolism 54
25 Amniotic fluid embolism 56
26 Disseminated intravascular coagulation 58

Section 11 Preterm labour

27 Prelabour rupture of membranes 60
28 Preterm labour and delivery 62

Part 4 Associated skills 65

Section 12 Instrumental and Operative deliveries

29 Instrumental vaginal delivery 66
30 Preparation and transfer to the operating theatre 68
31 Role of the scrub midwife or nurse 70
32 Receiving the baby in the operating theatre 72
33 Immediate care following surgery 74

Section 13 Fetal surveillance

34 Electronic fetal monitoring – actions following a suspicious or pathological trace 76
35 Fetal scalp electrode 78
36 Fetal blood sampling 80

Section 14 Maternal monitoring

37 Recognising the deteriorating woman 82
38 Examination *per vaginam* 84
39 Speculum examination 86
40 Urinary catheterisation 88

Section 15 Venous skills

41 Venepuncture 90
42 Intravenous cannulation 92
43 Blood transfusion therapy 94

Section 16 Augmentation

44 Artificial rupture of membranes 96
45 Oxytocic augmentation 98

Section 17 Perineal Trauma

46 Third- and fourth-degree tears 100
47 Perineal suturing 102

Section 18 Infection awareness

48 Maternal sepsis 104
49 Source isolation nursing 106
50 Group B streptococcus 108
51 Infection control 110

Self-assessment 113

Section 19 Revision and self-assessment

Multiple choice questions 114
Multiple choice answers 121

References 124
Index 131

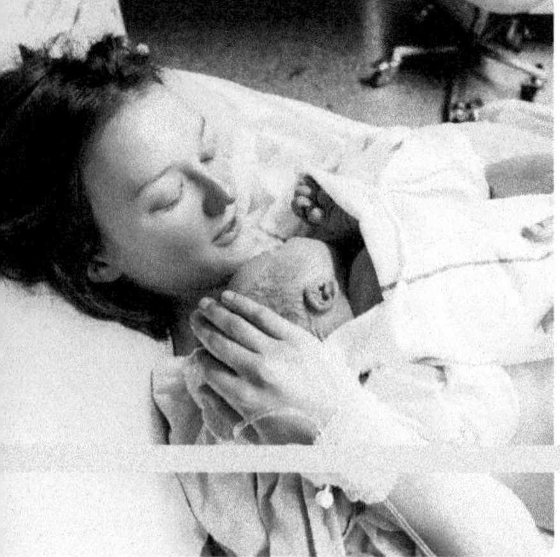

Preface

Statement 15 of The Code (Nursing and Midwifery Council, 2015) reminds us that a midwife 'must always offer help if an emergency arises in the practice setting or anywhere else' – the expectation is one of competent assessment and prompt actions in response to an obstetric or neonatal emergency. The intention of this book is to provide clear guidance on the factors which predispose to complications, so that preventative management can be employed whenever possible. Moreover, it should provide a concise, ordered overview which clearly directs the midwife through the management of an emergency in the specific order that the skills will be required. This is a resource that is intended to help guide the development of essential skills, but also to support the revision and maintenance of the skills during continuing professional development. In addition, many emergency situations may require additional, associated skills and so many of these are also included in this book. These may be useful in assisting in the progress of emergency management or to provide further review, screening or diagnostics.

The need to comply with the 'At A Glance' style, with chapters typically reduced to a double page, has presented its challenges. As midwifery lecturers, we have struggled to omit aspects that have previously been fundamental to our teaching sessions, such as the physiology behind the emergency and the evidence behind a particular management approach. We have had to reduce the detail to essentials only and become as succinct as was necessary. The result is a very pleasing, simple and clearly written guide, which gets straight to the heart of the skill, just as these books are intended to do. In addition, a page of varied figures provides additional information and/or improved clarity in a visual form. Its simplicity makes it a very useful tool – progressing directly to the specific management of the emergency.

For those with questioning minds who wish to increase their background knowledge, we have included, for your own analysis, many of the references that guide the management. Plus, the website contains the fully expanded answers to the multiple choice questions as not all the answers are to be found within the text – we hope this will encourage further reading.

This book is written predominantly with the midwife in mind – both for the student and for those already qualified. However, it would also support the education and continuing development of medical students, junior doctors, general practitioners and paramedics – any of whom may find themselves initiating emergency midwifery, obstetric or neonatal care.

Abbreviations

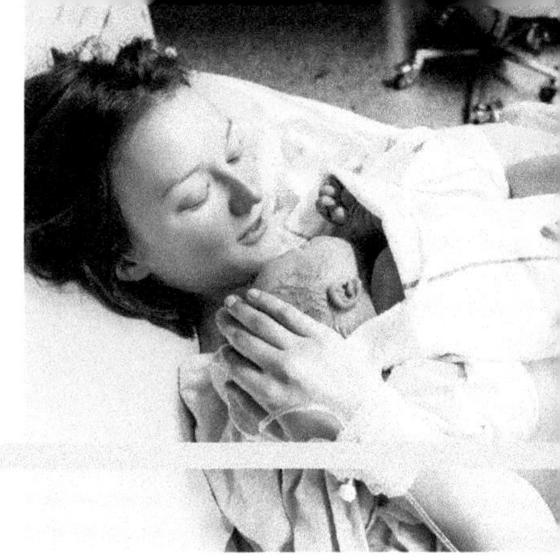

ACOG	American College of Obstetricians and Gynecologists
AED	Automated external defibrillator
AF	All fours
AFE	Amniotic fluid embolism
AP	Antero posterior
APA	American Psychiatric Association
APH	Antepartum haemorrhage
APTT	Activated partial thromboplastin time
ARM	Artificial rupture of membranes
BMI	Body mass index
BP	Blood pressure
bpm	Beats per minute
BVM	Bag, valve and mask
CODP	College of Operating Department Professionals
CPD	Cephalo-pelvic disproportion
CPD	Continuing Professional Development
CPR	Cardio-pulmonary resuscitation
CRP	C-reactive protein
CS	Caesarean section
CTG	Cardiotocography
CTPA	Computerised tomography pulmonary angiogram
DBP	Diastolic blood pressure
DIC	Disseminated intravascular coagulation
DTA	Deep transverse arrest
DVT	Deep vein thrombosis
ECG	Electrocardiography
ECT	Electroconvulsive therapy
ECTG	Electrocardiotocography
EPDS	Edinburgh Postnatal Depression Scale
FBC	Full blood count
FBS	Fetal blood sampling
FDP	Fibrinogen degradation products
fFN	Fetal fibronectin
FSE	Fetal scalp electrode
GAS	Group A streptococcus
GBS	Group B streptococcus
GMC	General Medical Council
HDU	High dependency unit
HELLP	Haemolysis, elevated liver enzymes, low platelet count (syndrome)
HVS	High vaginal swab
ICU	Intensive Care Unit
IM	Intramuscular
ISBT	International Society of Blood Transfusion
IV	Intravenous
IVF	*In vitro* fertilisation
JPAC	Joint United Kingdom Blood Transfusion and Tissue Transplantation Services Professional Advisory Committee
LFT	Liver function tests
LMWT	Low molecular weight heparin therapy
LSCS	Lower segment Caesarean section
LVS	Low vaginal swab
MDT	Multidisciplinary team
MEOWS	Modified Early Obstetric Warning System
MROP	Manual removal of the placenta
NEWS	National Early Warning System
NHLBI	National Heart, Lung and Blood Institute
NICE	National Institute for Health and Care Excellence
NICU	Neonatal intensive care unit
NMC	Nursing and Midwifery Council
NPSA	National Patient Safety Agency
OA	Occipito anterior
OASI	Obstetric anal sphincter injuries
OOB	Obstetric Observation Bay
OP	Occipito posterior
PE	Pulmonary embolism
PEEP	Positive end expiratory pressure
PET	Pre-eclamptic toxaemia
PP	Placenta praevia
PP	Presenting part
PPH	Postpartum haemorrhage
PPROM	Preterm premature rupture of membranes
PROM	Premature rupture of membranes
PTSD	Post-traumatic stress disorder
RCM	Royal College of Midwives
RCOG	Royal College of Obstetricians and Gynaecologists
REM	Rapid eye movement
SATS	Oxygen saturation
SBAR	Situation, Background, Assessment, Recommendation
SBP	Systolic blood pressure
SCBU	Special care baby unit
SHOT	Serious hazards of transfusion
SIRS	Systemic inflammatory response
SR	Semirecumbent
UKTIS	United Kingdom Teratology Information Service
VTE	Venous thromboembolism
WHO	World Health Organization

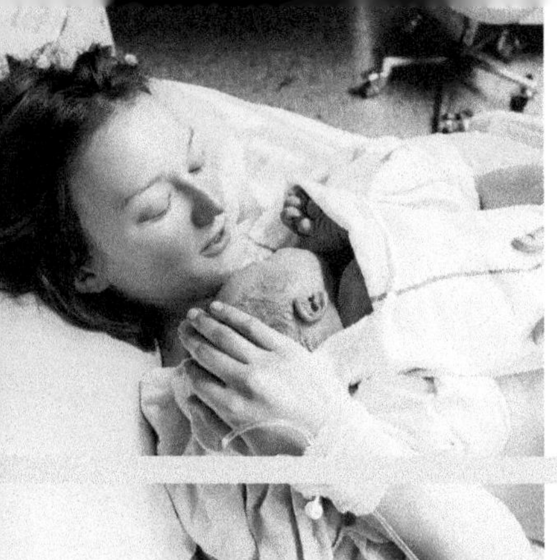

About the companion website

This book is accompanied by a companion website:

www.ataglanceseries.com/midwiferyemergencies

The website includes:

- Multiple choice questions (MCQs) and fully expanded answers

Professional issues

Chapters

Section 1 Professionalism

1 Professional standards 2
2 Communications during an emergency 4

1 Professional standards

Figure 1.1 Standards for pre-registration midwifery education. Source: https://www.nmc.org.uk/standards/additional-standards/standards-for-pre-registration-midwifery-education/. Reproduced with permission of NMC.

Figure 1.2 The Code. Source: https://www.nmc.org.uk/code/. Reproduced with permission of NMC.

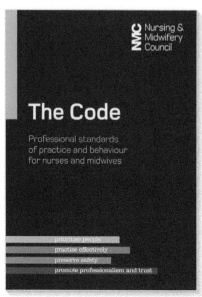

Figure 1.3 Standards to support learning and assessment in practice. Source: https://www.nmc.org.uk/standards/additional-standards/standards-to-support-learning-and-assessment-in-practice/. Reproduced with permission of NMC.

Figure 1.4 Standards for medicines management. Source: https://www.nmc.org.uk/standards/additional-standards/standards-for-medicines-management/. Reproduced with permission of NMC.

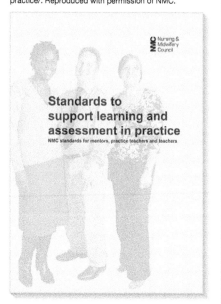

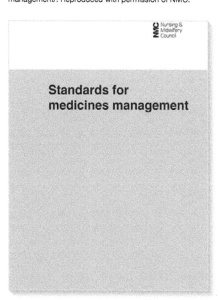

Figure 1.5 Standards for competence for registered midwives. Source: https://www.nmc.org.uk/globalassets/sitedocuments/standards/nmc-standards-for-competence-for-registered-midwives.pdf. Reproduced with permission of NMC.

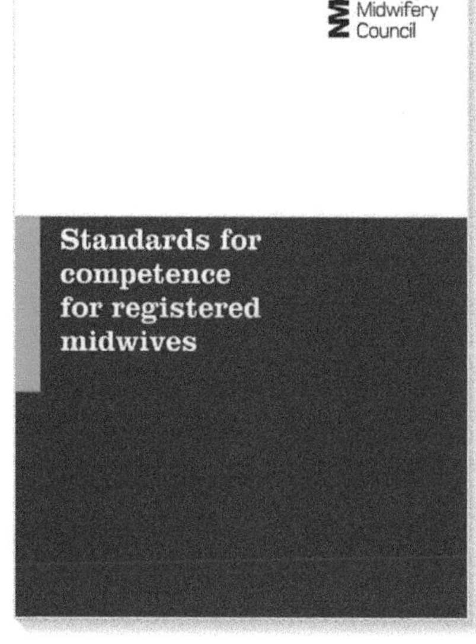

Figure 1.6 Revalidation. Source: http://revalidation.nmc.org.uk/. Reproduced with permission of NMC.

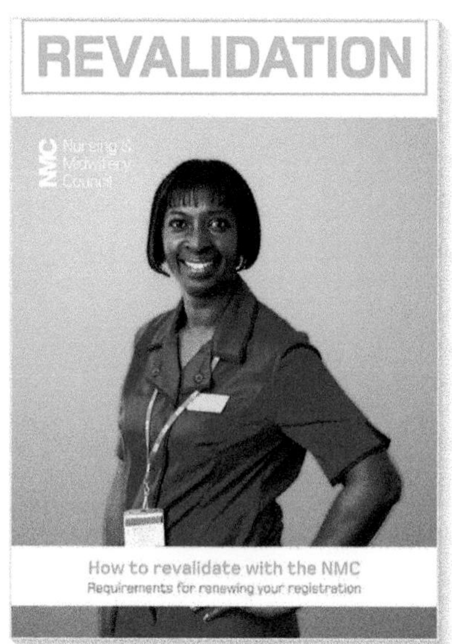

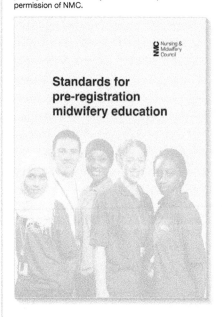

Midwifery Emergencies at a Glance, First Edition. Denise (Dee) Campbell and Susan M. Carr. © 2018 John Wiley & Sons, Ltd. Published 2018 by John Wiley & Sons, Ltd.
Companion website: www.ataglanceseries.com/midwiferyemergencies

This book is intended to inform and educate practitioners about the management of emergencies and the many associated skills. These emergencies may happen in a range of settings from fully equipped and staffed obstetric units to the stand-alone unit or homebirth. The practitioner has a professional responsibility to meet the standards necessary and to become so familiar with these skills that they can adapt them to any setting. They must be able to team work effectively and appropriately manage all the help available. In an ideal situation, the emergency will be supported by a full obstetric, paediatric, anaesthetic and operative team as required, with additional support from haematology, pathology, microbiology, blood bank, pharmacy and porters. When the practitioner is alone they must simultaneously initiate emergency management and call for assistance.

This chapter cannot cover all professional responsibilities associated with emergency management. It will concentrate on the need to achieve and maintain professional standards, continue professional development, maintain a high standard of record keeping, and show awareness of accountability.

Achievement and maintenance of professional standards

The standards of clinical expertise achieved by midwives are controlled by a number of training and monitoring processes. This begins at the interview and admission stage to midwifery training. The profession is looking not only for those academically able, but also for those whose personalities and ethical stance will enhance the profession and improve standards of care. Service users, clinicians, and midwifery tutors jointly decide on the selection approach to be used and which candidates have met these exacting standards. All training programmes align with stringent Nursing and Midwifery Council (NMC, 2009) guidelines and are variously quality monitored throughout (see Figure 1.1). The aim is to achieve clinical competency at the point of qualifying (alongside the skills of life-long learning).

With employment there comes a period of preceptorship (support, monitoring, and development). This is followed by regular employer and professional body review with standards monitored against local policies, as well as professional standards such as: The Code (NMC, 2015) (see Figure 1.2); Standards to support learning and assessment in practice (NMC, 2008) (see Figure 1.3); Standards of medicine management (NMC, 2007) (see Figure 1.4); Standards for competence for registered midwives (NMC, 2011) (see Figure 1.5); and, in addition, a great number of local hospital protocols. Periodic Revalidation (NMC, 2017) is required and this can only be met through a combination of clinical experience and continuing professional development (CPD) (see Figure 1.6).

Continuing professional development

In order to perform within expected standards of care, the professional has a duty to maintain skill competencies and knowledge levels. The process of Revalidation ensures that midwives engage in CPD, but most midwives will surpass any minimum levels set.

Midwives should maintain critical awareness of:

- Current research.
- Topical literature.
- Local and national statistics, case conferences, audits.
- E-learning material.
- Conference material.
- Local and national guidelines, for example NICE.
- New medications for use in obstetrics.
- Risk management reports.
- Evidence from the numerous reports produced by Mothers and Babies: Reducing Risk through Audits and Confidential Enquires across the UK (MBRRACE-UK).

They must attend clinical skills updates including:

- Interprofessional/multidisciplinary skills sessions in house.
- Local skills and drills requirements such as fire safety awareness, manual handling, blood products, documentation, etc.
- National/international skill courses, for example Advanced Life Support in Obstetrics (ALSO), Newborn Life Support (NLS), Practical Obstetric Multi-Professional Training (PROMPT).
- Limitations and capabilities including communication and referral.

Record keeping

A high standard of contemporaneous record keeping has long been understood to be an essential component of good practice. The NMC (2015) provides midwives with guidance on the principles of good record keeping. Yet, it can remain an issue during complaints investigations and is often included as a development requirement during supervised practice. During an emergency, record keeping becomes both a greater challenge and a greater necessity. Best practice would allocate the role of scribe to an individual best suited to the role – someone sufficiently experienced to know the important elements to include. Alongside this it requires:

- Clear, concise, accurate, factual, legible, and contemporaneous statements without abbreviations (unless explained).
- Records to follow local guidelines such that everyone knows where things are recorded.
- Observations of maternal, fetal, or neonatal health recorded.
- Date and time.
- Signatures and printed name.
- Medications recorded including dosage, time of administration, and any reactions.
- All actions taken are noted (including by whom) – whether successful or unsuccessful.
- Reference to any referrals made – the time and to whom, as well as the reason for the referral.

Accountability

Accountability is the taking of responsibility for ones own actions and ability to defend decision making. The professional may be questioned at any time (often years after an event) by a client, employer, professional regulatory body, or through a legal challenge. The professional is judged on whether they performed to the expected standard of care. This is based on the normal standards of professional practice typical at the time of the event. Expectations are also individualised to the circumstances of the incident and are expected to encompass:

- Identification of potential risk.
- Taking preventative measures.
- Competent practice.
- Support of the woman's informed choices.

2 Communications during an emergency

Box 2.1 Principles of good communication during an emergency.

- Taking appropriate turns at speaking and listening – one person as lead professional
- Active listening by all parties – ensuring the intended message is the one heard
- Seek clarification – that the true message has been understood; that you know what is expected
- Concentrate on what is being said whilst active in the care
- Respond appropriately to the lead professional – give updates on progress

Box 2.2 Potential barriers to good communication during an emergency.

- Heightened emotions – adrenaline during emergency, plus anxiety and stress (any party)
- Time limitations and pressures
- Numbers of professionals involved
- Terminology interpreted differently by professional groups
- Prioritising of emergency management over communications
- Personalities within the team
- Equipment noise and distractions

Box 2.3 Professionals potentially involved in emergency obstetric or neonatal care.

- Midwife
- Obstetrician
- Paediatrician
- Anaesthetist
- Delivery suite coordinator
- Students – midwifery or medical
- Specialist medical team
- Specialist midwife
- Operating department assistant
- Translator
- Porter
- Haematologist
- Blood bank staff
- Health care assistants
- Paramedic support (outside of the maternity unit)

Box 2.4 Barriers to collaborative working.

- Hierarchy may be less well defined
- Differing priorities – baby or mother
- Lack of clarity over responsibilities
- Lack of clarity over persons present – particularly when all wearing theatre 'blues'
- Confusing abbreviations and acronyms
- Varying levels of experience

Box 2.5 Enhancers to collaborative working.

- Skills and drills training involving interprofessional groups
- Clarity over people required to attend
- Clearly defined roles
- Identification used by everyone attending
- Clarity over lead professional
- Clarity over goal to be achieved
- Information sharing throughout

Companion website: www.ataglanceseries.com/midwiferyemergencies

Communication is considered to be a two-way interaction in which information is both given and received. This interaction is not only about the content of the communication but also about the process itself and the context in which it is being delivered (see Boxes 2.1 and 2.2). Communication is made up of verbal and non-verbal cues and is not a simple message exchange. It includes not only what is said but also how it is said (intonation), alongside the body language that accompanies it. Then, interpretation of the message by the recipient is influenced by numerous factors including: their own life-experience; knowledge level; socio-cultural issues; health and emotional state; disability; and the environment in which it is received. At the time of an emergency, there also may be anxiety, pain, shock, and fear to interfere with effective listening. Numerous heightened emotions will impact on both sides of the communication.

Informed consent

Informed consent may be gained verbally, in writing, and through the actions of the individual conveying consent. In some emergency situations, aspects of consent may have been gained even before the emergency occurred, for example gaining permission to use an oxytocic drug should a woman begin to haemorrhage. However, in most situations the emergency is unpredictable, unexpected, and the pace of change makes informed consent a challenge.

Achieving a holistic approach to communications between the professionals and the women they care for throughout an emergency is challenging. Whilst keeping the woman informed and gaining consent remain a priority, there are now multiple professionals involved (see Box 2.3) and time is limited. The priority for care becomes the management of the immediate emergency and associated pathophysiology. The concentration will be on emergency practical skills and interprofessional communications to achieve optimal outcomes (see Boxes 2.4 and 2.5). Additionally, the woman may be tired, medicated, frightened, and in pain, which affects her capacity to understand, retain information, appreciate the implications, and communicate her opinions (as expected by the Mental Capacity Act, 2005). All aspects of the management must be directed in the best interests of the woman.

This is not about underestimating the role of communication in general and informed consent in particular. It is about how much more challenging communications become in situations of uncertain outcomes, time limits, and rapidly changing management. It becomes essential that a member of the team takes the role of staying at the head of the bed, with the woman. They should explain and interpret events at an appropriate level. The speed at which the emergency management progresses may not always allow detailed explanations of evidence, discussions, and time for questions, but the essentials must still be applied, and the views of the woman passed back to the team. Communications should include full awareness of body language, good listening skills, and the ability to balance appropriately the information shared in the time available.

Clarification and ongoing communications

It is important that there is a full appreciation of how information is shared. Beware of using unfamiliar words without explaining their meaning, and appreciate that it is not only 'what is said' that portrays a message. Even the most skilful professional can unintentionally communicate through negative intonation or body language.

Be prepared for questions and anxiety. A balance is required between appropriate levels of honesty and realistic reassurances, without making guarantees that may not be achievable. Whilst some information needs to be shared immediately, the full extent of the problem in an emergency can only be determined retrospectively. Therefore, in most cases it is advisable to keep ongoing explanations simple, gaining permission to concentrate on the management of the emergency as the priority, but also giving reassurances that a full explanation of events will follow. This enables a full understanding of the concern to be known, and prevents the early sharing of misleading information (when the emergency may still change, reduce, or escalate). It also allows the woman time to digest the problem and begin to recover from the physical management and emotional shock associated with it.

Communications following the emergency

Following a traumatic episode such as an obstetric or neonatal emergency, adrenaline levels are raised and the woman may be in a state of further anxiety and stress. These are normal responses which will resolve naturally for the majority of women. It is important to appreciate that involvement in an emergency does not typically lead to a lasting stress disorder. Communications following the emergency are not intended as a debriefing exercise, particularly as evidence suggests a single-session may do more harm than good (Bastos *et al.*, 2015). Communications after an emergency are an opportunity to discuss the event in more detail, allow questions, then clarify any misunderstandings following a basic explanation of the emergency and its management. The woman must feel comfortable and be able to discuss aspects openly. Rather than a one-sided commentary by the professional, there should be a two-way conversation that fulfils the needs of the woman.

It is important to appreciate personal limitations and to not cross professional boundaries. Be honest about the limits of your expertise and involve the specialist or more senior practitioners in explanations of their role, as required. This is particularly relevant when breaking bad news – you may need to arrange for a more experienced, senior or specialist colleague to join you during the information sharing.

Every woman will have a different reaction to an emergency; there may be any number of aspects affecting her ability to assimilate information. Emotions can be affected by, for example, being in a postoperative state, in pain, sleep deprived, or hormonal. Cultural, ethnic, and social issues may also affect responses. It is important that any reactions to communications from you are received non-judgementally. It may be appropriate for you to offer to invite the husband/partner to attend and be available to answer any further questions once they have arrived.

At the end of the discussion, you should explain the care pathway and ongoing management that, with her consent, will follow the emergency. This should include specific information on:

- Any referral you will make for follow-up care (to whom, why, when, and how).
- Further screening or diagnostic investigations you will request (by whom, when, and what this will entail).
- Daily management (by whom, when, and what this will entail).
- Expected progress, side effects, and potential problems that may occur.
- How to make contact if she has any further questions.
- Alternative information sources available.

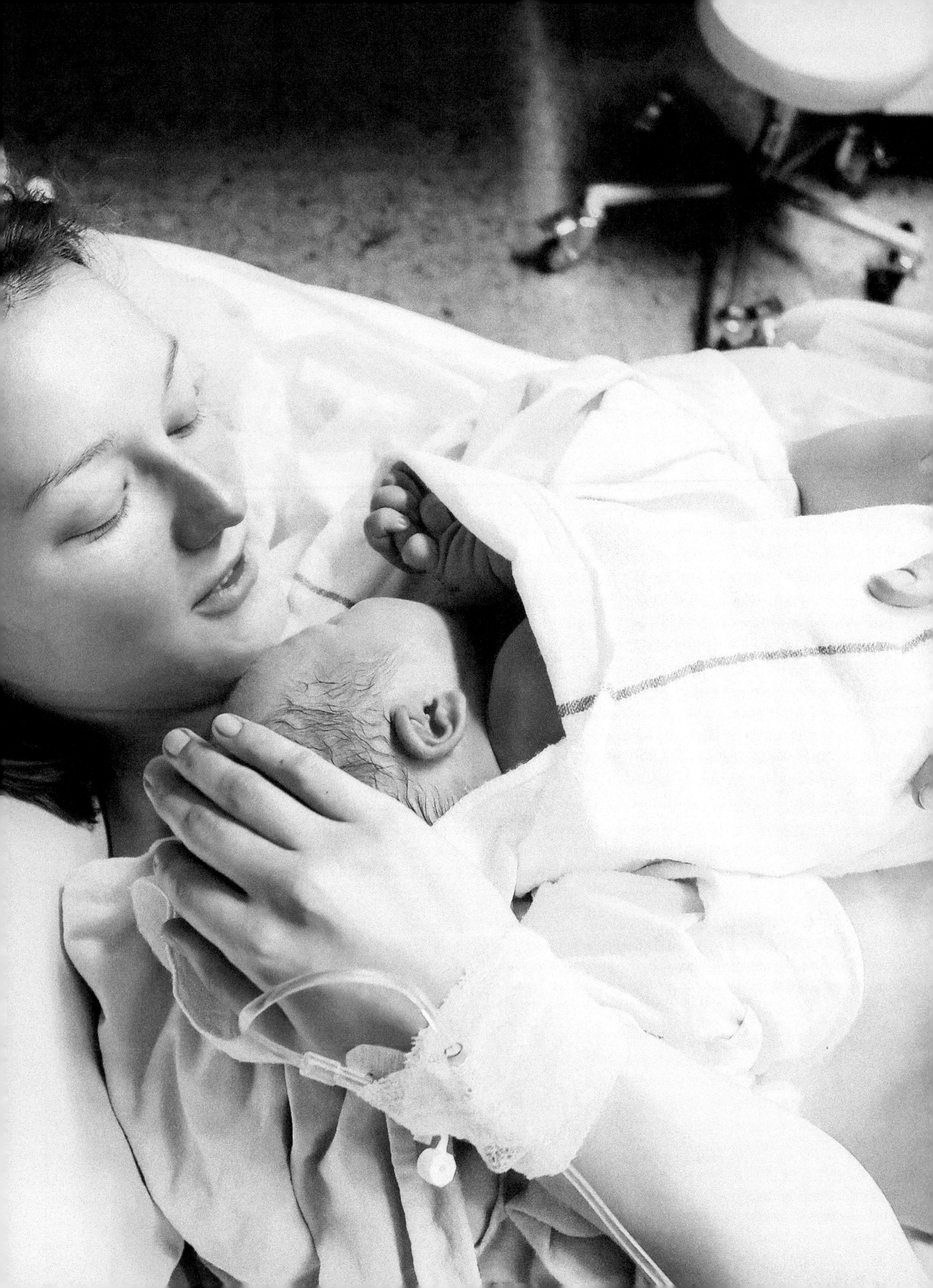

Emergency skills

Chapters

Section 2 Resuscitation

3 Maternal resuscitation 8
4 Neonatal resuscitation 10

Section 3 Haemorrhage

5 Antepartum haemorrhage 14
6 Primary postpartum haemorrhage 16
7 Secondary postpartum haemorrhage 18

Section 4 Malpresentations and multiple pregnancy

8 Occipito posterior positions 20
9 Face and brow presentations 22
10 Breech presentations 24
11 Cord presentation and prolapse 26
12 Twins 28

Section 5 Dystocia

13 Shoulder dystocia 30
14 Uterine dystocia – failure to progress 32

Section 6 Placental separation problems

15 Manual removal of the placenta 34
16 Adhered or partially adhered placenta 36

Section 7 Uterine emergencies

17 Uterine inversion 38
18 Uterine rupture and scar dehiscence 40

3 Maternal resuscitation

Figure 3.1 Logical sequence of events.

Is it safe to approach? – **secure the area before you become the next casualty**

↓

Is resuscitation needed? if the answer is **'yes'**, then THIS IS AN EMERGENCY

↓

Is the woman's airway clear? – Airway: head tilt, chin lift

↓

Is the woman breathing? – Breathing: look, listen and feel for breathing for no more than 10 seconds

↓

Call for help – be clear about who and what you need + location. If out of hospital identify any landmarks, access difficulties and problems, to guide the emergency services

↓

Circulation – reduce aortocaval compression manually or by tilting. Start chest compressions

↓

When help arrives – continue chest compressions and add inflation breaths

↓

AED – use as soon as it arrives

Prepare for – perimortem Caesarean section

Table 3.1 Physiological adaptations needed. Source: Data from Johnston & Grady (2011).

Physiological adaptation	Resuscitation modification
Gravid uterus:	
• Women can haemorrhage 1000–1200 mL before demonstrating signs of hypovolaemia	• Observe for concealed haemorrhage
• Aortocaval compression – up to 30% of the woman's blood volume can become sequestered in the lower extremities in a supine (collapsed) woman	• Displace the uterus to the woman's left to increase cardiac output by up to 25%
• Splinting of the diaphragm – may render inflation of the lungs more difficult	• Skilled midwives and obstetricians needed
20% increase in oxygen needed as a result of:	
• Haemodilution with resulting anaemia and reduction in oxygen-carrying capacity	• Rapid oxygenation of the woman using 100% oxygen
• Additional requirements of the fetal circulation	
Larger breasts than in non-pregnant state results in decreased chest wall compliance	• Greater force required when undertaking chest compressions
Oedema of the glottis, pharynx and nasal passages – difficult intubation	• Skilled anaesthetist in attendance
Relaxation of the cardiac sphincter – with risk of aspiration of the gastric contents	• Cricoid pressure and the use of a cuffed endotracheal tube for intubation

A maternal death is defined by the World Health Organization (WHO), as the death of a woman during pregnancy or up to 6 weeks postpartum as a result of conditions associated with, or made worse by, pregnancy (WHO, 2010). In the UK between 2011 and 2013, there were 214 maternal deaths, of which 69 were attributed to 'direct' causes such as amniotic fluid embolism, haemorrhage, sepsis, and thromboembolic disorders (Knight *et al.*, 2015). The remaining 145 women died as a result of indirect causes. While the need to resuscitate a young, fit, healthy woman is an increasingly rare occurrence, maternal collapse can and does happen and the outcome is dependent on effective and prompt action by those caring for her. Approximately 50% of maternal deaths are due to preventable and, therefore, treatable causes; the fact that the need to resuscitate a pregnant or recently delivered woman is a rarity suggests that regular drills for midwives and obstetricians should be undertaken if an individual's skills are to be maintained at a high standard.

Thus, the definition of maternal resuscitation is the support of a woman's life in the event of sudden collapse accompanied by apnoea and/or cardiac arrest.

Physiology

The systems of the woman's body adapt during pregnancy and therefore it is essential that these are understood so that effective resuscitation can take place (see Table 3.1).

Predisposing factors

- Thromboembolic disorders.
- Haemorrhage.
- Amniotic fluid embolism.
- Seizure – eclamptic and epileptic.
- Sepsis.
- Anaphylaxis.
- Accident.
- Pre-existing medical conditions.
- Psychiatric conditions.

Management (see Figure 3.1)

This is an emergency. It is essential to note that a woman who is not responding and whose breathing is abnormal is experiencing a cardiac arrest requiring early intervention and resuscitation. The sequence of interventions is as follows (Resuscitation Council (UK) 2015):

- Before approaching the woman make sure that it is safe for you to do so.
- Try to elicit a response from the woman by speaking to her in both ears. If she responds, try to find out what has happened.
- **Airway** – put a hand on the forehead of the woman and with two fingers under the point of her chin, tilt her head by lifting the chin to open the airway.
- **Breathing** – bend down close to the woman's face, turn to look towards the woman's feet and for **no more than 10 seconds:**
  - **Look** for chest rise – this may be shallow or absent.
  - **Listen** for the sound of breathing.
  - **Feel** for exhaled breath on your cheek.

If the woman is breathing, place her in the recovery position and call for help. Do not leave her and reassess the situation regularly.

If she is not breathing:

- **Call for help** – either call 999 if out of hospital and request a paramedic ambulance, or if in a clinical setting, pull/push the emergency buzzer and ask the person who responds to initiate a cardiac arrest alert and then return to help you with a pocket face mask or bag-valve–mask system if available) and an automated external defibrillator (AED). It has been shown that early use of an AED, within 3–5 minutes of collapse, may increase the victim's chances of survival by as much as 50–70%
- **Circulation**
  - If the woman is obviously pregnant, reduce aortocaval compression by manually displacing the uterus to the woman's left by either using two hands to pull the uterus towards you or one hand to push it away from you (Murphy & Cullinan, 2017). If this is not possible, or you are on your own, then tilt the woman onto her left side by placing whatever is at your disposal beneath her right side – ideally from her shoulder to her knee.
  - Commence chest compressions at a rate of 100–120 per minute, depressing the chest by 5–6 cm and allowing it to recoil between compressions without removing your hands, to encourage the refilling of the heart. Kneel beside the woman and place the heel of one hand in the centre of her chest with the heel of the second hand on top of the first. Interlace the fingers, lifting those of the lower hand off the woman's chest to avoid damage to the ribs. With your arms and back straight and your shoulders directly above your hands (perpendicular to her chest), deliver the compressions.
  - When assistance returns continue chest compressions but add two inflation breaths each lasting 1 second at a ratio of two breaths to 30 chest compressions, maintaining a head tilt and chin lift throughout.
  - As soon as the AED arrives, switch on the machine, attach the pads to the woman's chest, and follow the spoken instructions. If a shock is required, ensure all personnel stand away and oxygen is removed from the woman, then deliver the shock as instructed (Perkins *et al.*, 2015).
  - Immediately resume cardiopulmonary resuscitation.
- In the event of a pregnant woman requiring resuscitation, a perimortem Caesarean section must be performed by a trained medical practitioner within 5 minutes of the decision to resuscitate, or if the mother fails to respond with a return of spontaneous circulation within 4 minutes of commencing effective resuscitative measures.
- When to stop:
  - Qualified help arrives to take over.
  - The woman shows signs of spontaneous breathing.
  - You become exhausted.

Note: If more than one rescuer is present, alternate roles every 2 minutes to prevent fatigue, ensuring minimum delay during changeovers.

Following completion of the resuscitation, contemporaneous notes of the event must be completed, as well as an incident report form as per NHS Trust protocol. All present, including the parents, may require time to be debriefed.

Neonatal resuscitation

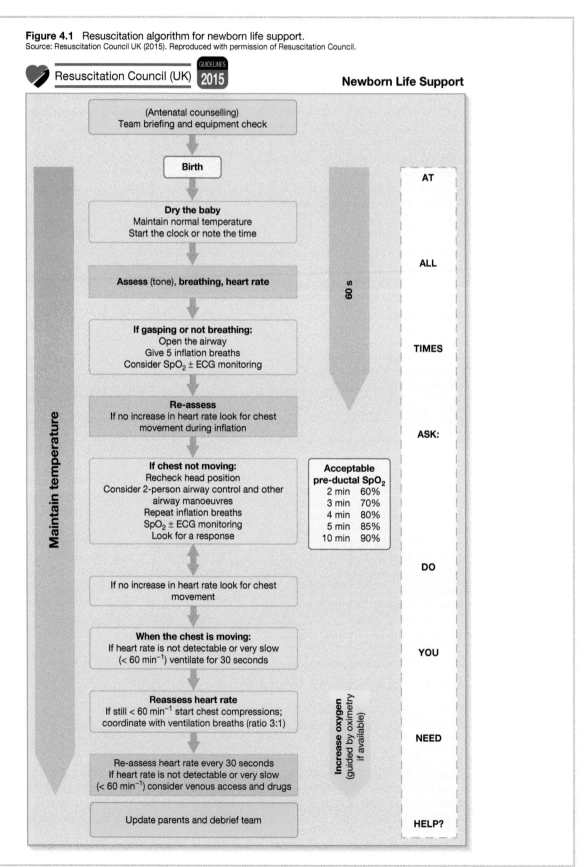

Figure 4.1 Resuscitation algorithm for newborn life support.
Source: Resuscitation Council UK (2015). Reproduced with permission of Resuscitation Council.

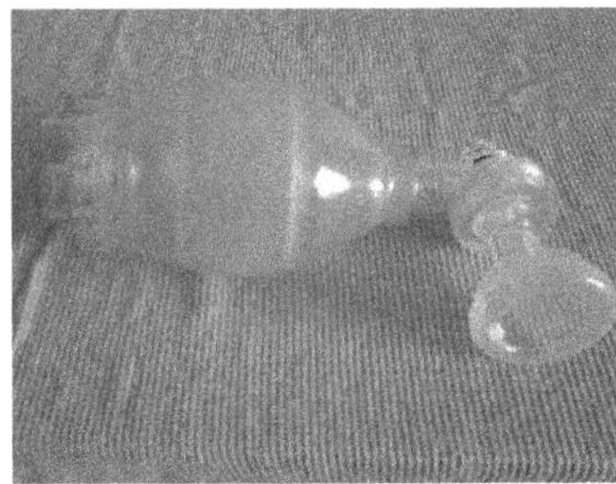

Figure 4.1 Mask ventilation via bag-valve-mask system.

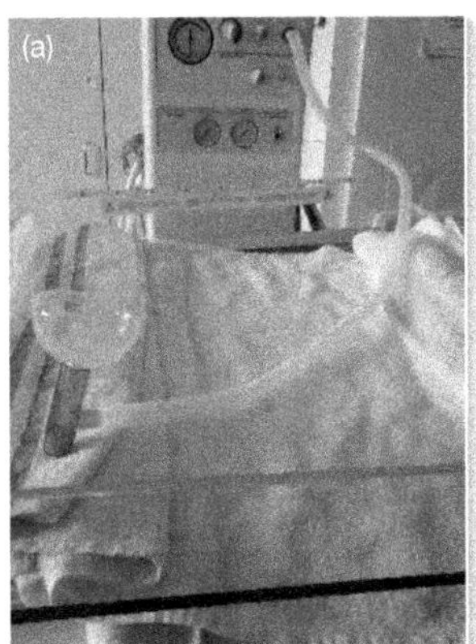

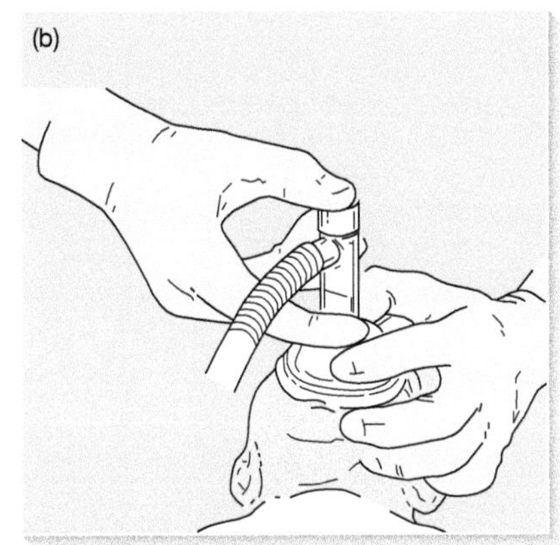

Figure 4.2 (a) T-piece mask connected to the air supply on the Resuscitaire (b) Mask ventilation. Source (b): From Lissauer & Fanaroff (2011). Reproduced with permission of John Wiley & Sons.

Neonatal resuscitation is a systematic approach to supporting the neonate in the transition from placental to pulmonary respiration (see Figure 4.1). The majority of neonates will make the transition to an extrauterine existence without requiring assistance. However, for those who have endured insults or stresses during the birth process, additional support, typified by the use of interventions to 'rescue' the sick neonate, may be required – this is then justifiably termed 'resuscitation'.

Physiology

The journey through the birth canal is a relatively hypoxic experience for the fetus as gaseous exchange through the placenta is interrupted during each contraction for between 50 and 75 seconds. If the hypoxia continues, the neural centres in the brainstem will no longer function and the fetus will experience **primary apnoea**, demonstrating no respiratory effort. This will result in the decreasing of the heart rate due to anaerobic metabolism and the release of lactic acid. Should this situation continue, **agonal gasping** will begin where the whole body shudders as a result of primitive spinal reflexes. If these gasps do not aerate the lungs, the neonate will enter **secondary** or **terminal apnoea** resulting in cardiac failure and neonatal demise.

Predisposing factors

- Multiple pregnancy.
- Obstetric emergency (antepartum haemorrhage, intrapartum haemorrhage, cord prolapse, shoulder dystocia, particulate meconium in the liquor amnii).
- Malpresentation (e.g. breech); malposition (e.g. occipito posterior position).
- Prolonged labour.
- Recent maternal sedation.
- Maternal disease.

Management (Wyllie *et al.*, 2015) (see Figure 4.1)

The approach to the management of resuscitating a neonate should be systematic in nature. This is an emergency situation in which a neonate's condition can deteriorate rapidly. Be prepared and anticipate the need to intervene.

The sequence of events is as follows:

- Start the clock/note the time and the time of birth and switch on the light and heater.
- Place the neonate on a flat surface and dry the neonate thoroughly discarding the wet towel and re-wrapping the neonate in a dry towel leaving the chest exposed. Apply a hat.
- Assess the neonate's condition: heart rate, respiratory effort, colour and tone. Repeat this every 30 seconds throughout the resuscitation and call for help.

Airway

- Place the neonate's head in the **neutral** position – that is, not flexed or extended. Remember the neonate has a large, rounded occiput which favours a flexed 'default' position – this can obstruct the airway if left unaddressed.
- Apply a pulse oximeter (neonatal) with the sensor placed on the right palm or wrist – this may take up to 90 seconds to start recording.

Breathing

- If the neonate is not breathing, give five **inflation** breaths, using a bag, valve and mask (BVM) system (see Figure 4.2) or a T-piece mask (see Figure 4.3) connected to the air supply on the Resuscitaire (size the mask to fit over the nose and mouth, but **not** eyes).
- Pressure should be 30 cm H_2O. Each inflation breath should take 2–3 seconds. If using a T-piece it is advisable to maintain a PEEP (positive end expiratory pressure) at 4–5 cm water if possible. Effective aeration will mean chest wall movement.
- If heart rate increases, that is, above 60 bpm but the neonate does not breathe spontaneously, continue with ventilation breaths each delivered over 1–2 seconds until the neonate breathes independently, or is intubated and ventilated mechanically.

Figure 4.4 Two-handed jaw thrust.
Source: From Lissauer & Fanaroff (2011).
Reproduced with permission of John Wiley & Sons.

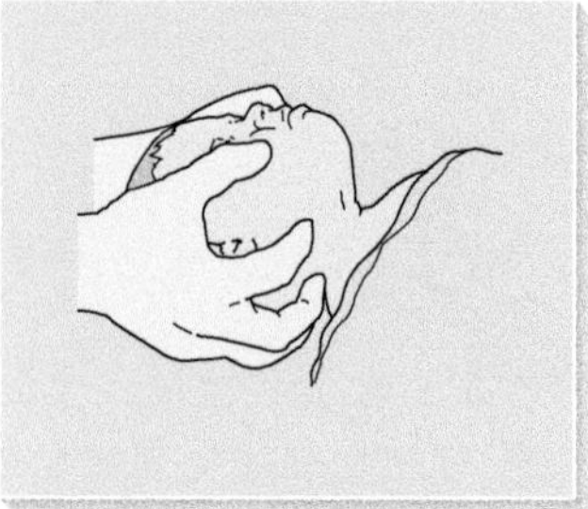

Figure 4.5 Two-person airway control.
Source: From Lissauer & Fanaroff (2011).
Reproduced with permission of John Wiley & Sons

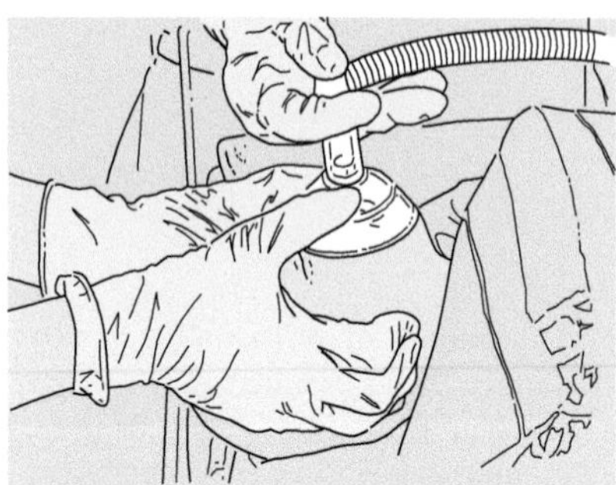

Consider using this if inflation breaths administered by mask, are ineffective. One person holds the mask in place having applied a jaw thrust and the assistant offers 5 inflation breaths to effect lung aeration.

Figure 4.6 (a-d) Methods of offering chest compressions.
Source: From Lissauer & Fanaroff (2011). Reproduced with permission of John Wiley & Sons.

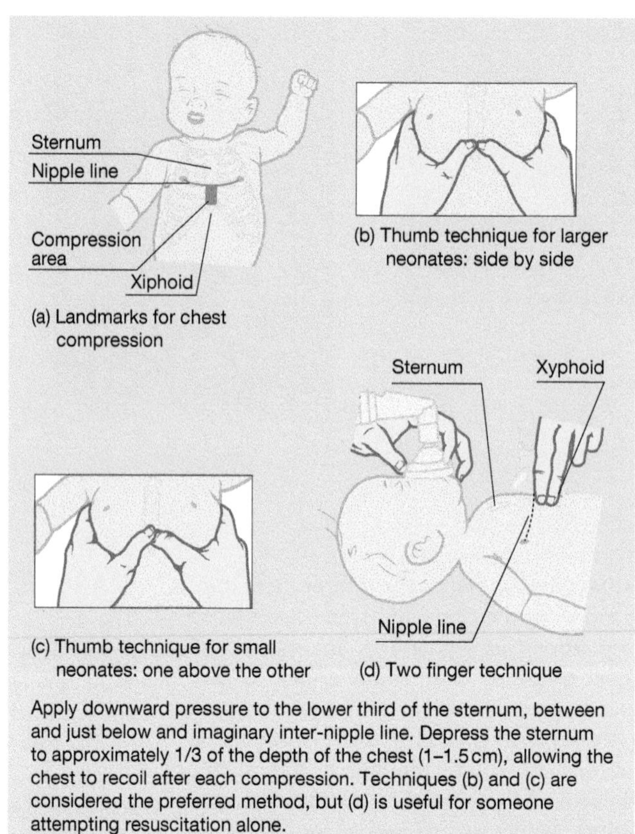

Apply downward pressure to the lower third of the sternum, between and just below and imaginary inter-nipple line. Depress the sternum to approximately 1/3 of the depth of the chest (1–1.5 cm), allowing the chest to recoil after each compression. Techniques (b) and (c) are considered the preferred method, but (d) is useful for someone attempting resuscitation alone.

Table 4.1 Drugs are rarely needed and are considered only if there is poor/reduced cardiac output despite effective lung inflation/aeration and chest compressions.

Drug	Concentration	Route of administration	Dose	Indication
Sodium Bicarbonate	4.2%	Intravenously via an umbilical vein catheter (UVC) or intraosseous route if UVC not an option	1–2 mmol per kg	Consider after a prolonged resuscitation
Adrenaline	1:10000	Intravenously via an umbilical vein catheter (UVC) or intraosseous route if UVC not an option	10 mcg per kg	After successful lung aeration and chest compression with heart rate of 60 beats per minute or less
Dextrose	10%	Intravenously via an umbilical vein catheter (UVC) or intraosseous route if UVC not an option	2.5 mL per kg	Hypoglycaemic
Volume 0.9% Sodium Chloride or similar crystalloid Whole blood		Intravenously via an umbilical vein catheter (UVC) or intraosseous route if UVC not an option	10 mL per kg given over 10–20 seconds	If the infant has lost a significant amount of blood and is therefore hypovolaemic

- If heart rate does **not** increase following inflation breaths, the most common cause is inadequate aeration of the lungs. Therefore, consider:
  - Position of head.
  - Need for jaw thrust/second person to help (see Figures 4.4 and 4.5).
  - An obstruction in the neonate's airway.
  - An oropharyngeal airway (Guedel).

Chest compressions

- Chest compressions are commenced **only if**:
  - **Lungs have been aerated successfully and the operator has seen the chest wall move.**
  - **Heart beat absent or rate is less than 60 bpm.**
  - **30 seconds of ventilation breaths have been given.**
- An oxygen supply is ready if oxygen saturation (SATS) remains low. Use only sufficient oxygen to restore the SATS to the level appropriate for its age and no more (see Figure 4.1).
- Method (see Figure 4.6):
  - Gold standard method is to encircle chest with two hands, with fingers over spine and thumbs overlapping one over the other on the sternum, just below an imaginary line between and just below the nipples. Remember – avoid compressing soft tissues.
  - Compress quickly and firmly to about one-third the depth of the chest at a ratio of three chest compressions to one ventilation breath.
  - Allow chest to recoil between compressions enabling the heart to refill.
- Ensure that the chest is still inflating with each breath.
- Re-assess heart rate, colour, tone and respiratory effort every 30 seconds throughout procedure.
- If two people are resuscitating the neonate together, one should count out loud to concentrate the effort.

Drugs – SAD (see Table 4.1)

Commonly used drugs include: **S**odium bicarbonate, **A**drenaline and **D**extrose. If volume is needed, then a bolus of sodium chloride may be given.

Use of suction

Suction is **not** recommended unless an airway obstruction is suspected in which case suction must only be attempted under direct vision with the aid of a laryngoscope.

Special situations

Preterm babies

Follow the approach as for any neonate with the following additions/changes in management:

- A delay in cord clamping of at least 1 minute from the complete delivery of the neonate is now recommended.
- Place the wet neonate straight into a food-grade plastic bag sealed at the neck with tape, under the radiant heater on the Resuscitaire. They should not be covered or wrapped. Apply a hat or plastic wrapping to the head.
- Reduce inflation pressures to 20–25 cm H_2O (dependent on gestational age). Use oxygen with great care and only with an oximeter.

Meconium

For babies born with a heavy covering of particulate meconium on their faces:

- If the neonate is crying and vigorous, treat as normal and observe.
- If particulate meconium is observed on or around the neonate's face, mouth, or nostrils, do not stimulate the neonate as this may cause the neonate to inhale the meconium.
- Wrap gently and place on a flat surface. Inspect the airway using a laryngoscope and remove any visible meconium with a Yankauer sucker. The neonate can then be resuscitated using the systematic approach already described, followed by transfer to a NICU for observation.

When to stop

The decision to stop resuscitation is multifactorial. Where there has been no detectable cardiac activity for more than 10 minutes, the decision to stop resuscitation is appropriate. However, the decision to withdraw resuscitative measures becomes far more complex if, for example, facilities are available for the therapeutic cooling of the neonate, intensive care accommodation is available, the reason for the collapse is known or if there are any subsequent complications, notwithstanding the parents' understanding of possible long-term morbidity issues for their baby. This demonstrates the need for senior personnel to be in attendance at the resuscitation as quickly as possible.

Following the resuscitation, the midwife will complete contemporaneous notes of the event plus an incident report form as required by local NHS Trust protocol. All present, including the parents, may require time to be debriefed.

5 Antepartum haemorrhage

Box 5.1 Placenta praevia.

Associated with:

- Previous placenta praevia
- Previous uterine surgery, including Caesarean section
- Head or presenting part is high
- The lie may be unstable
- Painless (unless in labour)
- Uterus not tender
- Uterus soft
- No uterine irritability or contractions
- Malpresentation
- Fetal heart usually normal
- Shock and anaemia correspond to apparent blood loss
- Coagulopathy very uncommon initially

Box 5.2 Placenta abruptio.

Associated with:

- Previous abruption
- Hypertensive disorders
- Abdominal trauma
- Presenting part may or may not be engaged
- Abdominal pain and/or backache (pain often described as 'exquisite')
- Uterine tenderness
- Increased uterine tone
- Uterine irritability or contractions
- Fetal heart may be abnormal or absent
- Shock out of proportion to visible blood loss
- May have coagulopathy
- Abruption may be seen on abdominal ultrasound

Antepartum haemorrhage (APH) is generally defined as bleeding from or into the genital tract from 24 completed weeks of pregnancy until the birth of the baby, and can affect between 3 and 5% of all maternities (Thomson & Ramsay, 2011; Chavan & Latoo, 2013).

Can antepartum haemorrhage be predicted?

Although a number of risk factors have been suggested, APH remains almost impossible to predict. Risk factors may include: increased maternal age (40 + years); previous Caesarean section; previous termination of pregnancy; pre-eclampsia; smoking and other substance misuse. However, it would appear that the most reliable predictor would be a history of previous pregnancy complicated by placental abruption.

Causes/predisposing factors

Potential causes are many and varied, but the most likely is placental abruption, that is, placenta praevia or placenta abruptio. However, genital tract and other non-specific causes can also be considered:

- Cervical disorders, for example cervicitis, cervical ectropion.
- Genital trauma, for example sexual intercourse, abuse.
- Genital varicosities, genital tumours – benign or malignant.
- Genital tract infection.
- Vasa praevia.

Placenta praevia (see Box 5.1)

Placenta praevia counts for approximately 30% of APHs and is defined as when the placenta is implanted in the lower segment of the uterus and may therefore be partially or wholly covering the internal cervical os. The severity of placenta praevia is graded as follows:

- Grade 1: the placenta encroaches on the lower uterine segment.
- Grade 2: the placenta abuts the internal cervical os.
- Grade 3: the placenta covers part of the cervical os.
- Grade 4: the placenta covers the cervical os when dilated.

Placenta abruptio (see Box 5.2)

Placenta abruptio refers to haemorrhage due to the premature separation of the placenta following bleeding into the decidua basalis layer of the uterus. This affects approximately 1–2% of all maternities. The fetal outcome will be directly related to the degree of separation.

Management

The management of APH is usually determined by evaluating a combination of the estimated blood loss and the clinical picture presented by the woman. However, the level of blood loss is frequently underestimated as only a small proportion of the total blood loss is visualised. Consequently, blood loss may be assessed as:

- 'Spotting' – when a woman's underwear or sanitary towel is stained with blood.
- Minor – where less than 50 mL blood have been lost and the bleeding has now settled.
- Major – where as much as 1000 mL have been lost, but the woman demonstrates no clinical signs of shock.
- Massive – where the blood loss is greater than 1000 mL.

Summon assistance by whatever means are available – shout for help, pull/press an emergency call bell, or send another person to call for help. In a maternity unit, the personnel required are a senior midwife, senior obstetrician, anaesthetist, neonatologist, haematologist, porter, and a scribe to record events. The midwife may wish to divide the woman into three zones so that as assistance arrives, specific tasks can be allocated to appropriate practitioners. However, it is essential that all treatment is delivered simultaneously and that observations, fluid balance, and drug, oxygen and fluid administrations are carefully recorded throughout on the Modified Early Obstetric Warning System (MEOWS) chart, fluid balance chart, and prescription charts respectively. Communication between all in attendance must be comprehensive. **Remember** – postpartum haemorrhage may follow an APH – be prepared. The three zones are:

- **Zone 1 – head**. While waiting for help to arrive, the woman should be laid with a left lateral tilt on the delivery bed and the head of the bed removed to ensure ease of access. The midwife should remember his/her underlying responsibilities, such as the reassurance of the woman and anyone accompanying her, throughout the resuscitation. The woman's airway and breathing will be assessed and high flow oxygen via a non-rebreathe face mask will be given (10–15 L/minute).
- **Zone 2 – arms**. Basic observations should be undertaken (blood pressure, pulse, respiratory rate) and a pulse oximeter applied. Two wide bore cannulae should be inserted – one in each antecubital fossa and blood taken for a full blood count, coagulation screen, grouping and crossmatching 4–6 units, urea and electrolytes, liver function tests, Kleihauer (in Rh negative women) (Thomson & Ramsay, 2011). Fluid replacement should initially begin with up to 2 L of a crystalloid fluid (for example, Hartmann's solution), followed by up to 1.5–2 L of a colloid solution if the blood pressure does not recover. O negative or uncrossmatched blood may be commenced while awaiting the arrival of type-specific blood for transfusion via a blood warmer. Administration sets with filters should not be used as these can slow down the infusion. Fluid replacement and the use of blood and blood products should be strictly monitored, and the amount given should be dictated by the lead clinician (consultant anaesthetist or consultant obstetrician) aided by the results of full blood count and clotting screen under the guidance of a haematologist and/or consultant in transfusion medicine.
- **Zone 3 – pelvis**. The bladder should be catheterised and a urometer attached for accurate measurement of urinary output.

Delivery

The status of the fetus and the degree of haemorrhage will determine:

- The decision to expedite delivery and the route.
- The anaesthesia required – however, regional anaesthesia remains the route of choice in the absence of any contraindications. A consultant anaesthetist is preferred.

Following the APH the midwife will complete contemporaneous notes of the event plus an incident report form as per NHS Trust protocol. All in attendance, including the woman and her supporter, may require time to be debriefed.

6 Primary postpartum haemorrhage

Figure 6.1 Management of major haemorrhage.

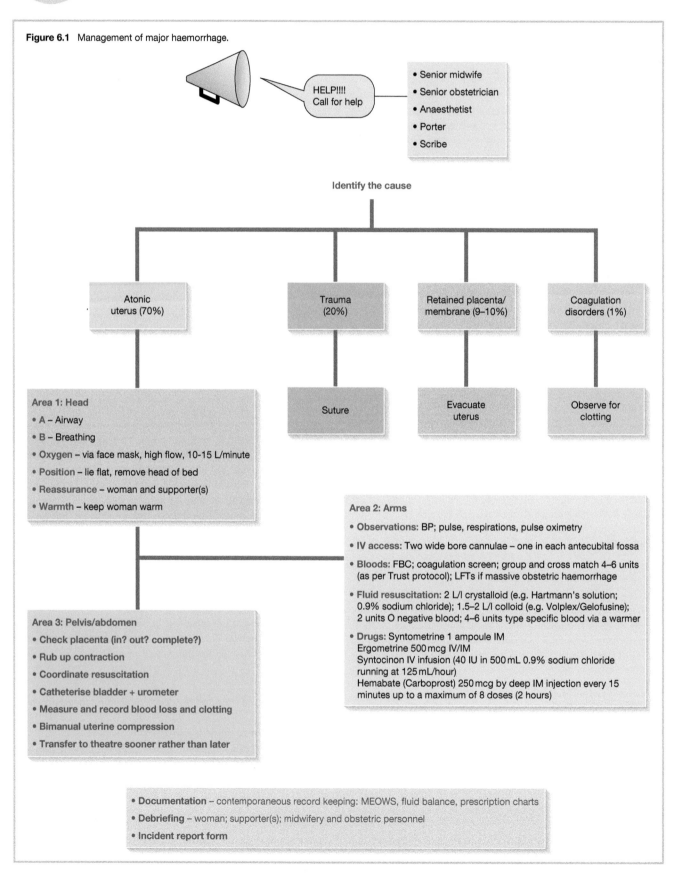

HELP!!!!
Call for help

- Senior midwife
- Senior obstetrician
- Anaesthetist
- Porter
- Scribe

Identify the cause

Atonic uterus (70%)	Trauma (20%)	Retained placenta/ membrane (9–10%)	Coagulation disorders (1%)
	Suture	Evacuate uterus	Observe for clotting

Area 1: Head

- **A** – Airway
- **B** – Breathing
- **Oxygen** – via face mask, high flow, 10-15 L/minute
- **Position** – lie flat, remove head of bed
- **Reassurance** – woman and supporter(s)
- **Warmth** – keep woman warm

Area 2: Arms

- **Observations:** BP; pulse, respirations, pulse oximetry
- **IV access:** Two wide bore cannulae – one in each antecubital fossa
- **Bloods:** FBC; coagulation screen; group and cross match 4–6 units (as per Trust protocol); LFTs if massive obstetric haemorrhage
- **Fluid resuscitation:** 2 L/l crystalloid (e.g. Hartmann's solution; 0.9% sodium chloride); 1.5–2 L/l colloid (e.g. Volplex/Gelofusine); 2 units O negative blood; 4–6 units type specific blood via a warmer
- **Drugs:** Syntometrine 1 ampoule IM
  Ergometrine 500 mcg IV/IM
  Syntocinon IV infusion (40 IU in 500 mL 0.9% sodium chloride running at 125 mL/hour)
  Hemabate (Carboprost) 250 mcg by deep IM injection every 15 minutes up to a maximum of 8 doses (2 hours)

Area 3: Pelvis/abdomen

- **Check placenta (in? out? complete?)**
- **Rub up contraction**
- **Coordinate resuscitation**
- **Catheterise bladder + urometer**
- **Measure and record blood loss and clotting**
- **Bimanual uterine compression**
- **Transfer to theatre sooner rather than later**

- **Documentation** – contemporaneous record keeping: MEOWS, fluid balance, prescription charts
- **Debriefing** – woman; supporter(s); midwifery and obstetric personnel
- **Incident report form**

Primary postpartum haemorrhage (PPH) is generally defined as blood loss ≥ 500 mL within 24 hours after birth, while severe PPH is blood loss ≥ 1000 mL within 24 hours and can be further defined as minor (500–1000 mL) or major (> 1000 mL). Major may be further divided to moderate (1000–2000 mL) or severe (> 2000 mL). Secondary PPH is defined as excessive bleeding from the genital tract between 24 hours and 12 weeks postpartum and is managed in a similar fashion to primary PPH (Evenson & Anderson, 2017; Mavrides *et al.*, 2016).

Risk factors

Antenatal risk factors

- Pre-eclampsia.
- Primigravid woman age > 40 years.
- Anaemia and blood coagulation disorders.
- Antepartum haemorrhage (placental abruption, placenta praevia, fibroids).
- Multiple pregnancy/polyhydramnios.
- Previous history of PPH, placenta praevia, Caesarean section.
- Asian ethnicity.
- BMI > 35.

Intrapartum risk factors

- Prolonged first, second, and third stage of labour.
- Precipitate labour.
- Augmentation/induction of labour.
- Assisted/instrumental delivery.
- Emergency/elective Caesarean section.
- Episiotomy/lacerations.
- Full bladder.
- Retained placenta/incomplete separation of placenta and/or membranes.

Causes

The causes of PPH fall into four basic categories: uterine atony (70%); trauma to the genital tract (20%); retained products of conception (placental/membrane tissue) (9–10%); blood coagulation disorders (1%).

Management: a holistic approach

The approach to the management of PPH should be holistic in nature. This is an emergency situation in which a woman's condition can deteriorate rapidly. Be prepared – treat any potential cause identified antenatally, for example anaemia. Prompt recognition and treatment is essential. Four basic principles should be applied:

- Summon medical assistance.
- Identify the cause (see Figure 6.1).
- Achieve haemostasis.
- Resuscitate the woman.

Summon assistance by whatever means are available – shout for help, pull/press an emergency call bell, or send another person to call for help. This is not an occasion to be alone with a woman who is haemorrhaging. In a maternity unit the personnel required are a senior midwife, senior obstetrician, anaesthetist, porter, and a scribe to record events. The midwife may wish to divide the woman into three zones so that as assistance arrives, specific tasks can be allocated to appropriate practitioners. However, it is essential that all treatment is delivered simultaneously and that observations, fluid balance, and drug, oxygen, and fluid administrations are carefully recorded throughout on the Modified Early Obstetric Warning System (MEOWS) chart, fluid balance chart, and prescription charts respectively.

- **Zone 1 – head** (see Figure 6.1). Whilst waiting for help to arrive, the baby should be removed to a place of safety if being cuddled by the woman at the time of her collapse; the woman should be laid flat on the delivery bed and the head of the bed removed to ensure ease of access. The midwife should remember his/her underlying responsibilities, such as the reassurance of the woman and anyone accompanying her, throughout the resuscitation. The woman's airway and breathing will be assessed and high flow oxygen via a non-rebreathe face mask will be given (10–15 L/minute).
- **Zone 2 – arms** (see Figure 6.1). Basic observations should be undertaken (blood pressure [automated], pulse, respiratory rate, and temperature) every 15 minutes plus a pulse oximeter and electrocardiogram applied. Two wide bore cannulae should be inserted – one in each antecubital fossa and blood taken for a full blood count, coagulation screen, grouping and cross matching 4–6 units, liver and renal function tests. It may also be appropriate to consider inserting an arterial line. Fluid replacement should begin initially with up to 2 L of a crystalloid fluid, followed by up to 1.5–2 L of a colloid solution if the blood pressure does not recover. O negative blood may be commenced while awaiting the arrival of type-specific blood for transfusion via a blood warmer. Infusion sets with filters should not be used as these may slow down the rate of infusion. Fluid replacement and the use of blood and blood products should be strictly monitored, and the amount given should be dictated by the lead clinician (consultant anaesthetist or consultant obstetrician) aided by the results of a full blood count and clotting screen under the guidance of a haematologist and/or consultant in transfusion medicine.

Medication should be given according to need and local protocol. If an oxytocic drug has not been administered at delivery, then oxytocin 5 IU can be given by slow intravenous injection. Ergometrine 500 mcg may also be given by slow intravenous injection unless contraindicated (e.g. in the presence of hypertension). It is likely that an intravenous infusion of 40 IU oxytocin added to 500 mL 0.9% sodium chloride/Hartmann's solution can be commenced at a rate of 125 mL/hour. Other options may include a deep intramuscular injection of a prostaglandin analogue intended for the treatment of PPH – 250 mcg every 15 minutes up to a maximum of eight doses. Local policy may also recommend the use of misoprostol 800–1000 μg sublingually or per rectum – side effects may include diarrhoea. Clinicians may consider the use of 0.5–1.00 g tranexamic acid administered intravenously. Move to the operating theatre sooner rather than later.

- **Zone 3 – pelvic area** (see Figure 6.1). The midwife will attempt to 'rub up' a contraction assuming that the placenta and membranes have been delivered. It is essential that the placenta and membranes are checked for completeness once delivered. If the placenta is still *in utero* then this must be delivered without delay. Once the bladder has been catheterised (and a urometer attached for accurate measurement of urinary output) and the midwife has identified the cause of the haemorrhage, in the presence of an atonic uterus he/she may wish to proceed to performing internal bimanual compression in order to achieve haemostasis. If trauma is the cause of the PPH, the episiotomy, tear, or other damage should be sutured as quickly as possible. Throughout, the volume of blood that has been lost must be measured accurately, including blood-soaked swabs, and it is essential that the ability of the blood to clot is assessed at regular intervals.

If the PPH is not brought under control, the management should continue in an obstetric theatre where operative measures may be required. Following the PPH the midwife will complete contemporaneous notes of the event plus an incident report form as NHS Trust protocol requires. All present, including the woman and her supporter, may require time to be debriefed.

Secondary postpartum haemorrhage

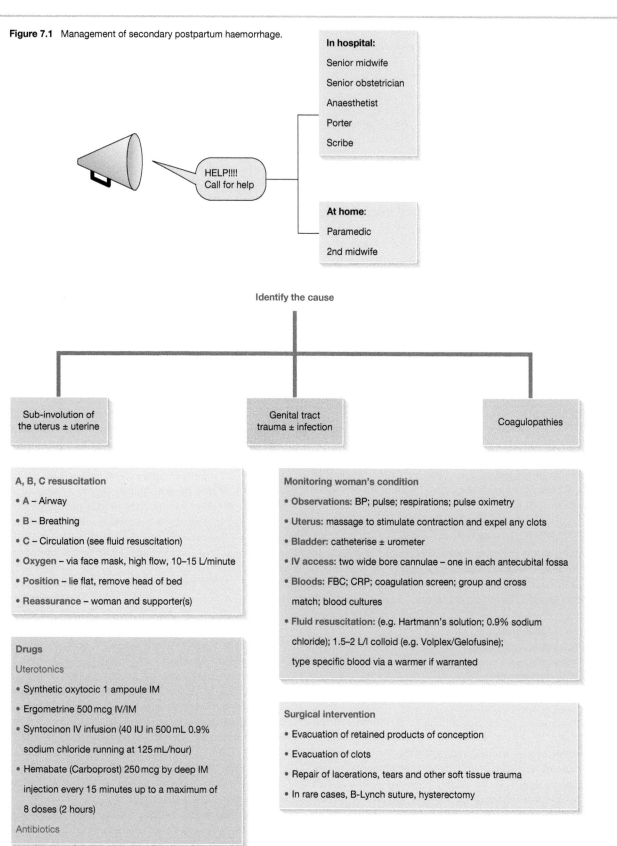

Figure 7.1 Management of secondary postpartum haemorrhage.

HELP!!!!
Call for help

In hospital:
- Senior midwife
- Senior obstetrician
- Anaesthetist
- Porter
- Scribe

At home:
- Paramedic
- 2nd midwife

Identify the cause

- Sub-involution of the uterus ± uterine
- Genital tract trauma ± infection
- Coagulopathies

A, B, C resuscitation
- **A** – Airway
- **B** – Breathing
- **C** – Circulation (see fluid resuscitation)
- **Oxygen** – via face mask, high flow, 10–15 L/minute
- **Position** – lie flat, remove head of bed
- **Reassurance** – woman and supporter(s)

Drugs

Uterotonics
- Synthetic oxytocic 1 ampoule IM
- Ergometrine 500 mcg IV/IM
- Syntocinon IV infusion (40 IU in 500 mL 0.9% sodium chloride running at 125 mL/hour)
- Hemabate (Carboprost) 250 mcg by deep IM injection every 15 minutes up to a maximum of 8 doses (2 hours)

Antibiotics

Monitoring woman's condition
- **Observations:** BP; pulse; respirations; pulse oximetry
- **Uterus:** massage to stimulate contraction and expel any clots
- **Bladder:** catheterise ± urometer
- **IV access:** two wide bore cannulae – one in each antecubital fossa
- **Bloods:** FBC; CRP; coagulation screen; group and cross match; blood cultures
- **Fluid resuscitation:** (e.g. Hartmann's solution; 0.9% sodium chloride); 1.5–2 L/l colloid (e.g. Volplex/Gelofusine); type specific blood via a warmer if warranted

Surgical intervention
- Evacuation of retained products of conception
- Evacuation of clots
- Repair of lacerations, tears and other soft tissue trauma
- In rare cases, B-Lynch suture, hysterectomy

Secondary postpartum haemorrhage (PPH) is defined as excessive or abnormal bleeding from the genital tract from 24 hours to 6 weeks postpartum, typically occurring 10–14 days after birth. Unlike primary PPH, the amount of blood loss is not generally specified and can therefore be open to subjective interpretation. The incidence of secondary PPH is approximately 1% of all births.

Risk factors

Antenatal risk factors

- Prelabour rupture of membranes at term.
- Prolonged rupture of membranes.
- Prolonged labour with repeated examinations *per vaginam.*
- Threatened miscarriage.
- Multiple pregnancy.
- Antepartum haemorrhage.
- Hospital admission during the third trimester.

Intrapartum risk factors

- Delivery by Caesarean section.
- Precipitate labour.
- Prolonged third stage of labour.
- Retained products of conception (i.e. incomplete placenta or membranes).
- Abnormal siting of the placenta (e.g. placenta accreta).
- Manual removal of the placenta.

Postpartum risk factors

- Primary postpartum haemorrhage.
- Sub-involution of the uterus.
- Postnatal sepsis.

Causes

Establishing a cause may be challenging. However, common causes are (Neill & Thornton, 2002; Frank *et al.*, 2017):

- Sub-involution of the uterus due to:
  - Retained placental tissue with consequent intrauterine infection.
  - Endometritis.
- Genital tract lacerations – haemorrhage may be concealed if there is haematoma formation following continued bleeding at the site of the injury.
- Coagulopathies, bleeding disorders, or use of anticoagulants. For example, women with congenital conditions such as von Willebrand's disease are at greater risk of delayed postpartum bleeding as the rise in maternal clotting factors during pregnancy then fall after birth. Often undetected in the antenatal period, conditions of this kind become apparent following the physiological challenge of childbirth.

Presentation

- Heavier vaginal loss than would be expected. Lochia would have changed from a pink–brown loss back to a bright red loss.
- Possible blood clots.
- Likely offensive lochia if infection is a causative factor.
- Maternal pyrexia and tachycardia, possible rigors.
- Suprapubic abdominal tenderness/pain.
- Uterine fundus higher than expected for the number of days postpartum with open cervical os.
- Possible uterine contractions/cramps.

Investigations

Blood tests should include the following:

- A full blood count.
- C-reactive protein.
- Clotting studies.
- Blood cultures if the woman is demonstrating signs of sepsis such as pyrexia and tachycardia.

Isolating the cause (see Figure 7.1) of possible infection would necessitate:

- High vaginal swab (HVS).
- Low vaginal swab (LVS).
- Possible pelvic ultrasound if retained placental or membrane tissue are suspected. However, the presence of clots on the uterus may create confusion when trying to differentiate between clots and retained products of conception. If a normal endometrial stripe is seen on ultrasound, it is unlikely that retained products will be the cause.
- Speculum examination to inspect the cervical os and lower genital tract.

Management (Frank *et al.*, 2017; Mavrides *et al.*, 2016)

- If the woman is still an in-patient, call a doctor – senior obstetric input for decision making and actions.
- Readmit to hospital via ambulance if the haemorrhage has occurred at home or transfer to a delivery suite or a close observation area/high dependency unit depending on hospital policy and condition of the woman if she is still an in-patient.
- As with any haemorrhage, the need for resuscitation is ever present (see Figure 7.1).
- Assess the blood loss by weighing any pads.
- Commence observations to include (see Figure 7.1):
  - Blood pressure, temperature, pulse rate.
  - Respiration rate and oxygen saturation monitoring.
- Administer facial oxygen.
- Cannulate using two wide bore cannulae.
- Draw blood for testing and take swabs to identify potential infecting organism.
- Commence crystalloid infusion to restore haemodynamic stabilisation, plus colloid infusion and the transfusion of blood if stabilisation is not achieved.
- Insert urinary catheter to monitor output and maintain an empty bladder – a full bladder may impede involution of the uterus.
- Massage the uterus per abdomen if palpable to encourage contraction and the expulsion of any retained clots.
- Consider the use of uterotonic medication as for PPH (see Figure 7.1).
- The use of a combination of antibiotics in the face of infection is recommended and is not contraindicated if the woman is breastfeeding her baby.
- Surgical intervention (see Figure 7.1) may be necessary if retained products of conception are suspected or if the bleeding becomes excessive or continuous.
- Maintain contemporaneous records.

8 Occipito posterior positions

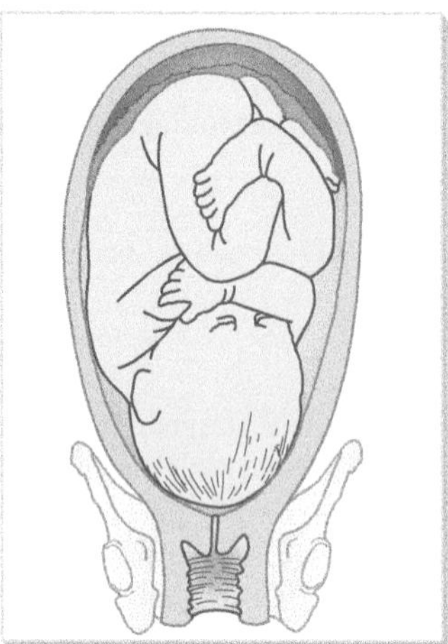

Figure 8.1 ROP position.

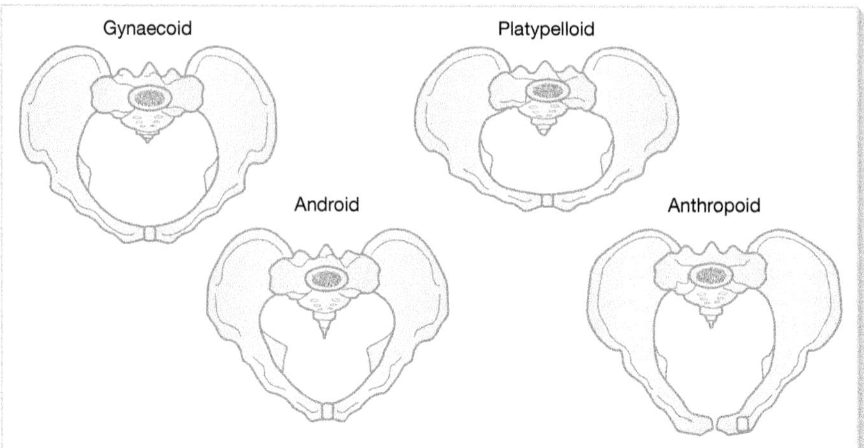

Figure 8.2 Pelvic shapes.

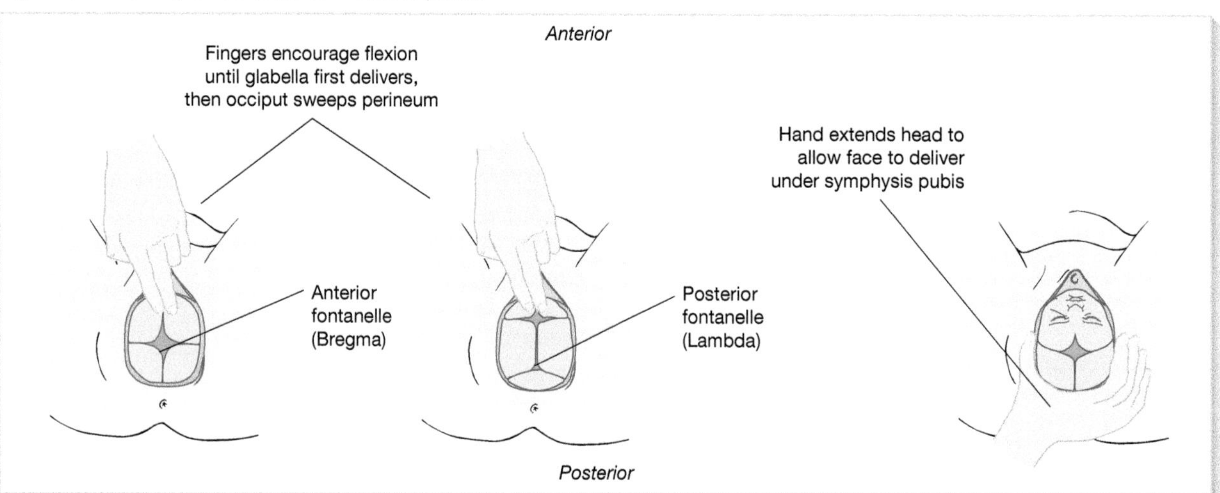

Figure 8.3 Delivery of the direct OP – face to pubis.

Box 8.1 Mechanism of ROP – long rotation to OA.

Lie = longitudinal
Presentation = cephalic/vertex
Denominator = occiput
Presenting part = occiput
Position = right occipito posterior
Attitude = flexed

- With contractions/descent the vertex flexes further
- The occiput reaches the pelvic floor and rotates three-eighths anteriorly to a direct OA; then descends below the symphysis pubis
- The head crowns then extends to deliver the face – sweeping the perineum
- Restitution occurs
- The shoulders reach the pelvic floor, rotate one-eighth to the direct AP
- The head rotates externally
- The anterior shoulder delivers under the symphysis pubis
- The posterior shoulder sweeps the perineum and the baby is born by lateral flexion

Box 8.2 Mechanism of ROP – short rotation and persistent OP.

Lie = longitudinal
Presentation = cephalic/vertex
Denominator = occiput
Presenting part = sinciput
Position = right occipito posterior
Attitude = deflexed

- With the deflexed head the sinciput reaches the pelvic floor first and rotates one-eighth anteriorly to a direct/persistent OP position
- The sinciput descends below the symphysis pubis up to the glabella
- The vertex/occiput sweeps the perineum by flexion
- The face delivers through extension of the head
- Restitution occurs
- The shoulders reach the pelvic floor, rotate one-eighth to the direct AP
- The head rotates externally
- The anterior shoulder delivers under the symphysis pubis
- The posterior shoulder sweeps the perineum and the baby is born by lateral flexion

Definition and incidence

The fetus has a cephalic presentation and longitudinal lie along the mother's axis but the occiput of the fetus is aligned with one of the maternal sacro-iliac joints. Hence the occiput bone is posterior and the fetus is facing forward (see Figure 8.1). The incidence is as high as 32% at the onset of labour, reducing to 5–10% at delivery. Of these persistent occipito posterior (OP) presentations only approximately 25% will deliver spontaneously: 50% will have an assisted vaginal delivery using ventouse or rotational forceps, and the remaining 25% will require Caesarean section (Reichman *et al.*, 2008).

Predisposing factors

The cause for the OP presentation may not be identified but a number of factors are associated with increased incidence:

- Android pelvis – the widest diameters of the heart-shaped brim are posterior, encouraging the wider diameters of the occiput to also lie posterior; then, the flat sacrum and prominent ischial spines prevent rotation to an anterior position (see Figure 8.2).
- Anthropoid pelvis – oval shape and narrow short transverse diameter. The vertex enters the brim in either a direct OA or direct OP position and the narrow transverse diameter prevents rotation (see Figure 8.2).
- Primigravida – increased uterine and abdominal muscle tone encourages OP and prevents rotation to occipito anterior (OA).
- Older mothers – greater rigidity of pelvic joints, impaired uterine action and increased premature births.
- Large babies – successful rotation to OA is less likely.
- Low maternal stature – associated with smaller bone structure generally and higher incidence of android-shaped pelvis.

Possible complications

The complications of OP labour are mostly associated with the deflexed head of the fetus and larger diameters, slowing or preventing the normal descent and mechanisms associated with labour and delivery. Additionally, the poor application of the presenting part (resulting from the high and/or deflexed head) reduces uterine stimulation, allows premature rupture of the membranes, and may fail to prevent possible cord presentation/prolapse. The longer labour, due to incoordinate uterine action and either the time required to rotate to the OA position or the greater degree of descent (to negotiate the pelvic curve) required before persistent OP delivery, is also associated with severe maternal backache (as the fetus pushes its spine into the mother's back). In addition, poor contractions and delayed progress may result in the need for oxytocic augmentation. Consideration must always be given to the labouring woman concerning back pain, longer labour, possible augmentation and all associated anxieties. A higher level of analgesia and/or anaesthesia is often beneficial, but unfortunately these may also bring further possible complications and side effects.

An attempt at long internal rotation may be arrested by loss of flexion of the head and the narrowed pelvic diameter associated with prominent ischial spines (android pelvis) resulting in a deep transverse arrest. Obstructed labour, resulting from cephalopelvic disproportion, is also possible if the practitioner misses the warning signs.

There is also increased likelihood of maternal and neonatal morbidity. In part this is because of the increased incidence of fetal hypoxia, and the necessity to expedite delivery via assisted vaginal delivery (ventouse or rotational forceps) or Caesarean section as a result of the complications already described. In addition, the upward direction of moulding associated with the deflexed fetal head can become excessive and increase the possibility of a tentorial tear or cephalic haematoma. Assisted deliveries are also known to increase maternal morbidity, but even the spontaneous vaginal delivery of a persistent OP fetus (with its wider diameters and need for greater descent before delivery) increases the risk of third and fourth degree perineal trauma. The long, painful labour, with its numerous possible complications, can also predispose to both acute and chronic psychological trauma for the woman.

Possible outcomes of labour

- Long internal rotation – to an OA position. The head flexes with pelvic descent and the occiput reaches the pelvic floor and rotates anteriorly. This is a three-eighths rotation within the pelvis into the antero posterior (AP) diameter with the occiput under the symphysis pubis (see Box 8.1).
- Short internal rotation – to a persistent OP. The head remains deflexed and the sinciput reaches the pelvic floor and rotates anteriorly to lie under the symphysis pubis. This is a one-eighth rotation into the AP diameter with the occiput lying against the sacrum (see Box 8.2).
- Deep transverse arrest.
- Extension of the direct OP head at the brim of the pelvis, into a face or brow presentation.
- Obstructed labour.

Delivery of the persistent OP fetus

The baby will be born facing the symphysis pubis ('face to pubis'). The second stage of labour will have been lengthened due to the greater degree of descent required for the deflexed head to pass the symphysis pubis. Anal dilatation and gaping of the vagina may occur well in advance of delivery due to the pressure of the wide diameters. Caput succedaneum and upward moulding may distend the perineum well in advance of the delivery. Consideration of an episiotomy will be based on: the previous obstetric history of the mother; size of this fetus; stretching of the perineum as the fetus descends; and knowledge that wider diameters will pass through the introitus than with an OA delivery.

The sinciput will be the first to appear from under the symphysis pubis. Pressure is applied to the sinciput by the practitioner to encourage and maintain flexion and support smaller diameters to pass through the introitus. This pressure prevents delivery of the face beyond the glabella and enables the occiput to descend, sweep the perineum and deliver (see Figure 8.3). Once the occiput has delivered, the practitioner grasps the head and assists the face to be born, easing it through under the symphysis pubis by extending the head.

Perineal lacerations (and extensions to episiotomies) are common due to the larger diameters and because the occiput lies posteriorly, requiring lower descent before delivery, causing increased pressure on the perineum.

9 Face and brow presentations

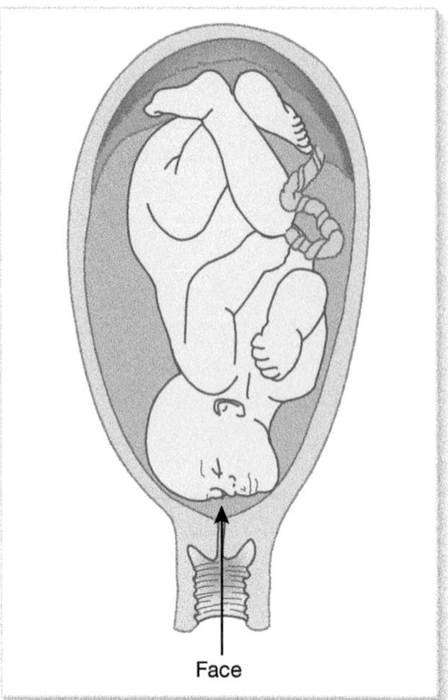

Figure 9.1 Face presentation.

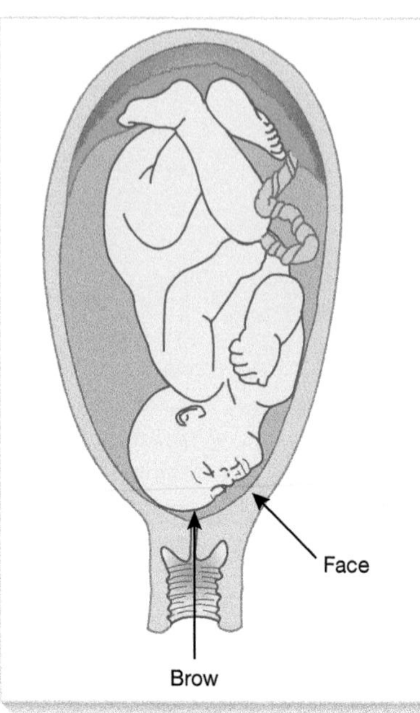

Figure 9.2 Brow presentation.

Box 9.1 Mechanism of a mento anterior face delivery.

Lie = longitudinal
Presentation = face
Denominator = mentum
Presenting part = malar bone (cheek)
Position = right mento anterior (RMA)
Attitude = full extension

- With descent the head fully extends and the mentum becomes the leading part
- The mentum reaches the pelvic floor first and rotates one-eighth anteriorly to a direct mento anterior position
- The mentum escapes from under the symphysis pubis
- The vertex and occiput sweep the perineum by flexion and the head is born
- Restitution occurs
- The shoulders reach the pelvic floor, rotate one-eighth to the direct AP
- The head rotates externally
- The anterior shoulder delivers under the symphysis pubis
- The posterior shoulder sweeps the perineum and the baby is born by lateral flexion

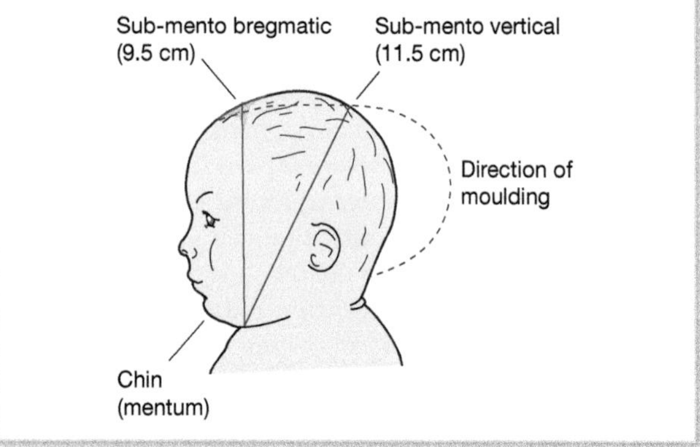

Figure 9.3 Diameters of a face presentation.

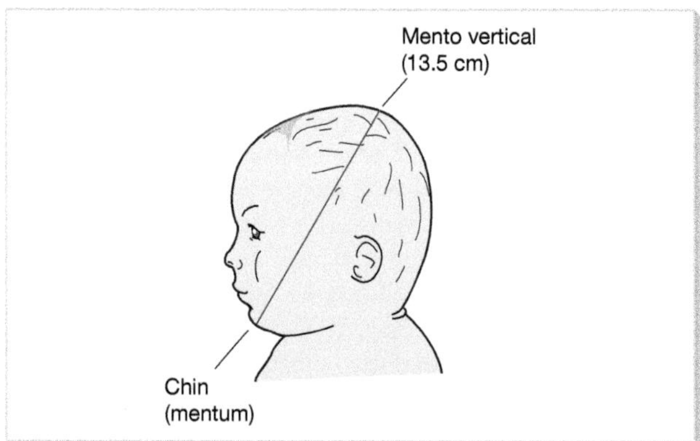

Figure 9.4 Diameters of a brow presentation.

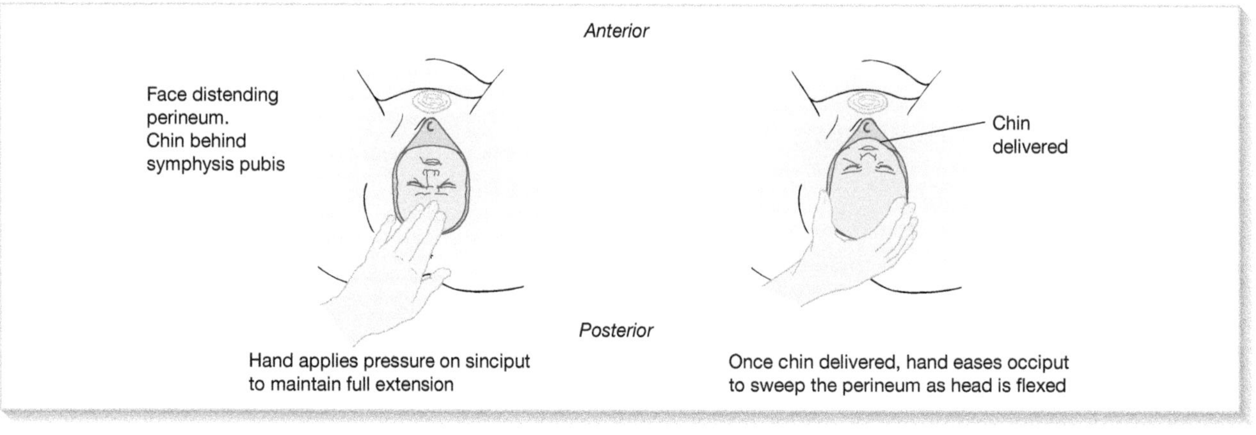

Figure 9.5 Delivery of a mento anterior face presentation.

When the head hyperextends to the degree that the occiput is against the fetal back, the face becomes the presenting part – face presentation (see Figure 9.1). If the head only partially extends (not reaching face presentation) the frontal bone leads – brow presentation (see Figure 9.2).

Incidence

The incidence for a face presentation is 1:500 with secondary face presentations being the most common. Secondary face presentations develop during an occipito posterior (OP) labour. A primary face presentation will have developed before labour commenced. Brow presentation is very rare at approximately 1:2000 deliveries. Most convert to a vertex presentation before labour or a face presentation with labour contractions.

Predisposing factors

The cause of a face or brow presentation may not be identified but a number of factors are associated with their increased incidence and they are particularly associated with an OP malposition:

- Poor abdominal tone and pendulous abdomen – more commonly associated with grand multiparity, the lack of tone allows the lie of the infant to fall forward and, with an OP position, tip the head back into a brow presentation. Contraction force may then exacerbate this position and result in a face presentation.
- Flattened pelvic brim – due to posture, trauma or may be a congenital development. An OP position particularly is affected, with the occiput resting on the brim of the pelvis rather than sliding through the brim. When contractions start, the force causes extension of the fetal head and a resultant brow or face presentation depending on degree of extension.
- Large fetal head – such that the occiput does not easily enter the pelvis and instead rests on the pelvic brim. Contractions extend the head to brow or face presentation.
- Abnormality of the fetal head – in cases where the vertex is damaged or absent (anencephaly) contraction force may push the face forward (brow presentation is not possible as there is no fetal vault).
- Abnormality of the fetal neck – tumours, webbing and long necks all increase the incidence of head extension to brow or face presentation.
- Polyhydramnios – associated with non-engagement of the vertex, sudden rupture of the membranes and a large flow of liquor, thus leading to increased malpresentation including brow and face.
- Oligohydramnios – restriction of the fetus from manoeuvring within the uterus and the greater degree of room posteriorly increases the likelihood of OP positions and malpresentations.

Complications – face presentation

There are six possible positions for a face presentation: right and left mento posterior, right and left mento lateral and right and left mento anterior. A persistent mento lateral or mento posterior position is not deliverable as the head becomes impacted. The head cannot deliver because it cannot descend low enough to pivot around the sacrum. Further descent is prevented as this would necessitate both the shoulders and head being in the pelvis at the same time. It cannot pivot anteriorly around the symphysis pubis because this would require extension and it is already fully extended. Labour becomes obstructed.

In some cases, a fully extended mento posterior/lateral position can rotate anteriorly when the mentum reaches the pelvic floor, and then become mento anterior and deliverable. Mento anterior positions do have a mechanism of labour possible. The diameter of the face presentation is the deliverable sub-mento bregmatic.

The face is typically bruised and swollen (particularly lips and eyelids) from the pressure of the cervix during birth, but this will be temporary. Significant neonatal morbidity is associated with the ill-fitting presenting part, early rupture of the membranes, and possible cord prolapse. Additionally, whilst the face itself cannot mould there may be rearward moulding and excessive compression at delivery, resulting in intracranial haemorrhage.

Maternal morbidity is associated with the increased likelihood of an assisted vaginal or operative delivery. Additionally, extension of the head to enable delivery increases diameters distending the perineum and may lead to increased perineal and vaginal trauma.

Complications – brow presentation

A brow presentation cannot even enter the brim of the pelvis because of the associated large mento vertical diameter (see Figure 9.4), let alone pass through the pelvis and be delivered. There are few exceptions to this and vaginal delivery of a brow presentation is extremely rare and limited to cases where the baby is small and the woman's pelvis is known to be adequate (typically prematurity). When detected in early labour without fetal compromise, the obstetrician may decide to allow labour to continue under close observation, to monitor the possibility of further extension to a face presentation. This trial of labour will be brief and monitored very closely. In all cases of brow presentation the most likely outcome will be Caesarean delivery to prevent obstructed labour.

Delivery of a face presentation

Spontaneous vaginal delivery of a face presentation can only occur with a spontaneous mento anterior position and adequate pelvis (see Figure 9.3). The second stage of labour will have been lengthened due to the greater degree of descent required before the face distends the vulva with the mentum under the symphysis pubis. Consideration of an episiotomy will be based on the previous obstetric history of the mother, size of this fetus, stretching of the perineum as the fetus descends and knowledge that wider diameters will pass through the introitus as the head is flexed following delivery of the mentum.

Pressure must be applied to the sinciput until the mentum has delivered – extension is maintained as any flexion of the head at this stage will increase delivery diameters to the undeliverable mento vertical. The sub mento vertical diameter is deliverable so, once the mentum has delivered, flexion is assisted and the occiput sweeps the perineum (see Box 9.1 and Figure 9.5).

Once the face presentation and head have delivered, management continues as for any vaginal delivery but with additional vigilance around perineal lacerations. Extensions to episiotomies or lacerations are common due to the larger diameters and posterior occiput.

10 Breech presentations

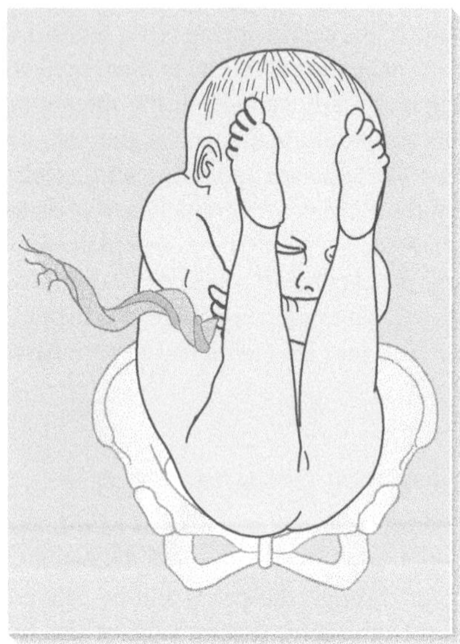
Figure 10.1 Frank breech.

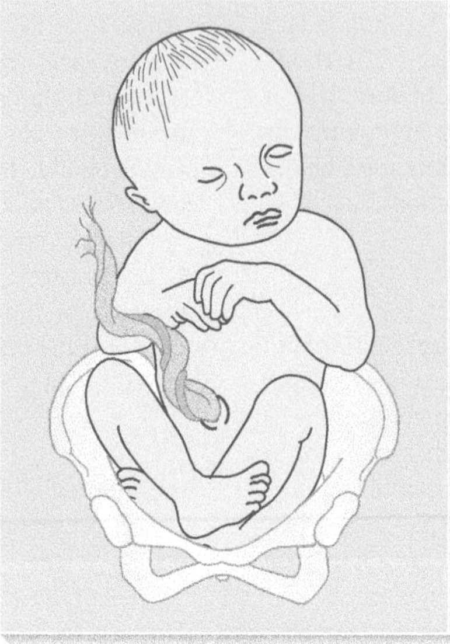
Figure 10.2 Complete (full) breech.

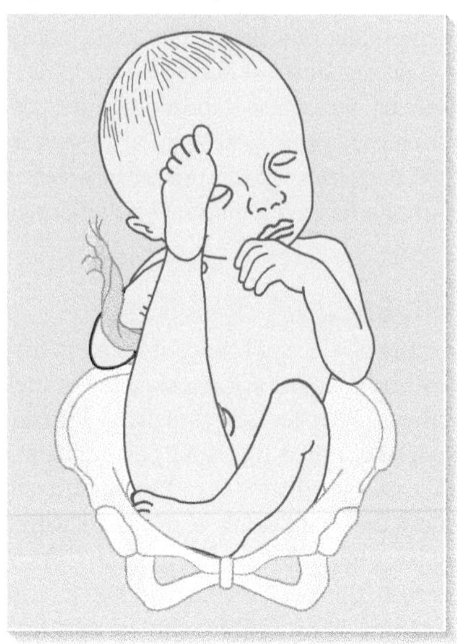
Figure 10.3 Incomplete breech.

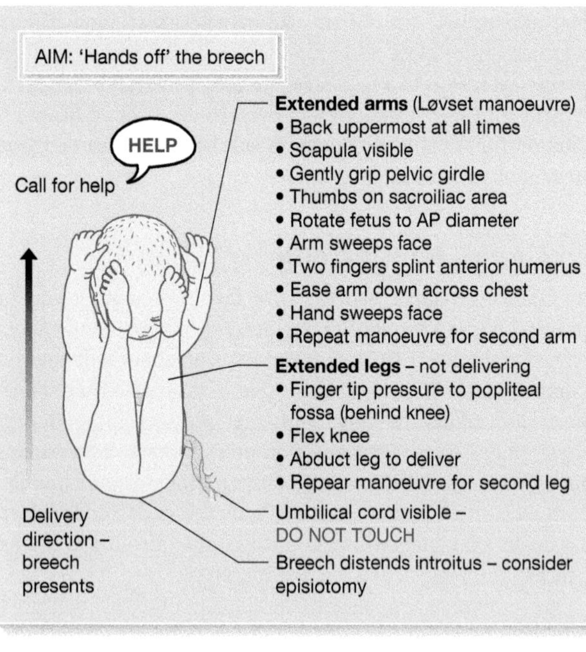

Figure 10.4 Breech delivery.

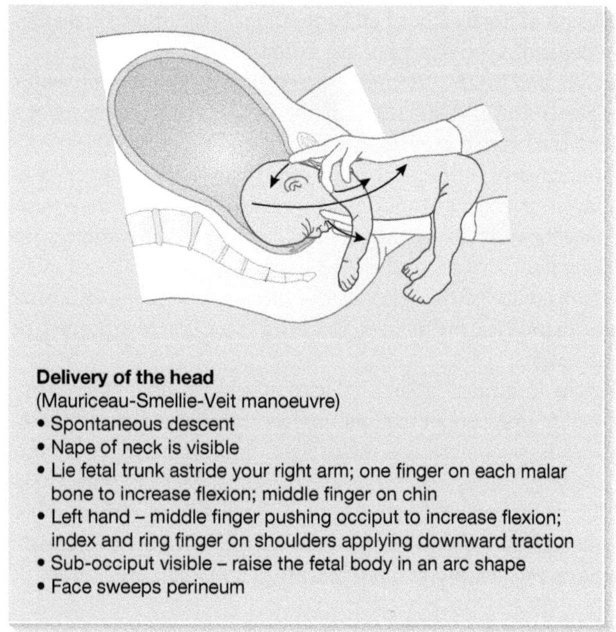

Delivery of the head
(Mauriceau-Smellie-Veit manoeuvre)
• Spontaneous descent
• Nape of neck is visible
• Lie fetal trunk astride your right arm; one finger on each malar bone to increase flexion; middle finger on chin
• Left hand – middle finger pushing occiput to increase flexion; index and ring finger on shoulders applying downward traction
• Sub-occiput visible – raise the fetal body in an arc shape
• Face sweeps perineum

Figure 10.5 Delivery of the head: Mauriceau – Smellie – Veit manouevre.

This chapter assumes that vaginal breech delivery follows an individualised decision-making process. Consideration will have been given to all the inherent risks and benefits of the options available (external cephalic version, vaginal breech delivery and Caesarean section – both planned and emergency). There will have been awareness of the predicted fetal size, pelvic capacity, progress in labour, fetal and maternal health – alongside informed maternal consent.

Definition

Breech is a malpresentation in which the buttocks of the fetus are the lowest presenting part. The incidence of breech presentation at term is 3–4%. The classification of the breech presentation is influenced by degrees of extension/flexion of the hips and knees, as follows:

- **Frank breech** (see Figure 10.1) – between 50 and 85% of breeches. Hips are fully flexed; knees fully extended; legs are straight and lie in line with the body; feet are in front or to the side of the face.

- **Complete (full) breech** (see Figure 10.2) – up to 15% of breeches. Both the hips and knees are flexed; feet are alongside the buttocks.
- **Incomplete breech** (see Figure 10.3) – up to 45% of breeches. Footling presentation may occur. Alternatively, one or both hips may be extended to a 'knee' presentation. If both the hip and knee are extended then the whole leg presents ahead of the breech.

Predisposing factors

The cause may not be identified but a number of factors are associated with increased incidence of breech presentation, often linked to unstable lie or the failure of an early breech presentation to rotate to cephalic:

- Older mothers.
- Prematurity – incidence is as high as 33% before 24 weeks gestation.
- Previous breech presentation.
- Multiple pregnancies.
- Reduced uterine/abdominal tone (e.g. grand multiparity).
- Polyhydramnios/oligohydramnios.
- Intrauterine growth restriction/low birth weight.
- Uterine abnormalities (septal defects, myomas).
- Fetal abnormalities (hydrocephaly, chromosomal disorders).
- Placenta praevia.
- Female fetus.

Vaginal breech delivery (Impey *et al.*, 2017) (see Figure 10.4)

Vaginal breech delivery must be performed by an experienced practitioner supported by a senior team in close proximity (midwife, obstetrician, paediatrician, anaesthetist, scribe and porter). Maternal positioning encourages gravitational forces and normal physiology – this may be either on all fours (AF) or semi recumbent (SR) with buttocks at the end of the delivery bed (either lithotomy position or with feet on two stools).

Spontaneous labour and delivery with minimal intervention is encouraged – 'hands off the breech'. Inappropriate traction or rotation could lead to complications such as extension of the fetal head or fetal arms. Monitor progress and descent throughout, alongside maternal and fetal health, to identify compromise or lack of progress.

Episiotomy

The head is the last part to deliver, with the greatest diameters and no time for moulding to occur. An episiotomy will not increase pelvic diameters, but it can make procedures easier and it is not easily performed once delivery begins. Selective rather than routine episiotomy occurs when the buttocks distend the perineum. This is influenced by fetal size and gestation, maternal parity and obstetric history, classification of the breech, and tightness of the perineum.

Delivery of the buttocks of the frank breech

This will normally happen spontaneously with the fetal hips in the antero posterior (AP) diameter. The anterior hip passes below the symphysis pubis, lateral flexion occurs, the posterior hip sweeps the perineum, external rotation occurs and the back turns uppermost if SR or lowermost if AF.

Delivery of the legs

Flexed legs will deliver automatically. For extended legs, wait until the popliteal fossa is visible at the vulva, then flex one knee by fingertip pressure on the popliteal fossa and deliver by abducting the leg. Repeat for second leg.

Management of the umbilical cord

Descent of the buttocks continues spontaneously to the height of the umbilicus supported by maternal effort (pushing). Do not touch the umbilical cord – any tension should ease with fetal descent.

Delivery of the trunk

Allow spontaneous descent. If there is failure to descend after delivery of the umbilicus, gentle downward traction is applied at an angle of 45 degrees. Thumbs must be on the sacroiliac area with fingers encircling the pelvis to avoid injury to internal organs. Keeping the back anterior (uppermost if SR or lowermost if AF), gently rotate the fetal body 90 degrees between the left and right oblique, continuing the downward traction until the anterior scapula can be seen. This also encourages the fetal arms to flex.

Delivery of extended arms (Løvset manoeuvre)

Flexed arms deliver spontaneously. If extended arms are present, wait until the scapula is visible, then continuing to keep the fetal back anterior (uppermost if SR, lowermost if AF), gently grip the pelvic girdle again and rotate the fetal body through 90 degrees, into the AP diameter. This encourages the anterior arm to sweep the face. Splint the anterior humerus with two fingers and ease the arm down across the chest allowing the hand to sweep the face. Keeping the back anterior now rotate the infant 180 degrees to bring the remaining extended arm anterior – deliver as for the first arm. Reposition into the transverse position (see Figure 10.4).

Head delivery (modified Mauriceau–Smellie–Veit manoeuvre) (see Figure10.5)

Management aims to flex the head (reducing diameters) as it passes through the pelvis. Allow spontaneous descent until the nape of the neck is visible. If SR, lie the baby astride your lower forearm – three fingers are in the vagina, one on each of the malar/cheek bones and one on the chin. Position your second hand above the baby – place the index and ring fingers on each of the fetal shoulders and insert the middle finger into the vagina onto the occiput. The finger on the occiput pushes upwards as the fingers on the malar bones apply downward pressure, jointly encouraging flexion of the fetal head and downward traction on the shoulders. As the sub-occiput becomes visible raise the fetal body in an arc shape to follow the curve of Carus and lastly, so that the face sweeps the perineum. When the woman is on AF, the fetal back lies along your lower arm; thumbs and little fingers wrap around the baby to hold it steady. The roles of the hands are reversed and the body will need to be lowered to follow the pelvic curve.

11 Cord presentation and prolapse

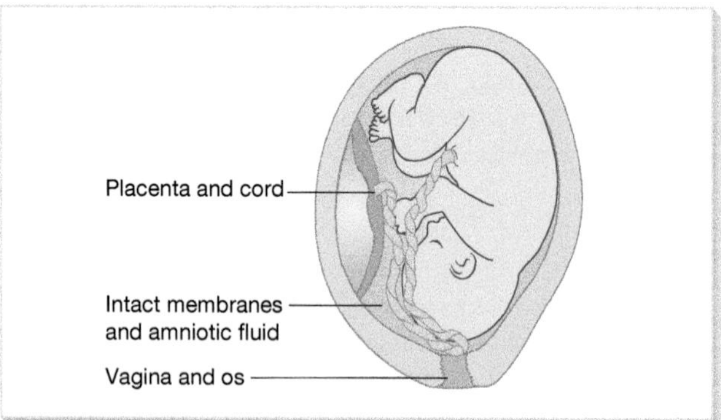

Figure 11.1 Cord presentation.

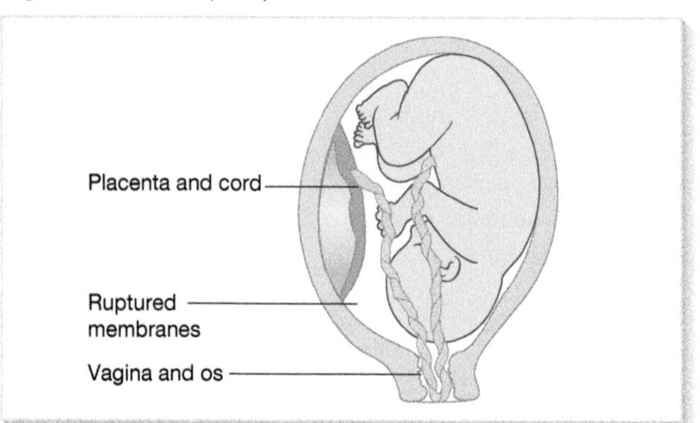

Figure 11.2 Cord prolapse.

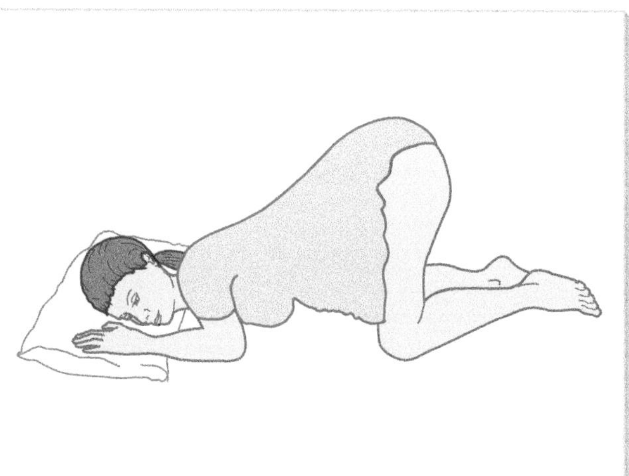

Figure 11.3 Knee – chest position.

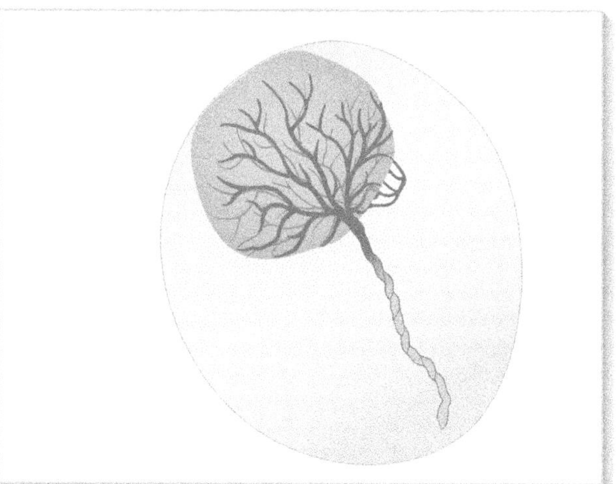

Figure 11.4 Loop of blood vessels within membrane.

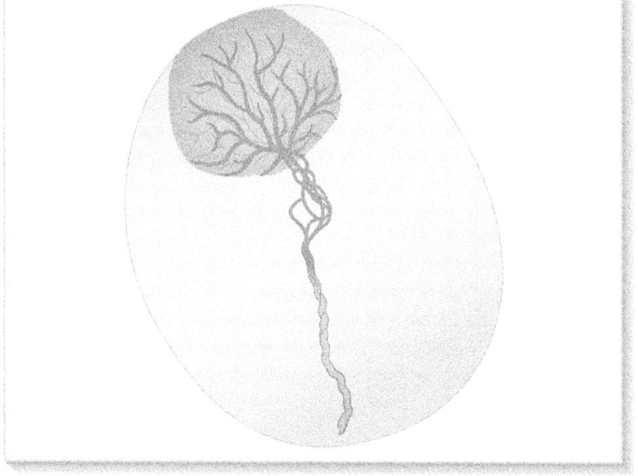

Figure 11.5 Velamentous insertion of cord.

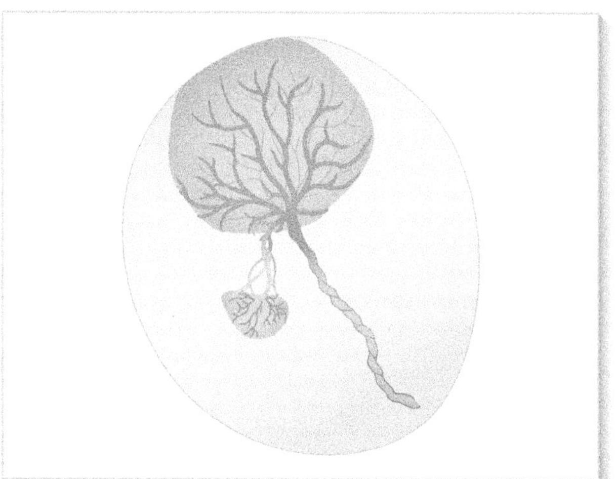

Figure 11.6 Vessels from a succenturiate lobe.

Definitions

Cord presentation is the presence of the umbilical cord, below the fetal presenting part (at the internal os) when the membranes are intact (see Figure 11.1). Cord prolapse is the presence of the umbilical cord, below the fetal presentation when the membranes have ruptured (see Figure 11.2). This may also be as a part of a compound presentation where the cord sits alongside the presenting part. The cord can prolapse to the extent of being visible hanging from the vagina. The incidence of cord prolapse is 0.5% of cephalic presentations, rising to 2% of breech presentations and 4% of multiple pregnancies (Permezel & Francis, 2015).

Predisposing factors

- Multiple pregnancies – increased cords, fluid and malpresentations.
- Premature labour – small baby and ill-fitting presenting part (PP).
- Small for gestational age – small baby and ill-fitting PP.
- Malpresentation – ill-fitting PP or breech presentation.
- Compound presentation that includes cord.
- Oblique or transverse lie – ill-fitting PP.
- Polyhydramnios – often high head and premature membrane rupture.
- Low lying placenta – cord leaves placenta low within uterus.
- Prelabour and premature rupture of the membranes.
- High PP – particularly with membrane rupture.

Recognition

Recognition of cord presentation may be by ultrasound or digital palpation during labour. With membrane rupture, the initial recognition may be by the woman feeling or visualising the cord. There may be suspicion of cord presentation or prolapse through the presence of predisposing factors and evidence of variable decelerations (or bradycardia) during contractions. These are a result of initial cord compression. Prolonged or total compression results in fetal demise.

Management

The following actions are written in order of priority where possible, but many will be happening simultaneously within a supportive, multidisciplinary team approach. When the fetal heart is heard in a viable fetus, the aim is to expedite delivery and maintain the most effective fetal oxygenation prior to birth. If the fetal heart is not heard (or the fetus is not viable), management is less urgent, allowing time to consider the best approach for delivery and greater involvement of the parents in decision making.

- Call for assistance (obstetric, anaesthetic, paediatric and senior midwife). Plan transfer to a delivery unit with full 24-hour cover (unless delivery is imminent) if not already there.
- Explain the emergency and prepare the woman for the additional staff and need for emergency delivery. Allocate a midwife to stay at the woman's head to explain the management and gain her consent.
- Immediate management requires the assessment of: the fetal heart; the stage of labour; the lie, station and presentation of the fetus; and awareness of any additional complications.
- If the cord is visible, replace it back within the vagina to maintain warmth and moisture, and support pulsation.
- Whilst preparing for delivery the pressure must be taken off the umbilical cord as much as possible. This is achieved through: maternal knee-chest positioning, with buttocks elevated (see Figure 11.3), or exaggerated Sims position for ambulance transfer; firm digital pressure against the PP using two fingers of a sterile gloved hand; stopping any oxytocic medication; filling of the maternal bladder with 400–700 mL of saline solution; and possibly tocolysis.
- Administer maternal oxygen – though evidence is limited about whether this benefits the fetus (Permezel & Francis, 2015).
- Caesarean section is recommended in the case of all labouring women where the fetal heart is still heard and delivery is not imminent. This includes:
  - primigravid women, even if in the second stage of labour
  - cases where the cervix is either not dilating or only partially dilated
  - cases where there are additional complications.
- Tocolytics may be administered by an obstetrician to reduce/stop contractions.
- In the case of full cervical dilatation of a multigravida woman, where there are no other complications and the cephalic presentation is descending well, vaginal delivery may be the quickest route. Pressure is held off the cord between contractions to enable fetal heart recovery, then the infant's delivery is expedited by maternal effort during contractions. This may be combined with an instrumental delivery as needed. Theatre should be prepared for a Caesarean section, in case of any delay with vaginal delivery.

Vasa praevia

Vasa praevia is similar to cord presentation in that fetal blood vessels appear in the lower uterine segment. In this case, they run through the amniotic membrane between the fetus and the internal os. They may occur:

- In a loop – out across the membranes and back into the placenta (see Figure 11.4).
- Between the placenta and a velamentous insertion of the umbilical cord (see Figure 11.5).
- Between a succenturiate placental lobe and the main placenta (see Figure 11.6).

These occur in approximately 1:2500 pregnancies with a perinatal mortality rate as high as 70% following rupture during either amniotomy or spontaneous rupture of the membranes (Israelsohn, 2015). Diagnosis by ultrasound during the antenatal period is more likely when a velamentous cord insertion (cord inserting into the membranes rather than the placenta) or succenturiate lobe (a lobe of placenta separated from the main placenta) have been identified and then a planned Caesarean section can occur at 36 weeks. Alternatively, the pulsation of vessels may be felt digitally on vaginal examination – this should always be checked for prior to amniotomy (see Chapter 44). Unfortunately, in most cases the problem first presents as antepartum or intrapartum haemorrhage with associated fetal demise.

12 Twins

Figure 12.1 Four most common twin presentations – transverse, oblique and compound presentations are also possible.

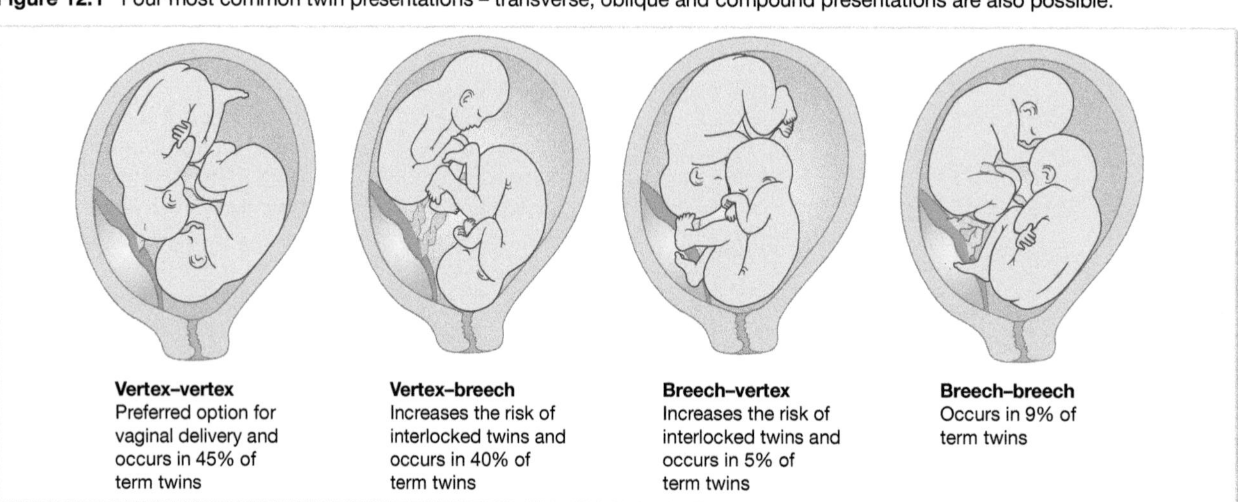

Vertex–vertex
Preferred option for vaginal delivery and occurs in 45% of term twins
Vertex–breech
Increases the risk of interlocked twins and occurs in 40% of term twins
Breech–vertex
Increases the risk of interlocked twins and occurs in 5% of term twins
Breech–breech
Occurs in 9% of term twins

Figure 12.2 Twins – options for placental, chorion, and amnion development.

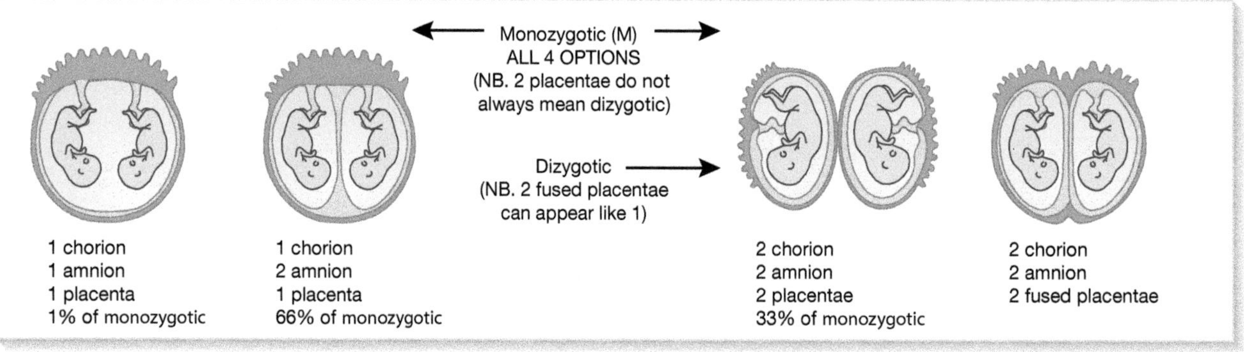

Box 12.1 Intrapartum complications requiring immediate emergency care.

- **Interlocked twins** – this occurs when the head of twin 2 sits lower in the abdomen than the head of the delivering twin 1. The chins interlock and it is no longer possible for twin 1 to deliver as its head cannot enter the pelvis. Most common with breech–vertex presentations but beware the breech–breech presentation where the second twin rotates to vertex as the uterus empties/during the delivery of twin 1.
- **Tangled umbilical cords** – this occurs with monoamniotic twins. The two fetuses and two umbilical cords are all contained within one bag of amniotic fluid. The umbilical cords can tangle around any part of either fetus – antenatally or during labour.
- **Prolapsed umbilical cord** – this can occur with the first twin due to the smaller baby and ill-fitting presenting part firstly making spontaneous rupture of the membranes more likely and secondly allowing the cord to flow past the fetus with the gush of amniotic fluid. It is even more likely with the second twin since the high presenting part may fail to engage and artificial rupture of the membranes may be necessary – in addition to the factors for the first twin.
- **Placental abruption** – this may occur following delivery of twin 1 when the decrease in size of the uterus may adversely affect the placental sites. Just as with a physiological third stage, the placenta may be sheared off the uterine wall. If this affects the placenta of the second twin, exsanguination may occur, as well as affecting maternal health.
- **Exsanguination of twin 2** – this may occur during placental abruption but can also occur if the umbilical cord of the delivered first twin is allowed to drain from a monozygotic, single placenta.

Midwifery Emergencies at a Glance, First Edition. Denise (Dee) Campbell and Susan M. Carr. © 2018 John Wiley & Sons, Ltd. Published 2018 by John Wiley & Sons, Ltd.
Companion website: www.ataglanceseries.com/midwiferyemergencies

The majority of twin pregnancies reaching term will spontaneously labour and more than 40% will deliver vaginally. Vaginal delivery is most appropriate for the healthy woman with a normally progressing pregnancy, where the first twin is in a cephalic presentation (see Figure 12.1) and there is no history of previous Caesarean section.

Incidence and complications

In 2016, the multiple pregnancy incidence in the UK was 1:63 (Office for National Statistics, 2016) and infant mortality rates were five times higher than for singleton pregnancies. Complications include pregnancy-induced hypertension, anaemia, gestational diabetes, placental abruption, placenta praevia, polyhydramnios, twin–twin transfusion, intrauterine growth retardation, premature labour (approximately one-third of twin pregnancies), fetal compromise, cord prolapse, and dysfunctional or obstructed labour.

Predisposing factors

Infertility treatment is the only predisposing factor for identical twins (monozygosity). However, there are numerous interrelated predictors for non-identical (dizygotic) twins:

- Fertility treatment – *in vitro* fertilisation and when medication is being used to ripen ova.
- Familial – linked to the maternal side.
- Heredity – female, non-identical twins have a 1:60 incidence of having twins; for male non-identical twins this is 1:125.
- Age – particularly in the > 31 age group and increasing with age.
- Race – increased for Nigerians; decreased for Chinese.
- Parity – increased for four and above.
- Body shape – increased for large and tall women; decreased for small and short women.
- Health – decreased during times of war and food scarcity.
- Diet – yam and dairy products believed to stimulate ova release.

Zygosity and chorionicity

Twins are either monozygotic (identical, developing from one ovum and one spermatozoon, splitting into two after fertilisation) or dizygotic (non-identical, developing from two ova and two spermatozoa quite separately but at the same time). Monozygotic twins can have a single placenta, two separate placentae, or two fused placentae. Two-thirds have a single placenta and single chorion (monochorionic). There can still be one or two amnions. Approximately one-third of twins born in the UK will be monozygotic. Dizygotic twins will always have two chorion and two amnion (one of each around each fetus) even when the two placentae fuse (see Figure 12.2).

Twin delivery

Contraindications to a vaginal delivery are excluded. Management must be by an experienced practitioner, supported by a senior team in close proximity (midwife, obstetrician, two paediatricians, anaesthetist, scribe and porter). Additional cord clamps and a second Resuscitaire must be available.

Episiotomy

Twin delivery alone is not an indication for an episiotomy. It may become necessary associated with labour complications.

Membrane rupture

Smaller babies, premature labour and the presence of two umbilical cords increase the likelihood of cord presentation/prolapse. This is less likely with an engaged, well applied vertex and two amniotic sacs. Vaginal examination is required to exclude these complications.

Delivery of twin one

The delivery of the first twin is the same as in a singleton delivery except **omit** the oxytocic administration completely. Following delivery, two clamps should be applied to the placenta end of the umbilical cord. This protects against blood loss from the placenta and exsanguination of a monozygotic twin (single placenta). Double clamping also identifies which cord is linked to twin one for any zygosity screening. The infant end of the cord has one clamp applied and identity bands are applied immediately.

Delivery of twin two – cephalic presentation

Twin two should deliver within 30 minutes. Palpation determines the presentation and lie, which should be stabilised within the pelvis by an assistant until the return of contractions and engagement of the presenting part. The fetal heart is auscultated. Vaginal examination is performed to confirm the presentation, degree of engagement and presence of membranes. Artificial rupture of the membranes (ARM) should only be considered if an uncomplicated presentation is below the ischial spines, there is no umbilical cord, and there are regular strong contractions. It should not be performed unless the practitioner is confident vaginal delivery is assured. ARM means there is limited time before delivery of the second twin. With maternal effort, the second twin delivers. Two umbilical cord clamps can be applied initially to identify the baby as twin two (removing one of these once identity bands are in place).

If the second twin is in a transverse or oblique lie, the obstetrician will need to correct this to longitudinal – either by performing external cephalic version or internal podalic version. See Figure 12.3 for other possible complications which may occur.

Management of the third stage

The enlarged uterus and placental site significantly increase the risk of postpartum haemorrhage. Consideration of individual obstetric history should enable informed choice. In a situation where physiological delivery has been decided upon, administration of oxytocic therapy can be agreed in advance of any emergency. Physiological delivery of the third stage follows the same procedure as with a single placenta.

Active management also follows the same procedure as for a single placenta, but with controlled cord traction applied to both umbilical cords simultaneously (following the administration of the oxytocic and contraction of the uterus). Dichorionic, same sex infants will require cord bloods and histological examination of the placenta/placentae for zygosity.

The smaller infants associated with twin deliveries make tissue trauma less likely, but the incidence of atonic uterus and retained membrane/placental tissue is increased and vigilance is required to ensure and maintain haemostasis.

13 Shoulder dystocia

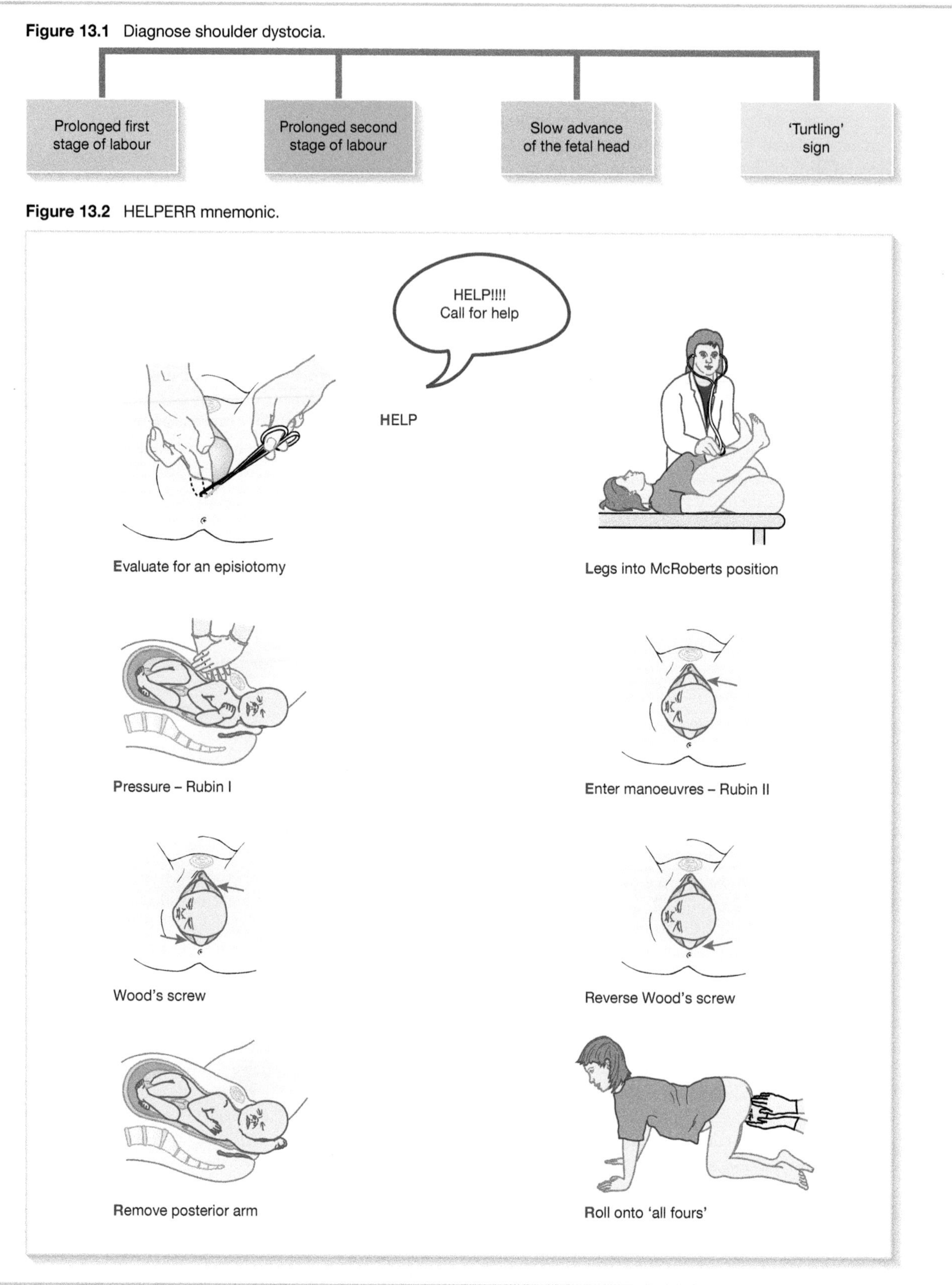

Figure 13.1 Diagnose shoulder dystocia.

Figure 13.2 HELPERR mnemonic.

Shoulder dystocia occurs in a vaginal, cephalic birth when either the anterior or very occasionally, the posterior, fetal shoulder becomes impacted behind the maternal symphysis pubis or sacral promontory respectively. As a result, the delivery of the fetal body may require additional manoeuvres, having first tried downward, axial traction. Shoulder dystocia may result in maternal and fetal morbidity and mortality (Crofts *et al.*, 2012).

Risk factors

It has been suggested that only 16% of cases of shoulder dystocia can be predicted by conventional risk factors and that it is a largely unpredictable and unpreventable event.

Antenatal risk factors

- Previous shoulder dystocia.
- Macrosomic fetus.
- Post-dates fetus.
- Maternal gestational diabetes mellitus.
- Short maternal stature.
- Abnormal maternal pelvic anatomy.
- BMI > 35.

Intrapartum risk factors

- Prolonged first stage of labour.
- Prolonged second stage of labour.
- Augmentation/induction of labour.
- Assisted/instrumental delivery.

Maternal and fetal complications

Maternal

- Third and fourth degree tears – anal sphincter damage.
- Psychological trauma.
- Postpartum haemorrhage.

Fetal

- Brachial plexus palsy.
- Fracture of clavicle or humerus.
- Hypoxic brain injury.
- Fatal acidosis.

Management – a systematic approach

The approach to the management of shoulder dystocia should be systematic, beginning with the most simple/least invasive strategies and working through to more complex manoeuvres (Gobbo *et al.*, 2017; Crofts *et al.*, 2012). This is an emergency situation in which the condition of the fetus can deteriorate rapidly (hypoxia may occur as a result of the fetal pH falling at a rate of 0.04 per minute). Prompt recognition and treatment are essential. Four basic principles should be applied:

- Diagnose the condition – 'turtling' sign (see Figure 13.1).
- Summon medical assistance.
- Systematic approach – the midwife will consider the use of the HELPERR mnemonic (Gobbo *et al.*, 2017).
- Summon a neonatologist as the baby may require resuscitative support at birth.

HELPERR (see Figure 13.2)

H – Call for help by shouting, activating the emergency call bell or sending another person to find help. In a maternity unit the personnel who are required are a senior midwife, a senior obstetrician, an anaesthetist, a paediatrician/neonatologist, and a scribe to record events. When the team arrives, inform the members that this is a shoulder dystocia.

E – Evaluate for/consider performing an episiotomy to increase space for possible internal manoeuvres. It will not resolve the bony impaction of the shoulders.

L – Legs elevated into the McRoberts' position. The legs may be straightened before being hyperflexed at the hip with the knees bent and positioned either side of the abdomen (if the fetal head has been delivered with the woman in the lithotomy position, her legs **must** be straightened before attempting the McRoberts' position). The woman must be lying flat on the bed to achieve this position. This increases the pelvic inlet while flexing the fetal spine. It also reduces maternal lumbar lordosis and flattens the sacral promontory. If any movement is seen, attempt delivery maintaining axial traction throughout.

P – Pressure. Apply suprapubic pressure constantly or intermittently using a CPR hand position, to the back of the anterior fetal shoulder towards the maternal groin on the opposite side, in an attempt to adduct the anterior shoulder thereby reducing the bisacromial diameter and enabling it to pass under the symphysis pubis. If any movement is seen, attempt delivery maintaining axial traction throughout.

E – Enter manoeuvres. Insert the fingers of one hand into the woman's vagina at either 5 o'clock or 7 o'clock depending on the position of the fetal back. Move the fingers upwards along the back until they are lying on the posterior aspect of the anterior shoulder and attempt to rotate the fetus into the oblique diameter. Suprapubic pressure can also be used externally to augment the internal manoeuvre. If no movement is seen, add the fingers of the other hand to lie on the anterior aspect of the posterior shoulder and attempt the Wood's screw manoeuvre. As before, external suprapubic pressure can also be used to augment the internal manoeuvres. If no movement is seen, remove the second hand and move the fingers of the other hand down the fetal back to lie on the posterior aspect of the posterior shoulder and attempt to rotate the fetus in the opposite direction through 180 degrees. It may be necessary to replace one hand with the other in order to complete the manoeuvre. If any movement is seen, attempt delivery maintaining axial traction throughout.

R – If no movement is seen, attempt to remove the posterior fetal arm by inserting a hand into the maternal sacral hollow and flexing the fetal arm at the elbow. This will then allow the arm to be drawn upwards across the fetal chest and be delivered, thereby reducing the bisacromial diameter and enabling the fetus to 'drop' into the sacral hollow resulting in the disimpaction of the anterior shoulder.

R – If none of the above has resulted in delivery of the fetus, roll the woman into an exaggerated 'all fours' position with the woman's head lower than her hips. It may now be possible to deliver the anterior shoulder, the posterior shoulder or remove the posterior arm.

If these manoeuvres fail, roll the woman back into the supine position and start again or consider surgical options (e.g. cleidotomy or the Zavanelli manoeuvre).

Following the resolution of the shoulder dystocia, contemporaneous notes of the event must be completed, plus an incident report form as per NHS Trust protocol. All present, including the parents, may require time to be debriefed.

14 Uterine dystocia – failure to progress

Figure 14.1 Uterine abnormalities.

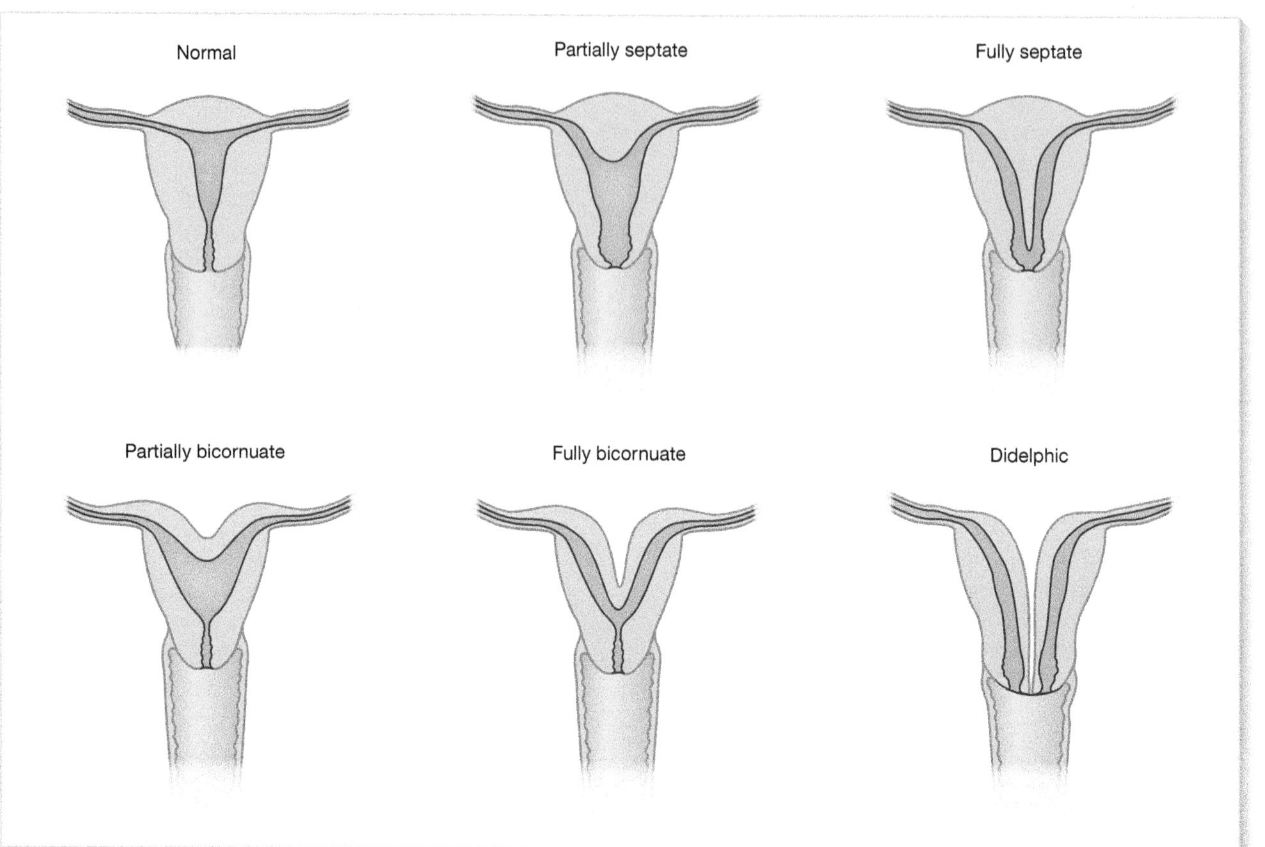

Box 14.1 Methods of augmentation.

- **Amniotomy –** NICE (2014) supports shortening of labour by approximately an hour when used for induction. Oxytocin alongside artificial rupture of the membranes (ARM) has greater support for augmenting labour.
- **Oxytocin –** a hormone which stimulates greater frequency, duration and strength of contractions (Gee, 2010). Effective for a hypotonic uterus or incoordinate contractions.

Box 14.2 Contraindications to oxytocin augmentation.

- An already optimally acting myometrium (Gee, 2010)
- Secondary arrest – unless due solely to uterine hypotonia
- Retraction ring evident
- Obstructed labour
- Pain and tenderness over Caesarean scar (or scar dehiscence)
- Monitoring opportunities and full obstetric, anaesthetic and paediatric cover are unavailable
- Lack of consent

Failure to progress can be a result of a problem associated with the contractions (power), fetus (passenger), pelvis and soft tissues (passage), or a combination of these factors occurring simultaneously. This results in the fetus being unable to descend normally through the pelvis.

Power

Contractions initiate at the fundus (fundal dominance) before a coordinated spread down through the muscles of the uterine wall (excitation wave). They gradually increase in strength, length and frequency through labour with retraction gradually shortening the muscle fibres. Interruption to this sequence may be a result of uterine inertia (failure to establish normal contractions), incoordinate uterine activity (failure to develop a regular pattern of contractions), hypotonia (weak or infrequent contractions), or uterine exhaustion (slowing or stopping of contractions). Aspects such as poor uterine tone (e.g. due to grand multiparity, polyhydramnios) and epidural anaesthesia can also slow labour and delay fetal descent (Cunningham *et al.*, 2014).

Passenger

In failure to progress linked to the fetus, there will be a complication affecting the enlargement of the delivering diameters. This may be due to size (e.g. macrocephaly), abnormality (e.g. hydrocephalus, conjoined twins), compound presentation (e.g. an arm next to the head, interlocked twins), malpresentation (e.g. brow, breech), abnormal lie (e.g. transverse), or resistance to normal moulding (e.g. postmaturity, craniosynostosis).

Passage

Complications of the passage relate to the diameters through which the fetus should pass – the overall pelvic capacity is reduced or contracted. This will more commonly be a direct cause of the pelvis (see Figure 8.4) or uterus (see Figure 14.1) but, in rare cases the vagina may be affected. It may be due to maternal size (e.g. small skeleton), congenital abnormality (e.g. bicornuate, septate or didelphic uterus, contracted pelvis, kyphosis, Naegele's pelvis), trauma (e.g. fractured pelvis), medical problem (e.g. pelvic tumour, osteomalacia), obstetric concern (e.g. fibromyoma, low lying placenta) or surgical complication (e.g. scar tissue, female genital mutilation).

Patterns of poor progress

- Prolonged latent phase.
- Primary dysfunctional labour.
- Secondary arrest.

Identifying failure to progress

Most often the identification of failure to progress will follow delayed cervical dilatation during the active first stage of labour (<1 cm/hour). This will continue despite interventions such as artificial rupture of the membranes and oxytocin augmentation. The lack of space and staff within many delivery suites increases the time pressures on the length of labour (Walsh, 2010). Be aware that this may influence unnecessary interventions during a physiological, latent phase of labour (Zhang *et al.*, 2002). These physiological variations for women are influenced by many factors including environment and their psychological state at the time and they are not a pathological failure to progress (Buckley, 2004). Therefore, midwives should consider all predisposing factors and signs of poor progress (not only delayed cervical dilatation). These include poor rotation, flexion or descent of the presenting part, prominent ischial spines, flat sacrum, narrow pubic arch, weakening of contractions (inertia likely with primigravida), coupling and incomplete relaxation between contractions (more forcible contractions likely with multigravida), increasing maternal distress, excessive caput or moulding, and fetal compromise. The identification of 'failure to progress' is individualised and based on all aspects of the labour, with full awareness of both the risks and reassuring features.

Complications

- **Cephalo-pelvic disproportion (CPD)** – the fetal head is unable to pass through the pelvis due to either an issue making the diameters of the presenting part unusually large, or the diameters of the pelvis being unusually small; or both.
- **Deep transverse arrest (DTA)** – fetal rotation is prevented through wider fetal diameters (e.g. deflexed head, abnormality) and/or reduced mid-pelvic diameters (e.g. prominent ischial spines).
- **Obstructed labour** – indicated by a combination of failure to progress in labour, fetal tachycardia, maternal tachycardia, pyrexia, haematuria, retraction ring.
- **Premature ruptured membranes** – due to ill-fitting presenting part, and further reduces stimulation of contractions.
- **Increased instrumental/operative deliveries.**
- **Fetal morbidity/mortality** – fetal compromise, shoulder dystocia, impacted fetus, trauma (e.g. intracranial haemorrhage, brachial plexus injury).
- **Maternal morbidity/mortality** – dehydration, blood loss, pain, infection, scar dehiscence, uterine rupture, perineal trauma, haemorrhage, fistula, psychological trauma.

Management considerations

- A normal latent phase is associated with satisfactory maternal and fetal conditions and reduced contractions – ensure this is the case when discounting failure to progress.
- Maintain empty maternal bladder – ensure no haematuria.
- Palpation and vaginal examination to determine cause (often multifactorial). Exclude vaginal bleeding, Bandl's contraction ring, hot and dry vagina, compound presentation, high presenting part, excessive moulding/caput, transverse arrest, and lack of progress.
- Maternal and continuous fetal monitoring in place – ensure neither maternal tachycardia or pyrexia nor fetal compromise.
- Intravenous fluid replacement as required – rehydration and prevention of ketosis to support muscle contraction.
- Augmentation – only if the failure to progress relates solely to 'powers' or there is adequate evidence that any failure in the passenger or passage can be safely overcome with improved 'power' (e.g. brow presentation extending to face). Confirm the health of the women and fetus prior to augmentation (see Box 14.1 and 14.2).
- Stop oxytocin administration in the presence of obstructed labour, fetal or maternal compromise (see Box 14.1 and 14.2).
- Antibiotics – if membrane rupture >18 hours.
- Consider instrumental delivery – during the second stage if presenting part neither impacted nor high; rotational forceps or ventouse for a non- occipito anterior position.
- Caesarean – in the presence of a non-fully dilated cervix or in preference to a difficult mid-forceps delivery; complicated by a very low presentation.

15 Manual removal of the placenta

Figure 15.1 Check uterus contracted.

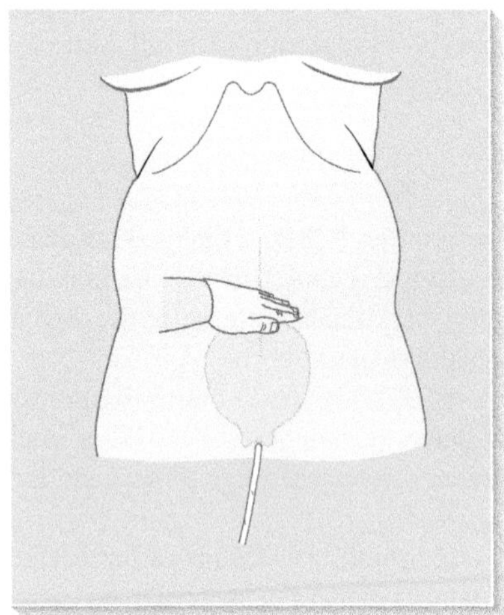

Figure 15.2 Hold umbical cord taut.

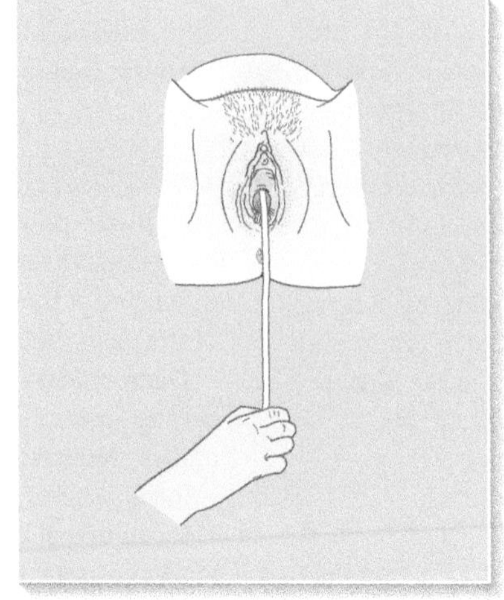

Figure 15.3 Cone-shaped hand.

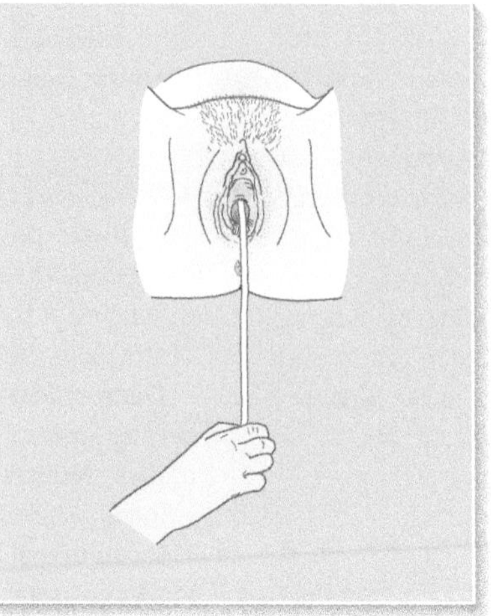

Figure 15.4 Follow cord to placenta.

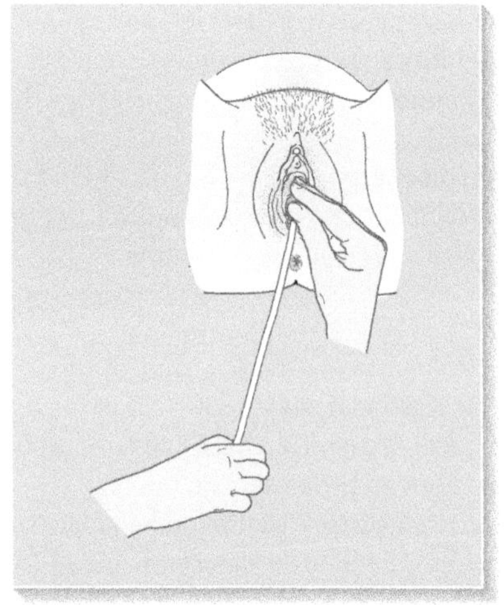

Figure 15.5 Apply counter pressure at fundus.

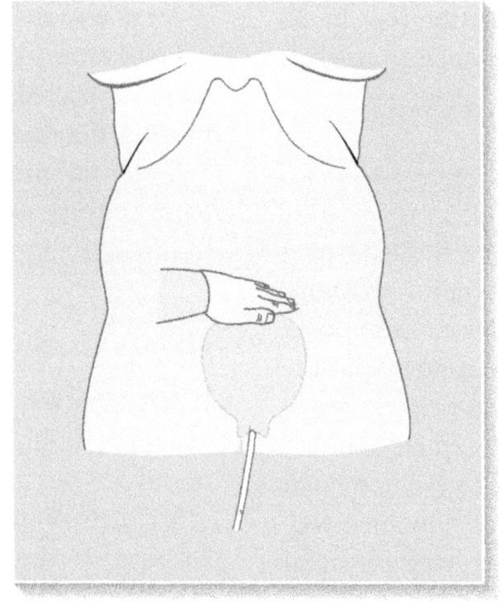

Figure 15.6 Finger tips behind placental edge.

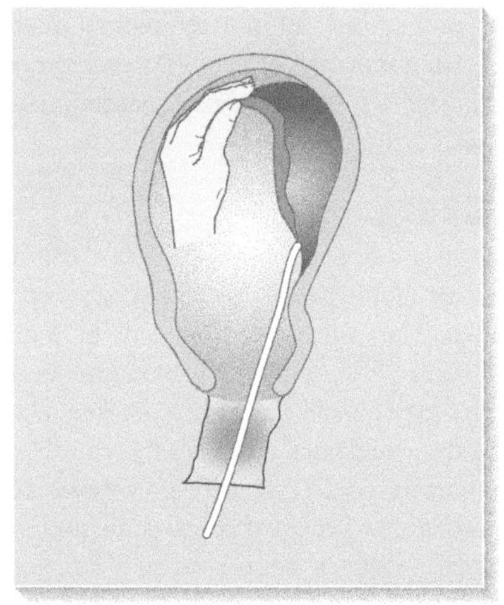

Figure 15.7 Fingers gently slice back and forth against placental edge.

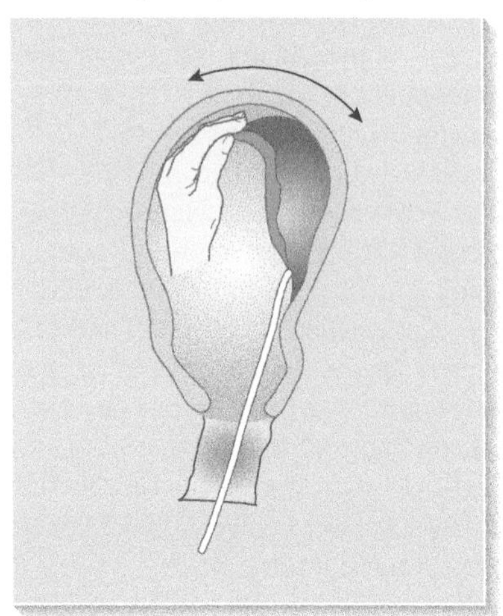

Figure 15.8 Rub up contraction once placenta separated.

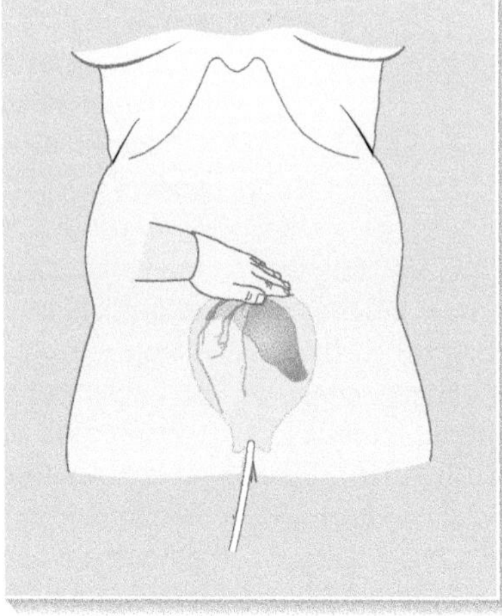

Figure 15.9 Placenta and hand expelled together.

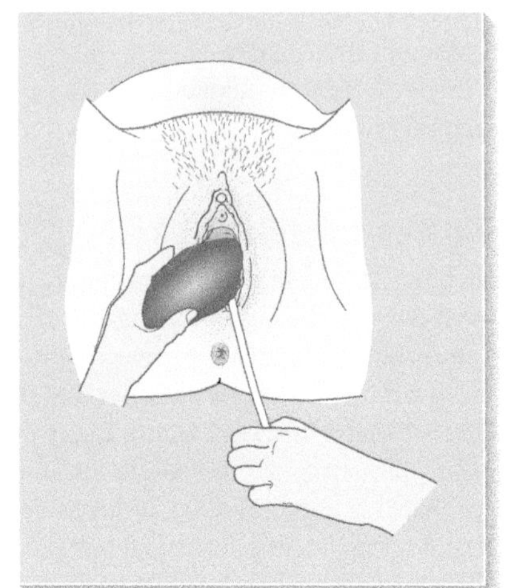

Manual removal of the placenta (MROP) is the physical removal of a placenta after it has been retained *in utero,* and following a prolonged third stage of labour. The physiological third stage should last no more than 60 minutes – NICE (2017a) suggests an actively managed third stage of labour is prolonged after 30 minutes.

Management of MROP should occur before or at the earliest onset of any significant bleeding in order to avoid haemorrhage. The risk of bleeding begins to increase from 10 minutes into the third stage and may necessitate immediate MROP. In the absence of an early haemorrhage, the arrangements for the MROP should commence 30 minutes into the third stage with all the management procedures completed before the infant is an hour old. This allows optimum time for normal expulsion of the placenta (expectant management) alongside the balance of MROP before haemorrhage risk becomes significant (Shinar *et al.*, 2016).

Incidence

A lack of conformity in the definition of prolonged labour has resulted in a 1–5.5% variation in the reported incidence. Applying the 30 minutes guidance, the incidence is 3% after which the balance of risk regarding haemorrhage outweighs the advantages of expectant management (Chongsomchai *et al.*, 2014; Urner *et al.*, 2014).

Causes

There are three causes of retained placenta:

- Adherens placenta – the retroplacental myometrium is insufficiently contracting to separate the placenta.
- Adherent placenta – invasive chorionic villi from all or part of the placenta are abnormally attached within the myometrium.
- Incarcerated placenta – a closed cervix has trapped the placenta *in utero.*

Predisposing factors (Urner *et al.*, 2014; John *et al.*, 2015; Shinar *et al.*, 2016)

- Short/snapped cord – may be only comparatively short due to entanglement around the neck, body or limbs of the fetus.
- Previous retained placenta.
- Previous dilatation and curettage.
- Low-lying placenta.
- Uterine scar.
- Premature birth.
- Stillbirth.
- Placental abnormalities (e.g. succenturiate lobe) – may lead to retention of just the succenturiate lobe.
- Primiparity.
- Multiparity – larger or multiple placentae.
- Grand multiparity – increases the risk of a low-lying placenta as the placenta can never embed in the same place twice.
- Older maternal age.
- Pyrexia in labour.
- History of abortion.
- Oxytocic use in labour – reduced or ineffective physiological uterine contractions.

Management (Chongsomchai *et al.*, 2014; Duffy *et al.*, 2015; Cummings *et al.*, 2016; Maher *et al.*, 2016; NICE, 2017a)

It should first be emphasised that the management of any postpartum haemorrhage (PPH), resultant shock or maternal collapse will take place alongside delivery of the retained products of conception (see Chapter 6).

- Explanation and informed client consent.
- Intravenous access – to maintain fluid balance and to administer oxytocics (only if haemorrhage begins). No pharmacological treatments are more effective in preventing PPH than MROP.
- Transfer to obstetric unit if necessary once haemostasis controlled.
- Adequate analgesia.
- Vaginal assessment to ensure placenta is not partially in the vaginal and also to assess cervical dilatation.
- Transfer to theatre.
- Effective anaesthesia for MROP.
- Aseptic procedure throughout.
- Ensure contracted uterus (see Figure 15.1).
- Non-dominant hand holds umbilical cord taut (see Figure 15.2).
- Insert dominant hand in a cone shape, through vagina, cervix and uterus to placenta, following cord (see Figures 15.3 and 15.4).
- Non-dominant hand releases cord and applies counter pressure at fundus as placenta is freed (see Figure 15.5).
- Dominant hand finger tips gradually apply increasing pressure under placental edge with a gentle slicing/sweeping movement (palm of hand inwards to uterus) (see Figures 15.6 and 15.7).
- Once the placenta has separated, a contraction is rubbed up (by the fundal hand) to deliver the placenta along with the hand holding it (see Figures 15.8 and 15.9).
- Ensure placenta and membranes are complete.
- Oxytocic therapy given intravenously to maintain uterine contractility.
- Ensure intact perineum or that any lacerations are appropriately sutured.
- Prophylactic antibiotic therapy is debated in the literature but without a strong evidence base for routine use.
- Ensure adequate analgesia is maintained post-delivery.
- In an emergency and life-threatening situation the procedure may need to be performed without anaesthetic.

Possible complications

- Endometritis.
- Endometriosis.
- PPH – massive haemorrhage.
- Sepsis.
- Uterine damage.
- Perineal infection.
- Death – fatality rates are high in less developed countries.

16 Adhered or partially adhered placenta

Figure 16.1 Focal placenta accreta.

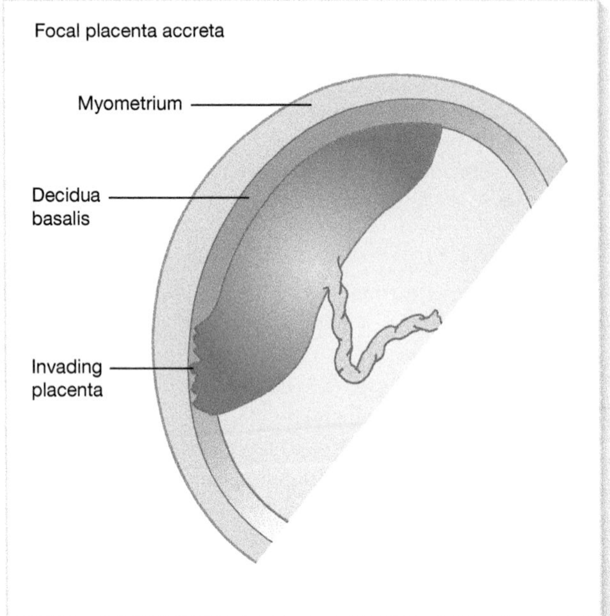

Figure 16.2 Placenta accreta.

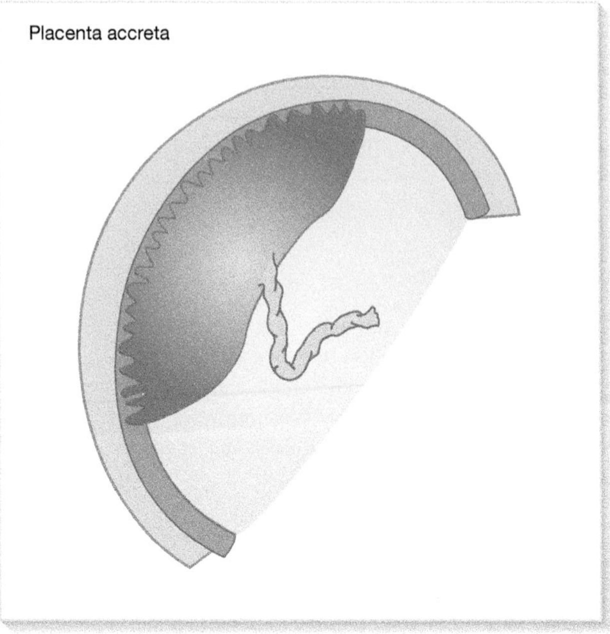

Placenta accreta

Figure 16.3 Placenta increta.

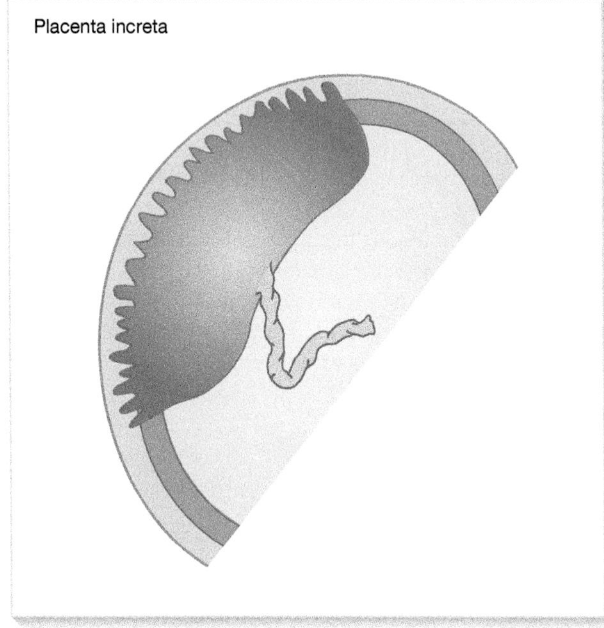

Figure 16.4 Placenta percreta.

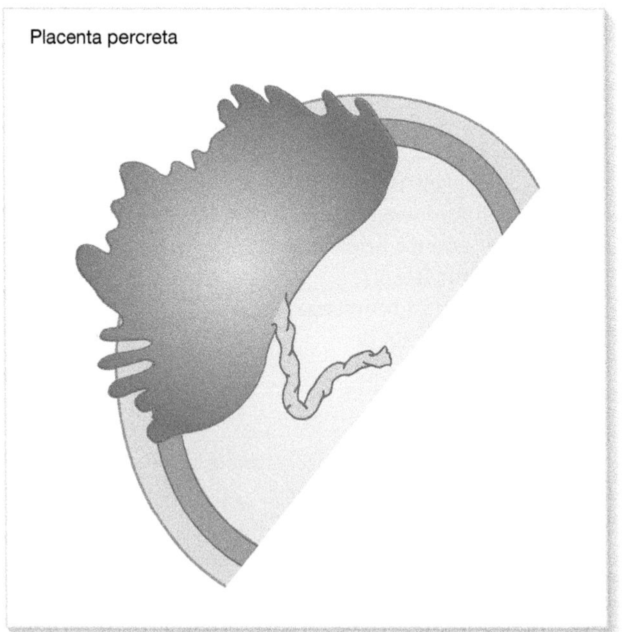

Definition

Placental tissue becomes adherent when chorionic villi invade the uterine wall and become too deeply embedded. The decidua basalis may be absent or incomplete allowing the placental cotyledons in that area to embed into the myometrium. The depth that the trophoblasts reach will vary in each case. There are a number of possibilities regarding adherent or partially adherent placentae – known as placenta accreta syndromes. The accreta syndrome may affect the whole or part of the placenta and to different depths within the myometrium.

- **Focal accreta** (see Figure 16.1) is a general term for when one or more parts are adherent. This may become apparent when inspection of the placenta reveals missing cotyledons which later prove adherent. More significantly, a partially adherent placenta will allow partial separation with the risk of massive haemorrhage.
- **Placenta accreta** (see Figure 16.2) may be applied as a general term when the full placenta is adherent. It may also be used more specifically to indicate that the chorionic villi invade to the decidua level of the myometrium.
- **Placenta increta** (see Figure 16.3) relates to the chorionic villi invading more deeply and within the myometrium.
- **Placenta percreta** (see Figure 16.4) relates to the chorionic villi penetrating through the myometrium to the visceral peritoneum lying over the fundus and posterior wall of the uterus (serosa). The villi may reach and embed into other internal organs such as the bladder.

Incidence

The UK incidence of accreta, increta and percreta is 1.7:10 000 of total maternity cases – lower when there has been no previous Caesarean section (CS) (1:33 000) and considerably higher (1:20) where there has been a previous CS and a current placenta praevia (PP) (Fitzpatrick *et al.*, 2012b). The incidence is increasing rapidly associated with higher CS or PP rates or age at onset of pregnancy (Fitzpatrick *et al.*, 2012b).

Countries such as the USA, where CS and PP rates are already higher, detail a 1:533 risk (American College of Obstetrics and Gynaecology, 2012). Accreta syndromes are becoming a major challenge with their associated maternal morbidity (haemorrhage and emergency hysterectomy) and mortality (8% of haemorrhage deaths are associated with accreta syndromes) (Berg *et al.*, 2010).

Predisposing factors (Fitzpatrick *et al.*, 2012b)

- Previous CS – not increasing with multiple CS.
- Low-lying placenta.
- Previous uterine surgery other than CS.
- Maternal age at delivery – risk increases with each additional year over the age of 35 years (without a history of CS).
- *In vitro* fertilisation (IVF) pregnancy.
- Uterine trauma.

Diagnosis

Ideally, accreta syndrome will be identified antenatally during ultrasound monitoring. A high level of suspicion, in cases of previous CS and current PP, should indicate colour Doppler screening, followed by confirmation by magnetic resonance imaging (Cunningham *et al.*, 2014). IVF, prior uterine surgery and maternal age are also associated with increased screening and may identify the complication. In cases where the problem is only identified in the third stage of labour, the first suspicion may be the retained placenta which, when totally adherent, rarely has a clear edge to allow manual removal procedures. More significant may be the degree of postpartum haemorrhage (PPH) (and maternal collapse) associated with a partially separated/partially adhered placenta.

Management (Johnston & Paterson-Brown, 2011; Walker *et al.*, 2013; Cunningham *et al.*, 2014; Fitzpatrick *et al.*, 2014)

Emergency

The haemorrhage must be treated as per primary PPH with a multiprofessional team (see Chapter 6). Here the cause is not just retained products but partially adherent ones. Stop attempts to deliver the placenta and apply bimanual compression. Surgery will be required. Percreta or increta will almost always require hysterectomy but haemostasis of a partial (focal) accreta may be achieved through management of individual bleeding points as the placenta is removed. Fluid replacement and airway management will need to be escalated. Maternal shock and blood transfusion is likely.

Expectant

Expectant management is possible when the accreta syndrome is recognised antenatally, when there is natural haemostasis after delivery and when the placenta has delivered but focal adherent lobes have been retained. If identified after a vaginal delivery, leaving the placenta *in situ* is a possibility – this allows time for further investigation and decisions for optimal care, or for the placenta to reabsorb.

When identified antenatally, management may include:

- Detailed screening and diagnostic tests to confirm diagnosis and determine degree of accreta.
- Explanation, information and psychological support.
- Preoperative assessment and maternal tour of obstetric observation bay (OOB) or intensive care unit (ICU).
- Management and delivery by multiprofessional team (invasive placenta surgical team) – planned, 36 week CS.
- Minimum of two units of cross-matched blood available.
- Preoperative placement of balloon catheters in the internal iliac arteries – becoming less popular as recent studies suggest they do not significantly reduce blood loss (Salim *et al.*, 2015).
- Postoperative management in OOB or ICU.

Complications and outcomes (Cunningham *et al.*, 2014)

- Placenta left *in situ* and hysterectomy performed.
- Thrombosis of iliac arteries from incorrect use of balloon catheters.
- PP may limit anterior wall and lower segment incision possibilities.
- Spontaneous bleeding from partial separation – life-threatening haemorrhage requiring immediate hysterectomy.
- A placenta left *in situ* may become infected or begin to bleed and necessitate medical intervention or hysterectomy at a later stage.
- Increased risk of reoccurrence.

17 Uterine inversion

Figure 17.1 Uterine inversion.

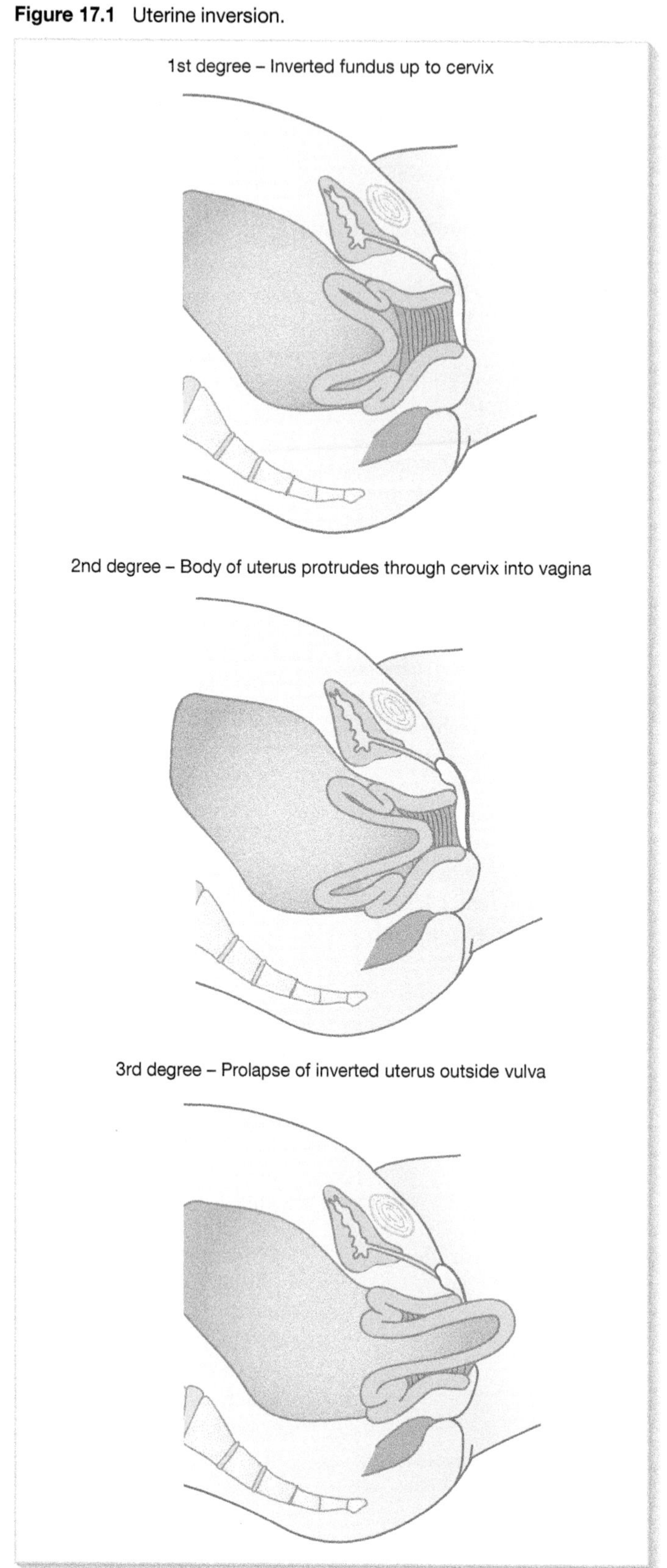

Midwifery Emergencies at a Glance, First Edition. Denise (Dee) Campbell and Susan M. Carr. Published 2018 by John Wiley & Sons, Ltd.
Companion website: www.ataglanceseries.com/midwiferyemergencies

Usually the placenta and membranes detach from the wall of the uterus and are delivered via the cervix and through the vagina within 60 minutes of the birth of the baby. However, acute inversion of the uterus, a rare event, may occur in the third stage of labour, when the uterus is turned partially or completely inside out. The incidence varies greatly from one in 1500–2000 maternities, to one in 20 000 – 50 000 maternities. This is potentially life threatening. However, it is estimated that the maternal survival rate is between 85 and 95%.

Risk factors and causes

Acute inversion of the uterus is associated with conditions which may render the uterus atonic in the presence of cervical dilatation.

Predisposing risk factors

- Previous history of uterine inversion.
- Primiparity or grandmultiparity.
- Prolonged labour or a precipitate delivery.
- Short umbilical cord (Dawn *et al.*, 2000).
- Congenital uterine abnormality (e.g. unicornuate uterus).
- Macrosomic fetus.
- Polyhydramnios.
- Maternal connective tissue disorder (e.g. Marfan's syndrome – rare).

Causes

- The most common cause of uterine inversion is mismanagement of the third stage of labour when the uterus is atonic and excessive traction on the umbilical cord has been applied with or without fundal pressure prior to the separation of the placenta.
- Retained placenta in the presence of over-zealous traction on the umbilical cord.
- Fundal pressure prior to separation of the placenta.
- Abnormally adherent placenta (e.g. placenta accreta where the placenta has invaded the uterine wall too deeply in the embryonic stage of development).
- Manual removal of the placenta (i.e. if the internal hand of the operator is removed rapidly while the external hand is still applying fundal pressure).
- Spontaneous inversion of the uterus with an unknown aetiology.

Classification (see Figure 17.1)

In general, inversion of the uterus is classified according to:

(i) The severity of the prolapse of the uterus:
- **First degree or incomplete inversion** – when the fundus of the uterus indents or collapses into the cavity of the uterus, but does not pass through the cervical os.
- **Second degree or complete, prolapsed inversion** – when the uterus is inside out and has passed through the cervical os, but remains within the vagina.
- **Third degree or total inversion** – when the uterus, cervix and vagina are visible inside–outside.

(ii) The timing of the inversion in relation to the birth of the baby:
- **Acute** – within 24 hours of the birth.
- **Sub-acute** – between 24 hours and 4 weeks after the birth.
- **Chronic** – more than 4 weeks after the birth.

Signs and symptoms

- Severe abdominal pain.
- Uterine palpation may reveal an indent in the fundus of the uterus, or the absence of the uterus depending on the severity of the inversion.
- Major postpartum haemorrhage after the separation of the placenta.
- Cardiovascular collapse due to haemorrhage and neurogenic shock due to the pressure from traction on the round and infundibulopelvic ligaments.
- Appearance of the uterus at the vulva.

Management

Management will depend on the degree of severity and the condition of the woman. Speed is of the essence when replacing the uterus, as delay may cause it to become oedematous, thus impeding its replacement.

Reduction of the inversion

- Summon emergency help to include: senior midwife, a senior obstetrician, an anaesthetist, a porter and a scribe to record events.
- Manual re-insertion of the uterus if possible with or without a general anaesthetic by applying digital pressure working up from the sides of the uterus so that the fundus is replaced last. Tilting the delivery bed into a head-down position may assist the operator and reduce the traction on the round and infundibulopelvic ligaments.
- Hydrostatic replacement of the uterus under general or spinal anaesthetic: 2–3 L of warmed 0.9% normal saline are instilled into the uterus through an intravenous infusion set via the vagina. This will fill the vagina and fornices before inflating the uterus and restoring it to its rightful position. The operator may then seal the introitus with either their hand or a soft cup used for vacuum extraction. Tilting the delivery bed into a head-down position may assist the operator and reduce the traction on the round and infundibulopelvic ligaments (Gupta *et al.*, 2014).
- If these measures are unsuccessful, surgical intervention may be attempted.
- Tocolytic therapy may be required to relax the uterus.

Resuscitation of the woman

- An intravenous cannula should be inserted and blood taken for group and cross-matching.
- Catheterisation of the urinary bladder should be performed.
- Remedy hypovolaemic shock with a rapid infusion of warmed crystalloid fluid and/or blood products depending on the degree of haemorrhage.
- If the placenta is still adhered to the wall of the uterus, it should be left *in situ* until the uterus has been replaced.
- Oxytocic therapy may need to be commenced to achieve and then maintain the contraction of the uterus. Only then may delivery of the placenta be attempted.

18 Uterine rupture and scar dehiscence

Figure 18.1 Uterine rupture.

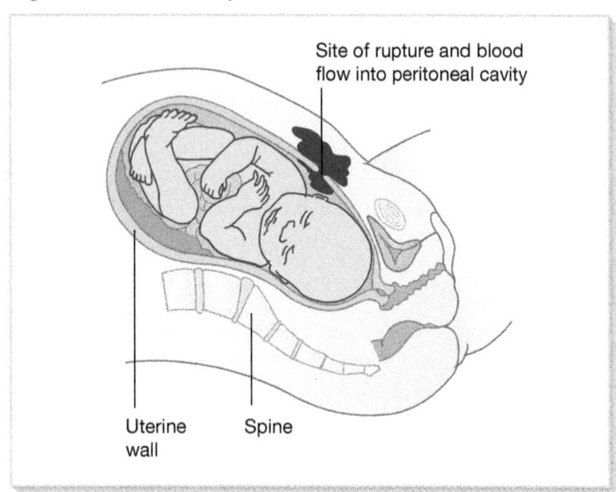

Figure 18.2 Scar dehiscence.

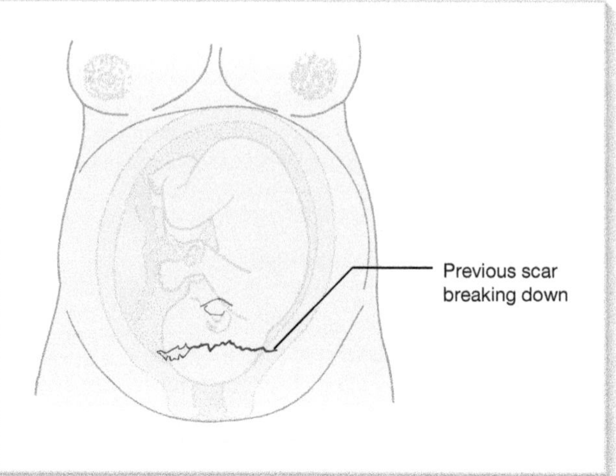

Previous scar breaking down

Figure 18.3 Maternal mortality – direct and indirect deaths.

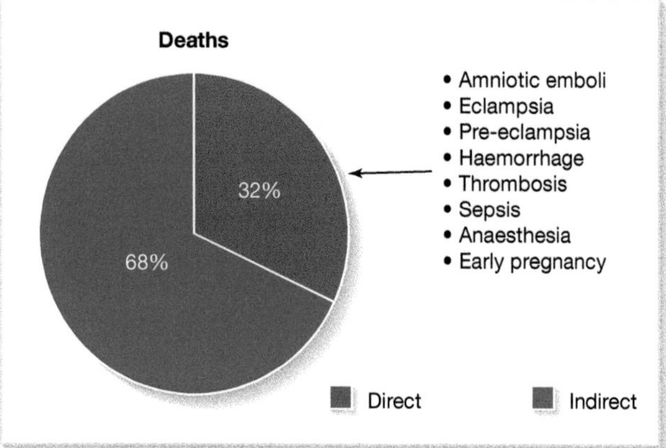

Figure 18.4 Deaths associated with haemorrhage.

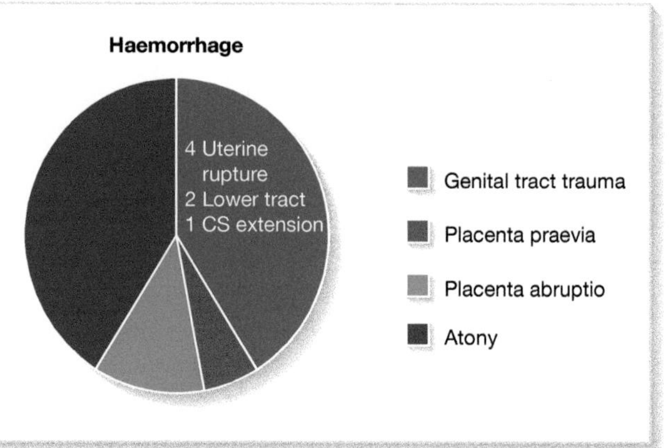

Figure 18.5 Fetal heart may have reduced beat to beat variation, variable then late decelerations, plus fall in baseline.

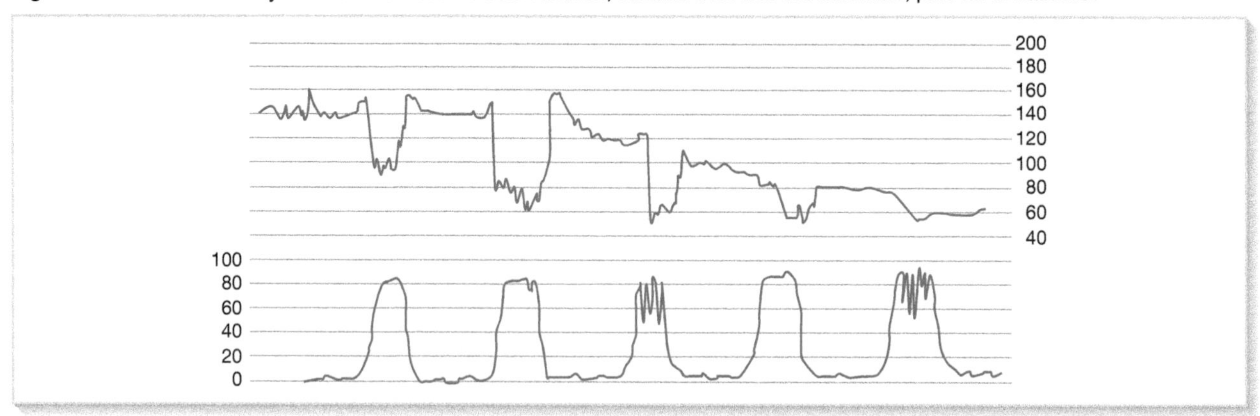

Midwifery Emergencies at a Glance, First Edition. Denise (Dee) Campbell and Susan M. Carr. © 2018 John Wiley & Sons, Ltd. Published 2018 by John Wiley & Sons, Ltd.
Companion website: www.ataglanceseries.com/midwiferyemergencies

Definition

The definitions for uterine rupture can vary in the literature from being the 'direct communication between the uterine and peritoneal cavities occurring when there is full thickness disruption of the uterine wall' (Porecco *et al.*, 2009) to more staged degrees of complete or incomplete rupture. When stages are described, the definition by Porecco *et al.* (2009) aligns with a 'complete rupture', whereas incomplete rupture involves separation of the uterine muscles without involvement of the visceral peritoneum. When an incomplete rupture affects previous scarring this is known as dehiscence (see Figures 18.1 and 18.2) (Cunningham *et al.*, 2014). In addition, uterine rupture may be described as primary if there has been no previous uterine damage (traumatic or operative), and secondary when the uterus has a history of previous incision, injury and scarring (Cunningham *et al.*, 2014).

Incidence

Uterine rupture is a relatively rare condition associated with increased morbidity and mortality for both mother and fetus/infant. Between 1976 and 2012 the incidence of uterine rupture was 1:1416 pregnancies across both developed and non-developed countries (Nahum, 2015); 1:4800–5000 for developed countries alone (Fitzpatrick *et al.*, 2012a; Getahun *et al.*, 2012); and only 1:8434 in developed countries when scarred uteri are excluded (Nahum, 2015). However, when there has been one previous Caesarean section (CS) and no vaginal birth, uterine rupture may be as high as 2.1–5:1000 – rising to 1:70 after a second CS (Fitzpatrick *et al.*, 2012a; Permezel, 2015a).

Maternal mortality studies between 2009 and 2012 across the UK identified five maternal deaths where uterine rupture played a part – four (22.8%) within the postpartum haemorrhage statistics and one following a termination of pregnancy (see Figures 18.3 and 18.4) (Paterson-Brown & Bamber, 2014). The overall risk of perinatal deaths following uterine rupture varies in the literature from 6.2 to 12.4% (decreasing to 2.8% for term infants) but with an additional 13% having significant morbidity issues (Guise *et al.*, 2010; Fitzpatrick *et al.*, 2012a).

Predisposing factors (Permezel, 2015a)

- Upper uterine scars – hysterotomy, classical incision CS.
- Lower uterine section scar – CS.
- Induction of labour or inappropriate/excessive use of oxytocin.
- Obstructed labour – lower uterine segment progressively thinning.
- Blunt-force trauma – such as from a fall, road traffic accident, internal podalic version, or an instrumental delivery.
- Invasive trauma – accidental (impalement injury) or nonaccidental (knife attack).
- Internal version – second twin, malpresentation.
- Prolonged labour or dystocia – cephalopelvic disproportion.
- Abnormalities of the uterus.
- Uterine distension – multiple pregnancy, polyhydramnios.
- Myometrial placentation – placenta accreta or hydatidiform mole.

Recognition

The number of symptoms relates to the degree of rupture/dehiscence, and degree of protuberance of the fetus and/or placenta into the peritoneal cavity. Recognition and diagnosis of uterine rupture is challenging in its earliest stages and when damage is minimal. Holmgren (2012) identified that signs of fetal compromise were the most common feature found in 24 cases (66.7 %), maternal symptoms were found in eight cases (22.2%), and three cases had symptoms in both mother and fetus (8.3%); there were no symptoms in one case (2.8%). Symptoms include:

- **Variable heart rate decelerations** worsening to **late decelerations** as fetal hypoxia increases – severity increasing with degree of placental abruption (see Figure 18.5).
- **Pain** over the site, or referred to higher in the chest/shoulders – referred along the phrenic nerve to the shoulder area when intraperitoneal bleeding causes diaphragmatic pressure (may be mistakenly taken for abruption, pulmonary or amniotic emboli).
- **Shortness of breath** – due to diaphragmatic and peritoneal pressure.
- **Unexplained bleeding** – uterine haemorrhage or haematuria.
- **Palpation of fetal parts** – if fetal parts are now within the abdomen.
- **Maternal collapse** – hypovolaemic shock and maternal death.
- **Fetal death** – from anoxia.

Management (Cunningham *et al.*, 2014)

- In emergency management there needs to be simultaneous management of:
  - Resuscitation – airway, breathing, circulation.
  - Haemorrhage – haemostasis, hypovolaemic shock.
  - CS delivery.
  - Uterine damage repair (hysterectomy is the most likely course to control haemostasis).
- A multiprofessional approach is used that aims to minimise the decision to delivery time as the hypoxia risks to the fetus increase with delivery delay.
- Postoperative care within an obstetric observation bay.

When haemostasis is controlled and the fetus either shows no signs of hypoxia or has delivered vaginally there may be:

- Routine scar exploration following vaginal delivery – becoming less common but may be performed following instrumental deliveries.
- Surgical correction of scar dehiscence – generally not necessary unless there is significant bleeding.
- Uterine repair – high risk of rupture reoccurrence in future pregnancy.

Outcomes and complications

- Placental abruption – as a result of rapid reduction in uterine size.
- Anaesthetic or operative complications – linked to emergency situation and deteriorating maternal condition.
- Laceration to fetus – linked to unpredictable positioning.
- Fetal hypoxia – depends on degree of abruptio, haemorrhage and fetal protrusion into the peritoneum.
- Placenta accreta in a future pregnancy.
- Reoccurrence in any future pregnancy if repair carried out.
- Sepsis – maternal and neonatal.
- May extend through cervix and vagina or into the active uterus.
- Planned CS required for future pregnancies.

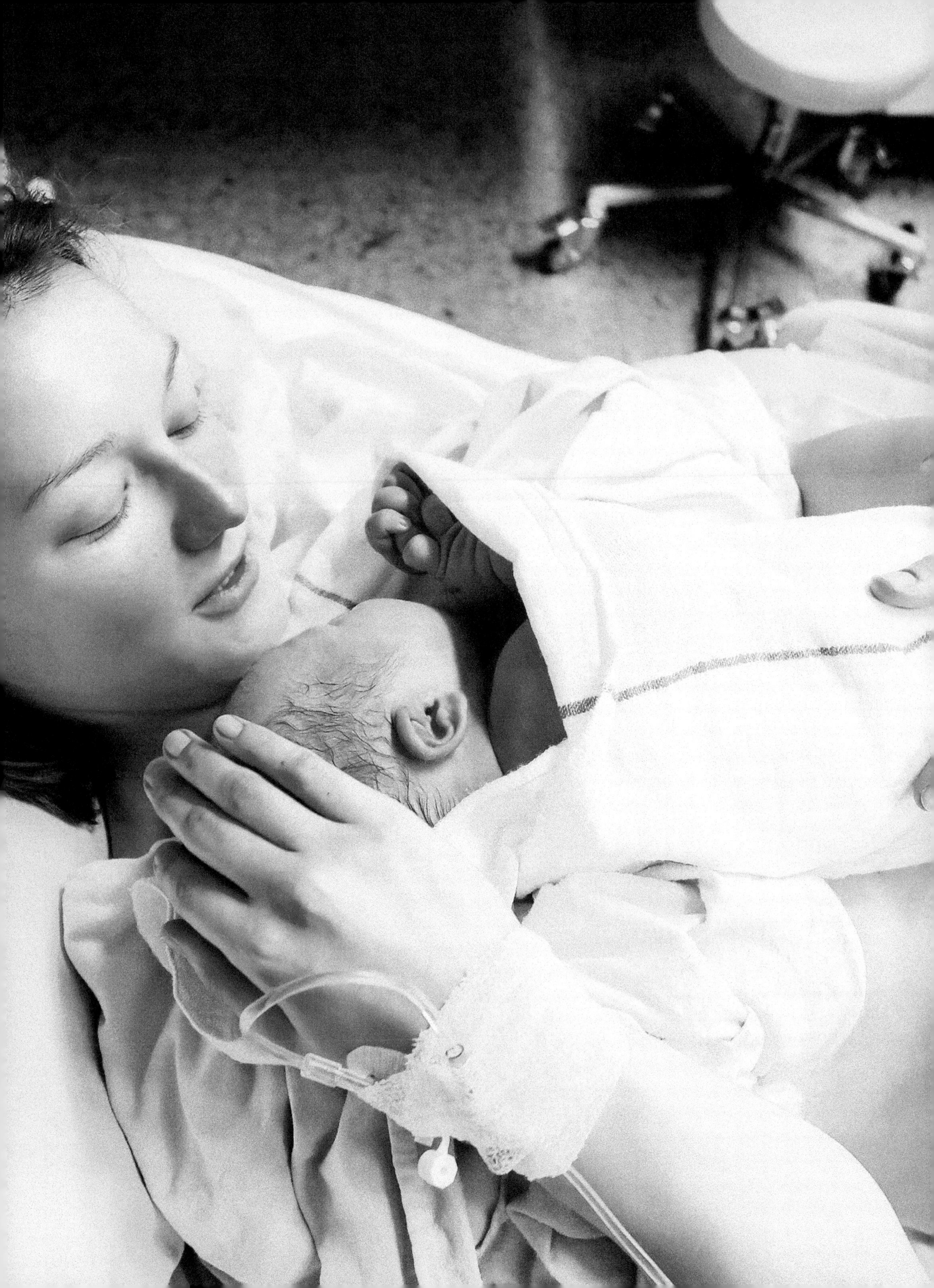

Medical and psychological emergencies

Chapters

Section 8 Psychological disorders
19 Post-traumatic stress disorder 44
20 Postnatal depression (mood disorder) 46
21 Puerperal (postpartum) psychosis 48

Section 9 Hypertensive disorders of pregnancy
22 Pre-eclampsia 50
23 Eclampsia 52

Section 10 Embolic and coagulation disorders
24 Venous thromboembolism 54
25 Amniotic fluid embolism 56
26 Disseminated intravascular coagulation 58

Section 11 Preterm labour
27 Prelabour rupture of membranes 60
28 Preterm labour and delivery 62

19 Post-traumatic stress disorder

Figure 19.1 Signs and symptoms of complex PTSD. Source: Flickr, https://www.flickr.com/photos/traumaanddissociation/10269350356/. Licensed under CC BY ND 2.0.

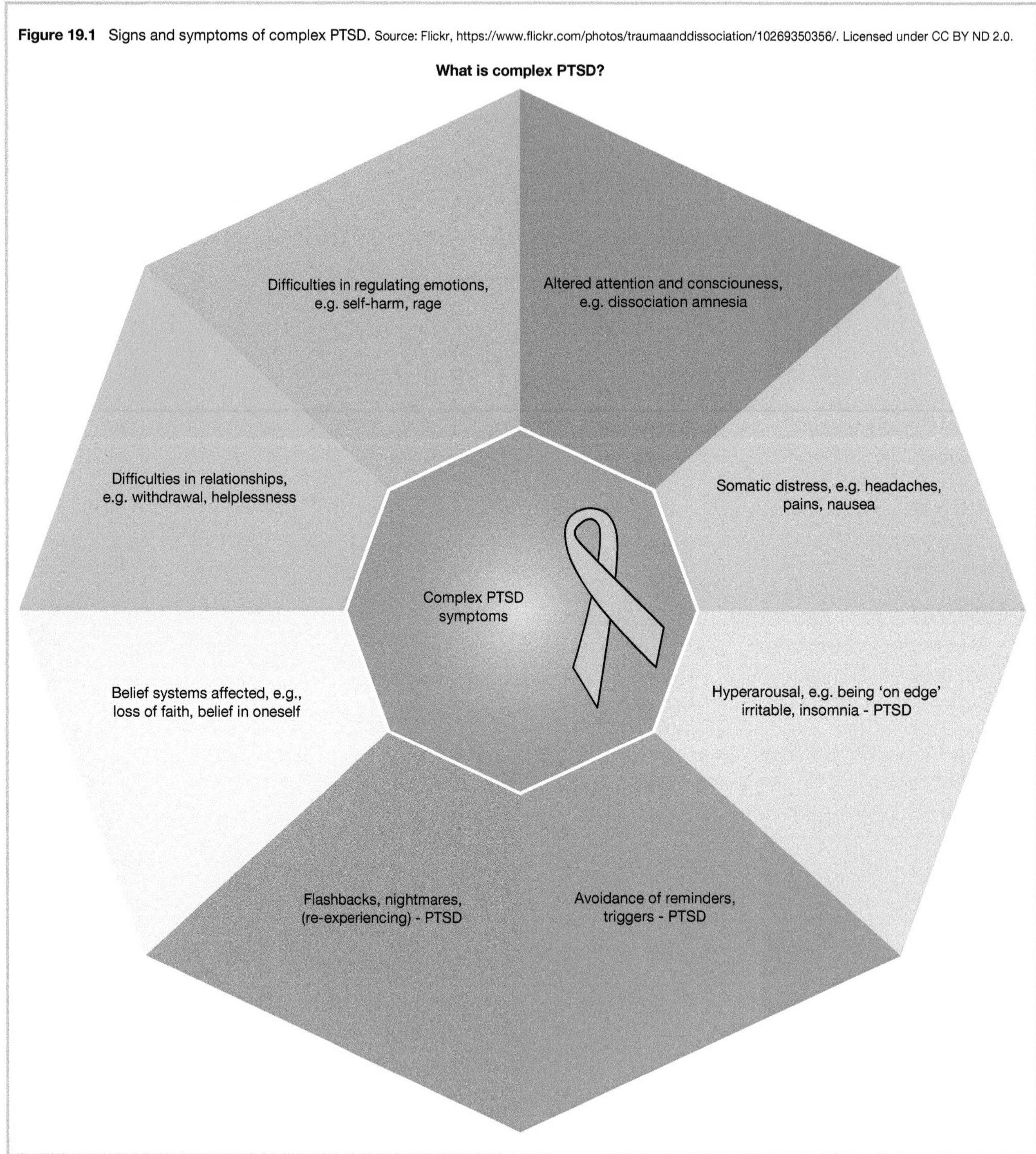

Midwifery Emergencies at a Glance, First Edition. Denise (Dee) Campbell and Susan M. Carr. © 2018 John Wiley & Sons, Ltd. Published 2018 by John Wiley & Sons, Ltd.
Companion website: www.ataglanceseries.com/midwiferyemergencies

The incidence of postpartum post-traumatic stress disorder (PTSD) ranges from 1 to 30%, but more typically it is around 3.1% for the general population rising to 15.7% for those considered higher risk (Grekin & O'Hara, 2014). These are worrying figures for a pregnancy-related condition since this is a psychiatric disorder believed to result from traumatic or life threatening attacks and violent personal assaults (Iribarren *et al.*, 2005). Stress at these levels can cause psycho-emotional and pathological problems, with significant impact on daily life and the possibility of becoming life threatening (Iribarren *et al.*, 2005).

Predisposing factors (Lev-Wiesel, *et al.*, 2009; Andersen *et al.*, 2012; Grekin and O'Hara, 2014; Ayers *et al.*, 2016)

- Previous history of PTSD.
- Experience of personal childhood sexual abuse.
- Traumatic labour experiences or interactions with medical staff.
- A history of psychopathology.
- Current depression or in pregnancy.
- Newborn complications.
- Subjective distress and negative experience in labour.
- Inadequate support during labour and delivery.
- Psychological difficulties in pregnancy.
- Previous traumatic experiences.
- Obstetric emergencies.
- Tocophobia – fear of childbirth.
- Poor health or complications in pregnancy.
- Operative birth (assisted vaginal or Caesarean).
- Postnatal problems coping with newborn.

Diagnosis

The *Diagnostic and Statistical Manual of Mental Disorders* (DSM-5) (American Psychiatric Association, 2013) suggests diagnosis of PTSD can link to a number of factors – the one that would appear relevant to the postnatal period would be direct experience of the trauma. In addition, they propose that diagnosis requires exposure to one or more of the following:

- Actual or threatened death.
- Serious injury.
- Sexual violation.

In the postnatal period these could relate to events that are actual (e.g. from previous child abuse, rape or a life threatening obstetric emergency), or a sensed experience (e.g. linked to an obstetric emergency, operative delivery, perineal trauma, vaginal examination).

Furthermore, the DSM-5 describes four diagnostic clusters for PTSD:

- Re-experiencing – in flashbacks or in dreams.
- Avoidance – of memories and external reminders.
- Negative cognitions and mood – blame of self or others, significantly reduced interest in activities, unable to remember aspects of the event.
- Arousal – aggression, self-destructive behaviour, disturbed sleep or apnoea, 'fight or flight' emotions.

Resultant risks to mother and newborn

Iribarren *et al.* (2005) highlight a spectrum of disorders associated with difficulties functioning and daily living often compounded by depression and the possibility of developing substance abuse (alcohol, smoking or drugs) alongside PTSD. These include:

- Problems of memory and understanding.
- Difficulties functioning as a parent.
- Difficulties functioning socially, including marriage problems.
- Difficulties functioning at work.
- Suicidal thoughts/attempts/achievement.

For the newborn there may be problems of:

- Prematurity (Yonkers *et al.*, 2014).
- Inability of the mother to react appropriately to newborn emotions (Webb and Ayers, 2014).

Preventative management of known risk

It was once hoped that debriefing of women following traumatic pregnancy events would help prevent PTSD, but evidence has not supported this approach (Bastos *et al.*, 2015). Some non-obstetric trials have identified benefits in hydrocortisone treatment for preventative care (Amos *et al.*, 2014). These would have to be used with great caution during pregnancy due to associations between corticosteroids and cleft palate abnormalities. Postnatally there is also a risk of possible toxicity if breastfeeding.

Acute management in an emergency

The acute, emergency management will depend on the health risk to the mother and newborn and any comorbidity that develops with depression and/or substance abuse. Management may involve:

- Assess and minimise immediate risk of harm (to self or newborn).
- Consider duty of care and escalation of safeguarding responsibilities.
- Referral to mental health services – preferably a specialist perinatal team (see Figure 21.3 which is also relevant here).
- Liaise with obstetrician, paediatrician and GP.
- Consider admission to psychiatric care – a specialist mother and baby unit where available (see Figure 21.4 which is also relevant here).
- Mood stabilisation – selective serotonin reuptake inhibitors (SSRIs) alongside cognitive-behavioural therapy (Song and Chae, 2016).
- Ongoing care with psychological therapies (Roberts *et al.*, 2010; Bisson *et al.*, 2013; Roberts *et al.*, 2016).
- Regular monitoring and coordinated on-going care with information and advice – intervention as required.
- Safe mother and newborn interaction and relationship building.
- Communications across midwife, health visitor, obstetrician, paediatrician, GP and psychiatry teams.

Iribarren *et al.* (2005) suggest recovery is slow and frequently delayed by traumatic memories. Symptoms can become complex (see Figure 19.1) and may never completely disappear. Treatment is therefore aimed at:

- Reducing reactions.
- Diminishing the acuity of the reactions.
- Increasing ability to manage trauma-related emotions.
- Greater confidence in coping abilities.

Postnatal depression (mood disorder)

Figure 20.1 Incidence of postnatal depression. Source: Data from Haskett (2010).

10–15% (1:7–10) of women develop postnatal depression

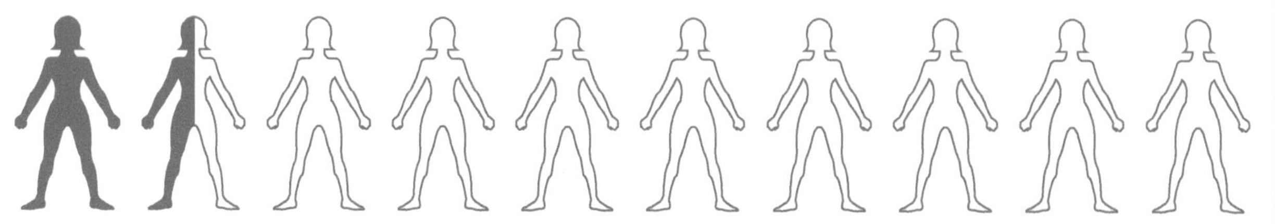

Box 20.1 Edinburgh postnatal depression scale (EPDS). Source: Data from Cox *et al.* (1987).

General guidelines

- The mother is presented with ten questions and all of them need to be answered
- She must underline the response which comes closest to how she has been feeling in the previous 7 days from the four answers offered
- The mother completes the scale herself
- Translations should be made available for anyone who has limited English
- Support may be given for anyone with reading difficulties
- The answers need to be her own opinion and so should not follow discussion with others
- Screening should occur between 6 and 8 weeks postnatal

Question topics all relate to the previous 7 days associated with the mother's:

- Ability to laugh and appreciate humour in things
- Ability to positively look forward to things
- Levels of inappropriate self blame
- Frequency of unreasonable anxiety and worry
- Frequency of unreasonable fear, or feelings of panic
- Frequency with which they feel unable to cope
- Frequency of difficulties sleeping (linked to unhappiness)
- Frequency of feeling sad or miserable
- Frequency of crying due to unhappiness
- Frequency of thoughts about self harm

Scoring

- Response categories are generally scored 0, 1, 2 and 3 according to increased severity of the symptom
- Three of the ten questions are reverse scored to ensure that completion is not by a recognised pattern (i.e. 3, 2, 1 and 0)
- The total score is calculated by adding together the scores for each of the ten items

Relevance of results

- Final scores can range from 0 to 30
- The validation study showed that mothers who scored above a threshold 12/13 were likely to be suffering from a depressive illness
- This can be of varying severity
- The EPDS score should not override clinical judgement
- A careful clinical assessment should be carried out to confirm the diagnosis before considering management

Postnatal (postpartum) depression is the onset of a major depressive illness or mood disorder following childbirth. Literature on the topic describes a time frame which can range from 4 weeks after the delivery up until the child reaches 1 year old. It is distinguished from the 'blues' by its persistence beyond the first week postnatally, the degree of effect on the woman's ability to function normally, persistent depressed mood beyond 2 weeks, and the increased risk to the mother and newborn (Haskett, 2010). Major unipolar depression (covered in this chapter) affects 10–15% (1:7–10) of mothers and is the most common complication of childbirth (Haskett, 2010) (see Figure 20.1). Mood disorders may occur as a singular condition or alongside domestic violence and/or alcohol or substance misuse.

Ensure this is not the depressive stage of a bipolar disorder

It is important to assess the woman fully and consider mood lability. Depression may be a symptom within bipolar disorder (manic depression) where the mood will swing between mania and depression. Missing a diagnosis of first episode, bipolar disorder in postnatal women can have significant and even tragic consequences (Sharma & Burt, 2011). In bipolar disorder, the depression may follow an episode incorporating feelings of elation, increased goal-directed activity, over-talkativeness, racing thoughts, decreased sleep requirement, distractibility and irritability (Sharma & Burt, 2011, p. 68).

Predisposing factors (Haskett, 2010; Cunningham *et al.*, 2014)

- Past history of postpartum depression.
- Past (or first degree relative) history of depressive illness.
- Antenatal depression or depressive symptoms.
- Lack of or poor social support including being a single parent.
- Increased stress – social, economic, physical or obstetric.
- An elevated score on the Edinburgh Postnatal Depression Scale (EPDS) – see Box 20.1.

Signs and symptoms

The *Diagnostic and Statistical Manual of Mental Disorders* (DSM-5) (American Psychiatric Association, 2013) supports that postpartum depression aligns with its normal criteria for major depression but with postnatal commencement. There must be 2 weeks of the following symptoms:

- A depressed mood or a loss of interest or pleasure in daily activities which represents a change from normal mood.
- A clinically significant distress or impairment in social, occupational, educational or other important areas of functioning.

In addition, five or more of the following symptoms must also be present almost every day:

- Depressed mood most of the day, indicated by subjective report or the observations of others.
- Reduced interest or pleasure in all (or nearly all) activities for most of the day.
- Significant weight loss or gain, or decrease or increase in appetite.
- Insomnia or hypersomnia.
- Psychomotor agitation or retardation.
- Fatigue or loss of energy.
- Feelings of worthlessness or excessive or inappropriate guilt.
- Diminished ability to think or concentrate, or indecisiveness.
- Recurrent thoughts of death, recurrent thoughts of suicide without a plan, a plan for committing suicide or a suicide attempt.

Risks to mother and newborn

- Thoughts about or complete suicide risk (Cantwell *et al.*, 2015) becomes 70 times greater than mortality amongst women of the same age (Haskett, 2010).
- Adverse effects on infant which continues into adulthood – on emotional and physical development, including brain development and reactions to stress (Lupien *et al.*, 2011).
- Infanticide or guilty thoughts around committing infanticide even when not fulfilling the act (Barr & Beck, 2008).
- Inability to provide adequate self or newborn care.

Preventative management

Women with a known high-risk status with early signs of depression or a previous incidence may be medicated with antidepressants postdelivery. Antenatal administration has been linked to possible fetal heart defects, neonatal withdrawal syndromes and hypertension (Cunningham *et al.*, 2014). A number of other therapies may also be used such as increased midwife input, hormonal replacement, psychotherapy, hypnosis and dietary enhancement, but there is limited supporting evidence for these (Morrell *et al.*, 2016). Similarly, a number of screening tools are available to attempt to identify those at greatest risk – the EPDS remains the most widely used of these (see Figure 20.2). It has limited diagnostic value but continues to be used in the absence of any better tool because it provides enough information to support referral for further investigation (Gibson *et al.*, 2009).

Acute management in an emergency

Postpartum depression is rarely an emergency unless it is associated with thoughts or attempts at self or infant harm. In these situations:

- Assess and minimise immediate risk of harm (to self or newborn).
- Consider duty of care and escalation of safeguarding responsibilities.
- Refer to mental health services – preferably a specialist perinatal team (see Red flag box in Chapter 21 which is also relevant here).
- Liaise with obstetrician, paediatrician and GP.
- Consider admission to psychiatric care – a specialist mother and baby unit where available (see Box 21.1 which is also relevant here).
- Stabilise mood – medication (e.g. antidepressants).
- Consider long-term therapy – medication (including oestrogen replacement), psychotherapy (cognitive-behavioural therapy).
- Monitor regularly and coordinate on-going care with information and advice – intervention as required.
- Encourage safe mother and newborn interaction and relationship building.
- Communications across midwife, health visitor, obstetrician, paediatrician, GP and psychiatry teams.

Oestrogen and antidepressant medications both impact on breastfeeding. Oestrogen inhibits lactation (if it is not already established) and antidepressants are excreted at low levels in breast milk. Little is known about the toxicity and side effects, but current beliefs are that the advantages of breastfeeding are likely to outweigh any disadvantages during the postnatal period (Gentile, 2015). Mothers should be made aware of the best evidence available and be prescribed the lowest risk, effective antidepressants.

21 Puerperal (postpartum) psychosis

Figure 21.1 Mortality statistics. Source: Data from Cantwell *et al.* (2015).

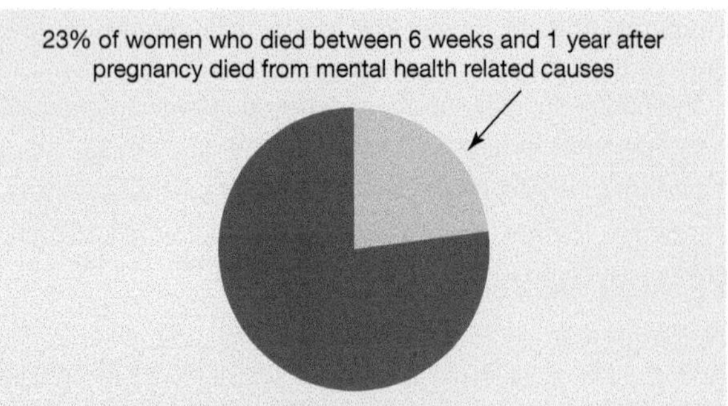

23% of women who died between 6 weeks and 1 year after pregnancy died from mental health related causes

Figure 21.2 Suicide rates. Source: Data from Cantwell *et al.* (2015).

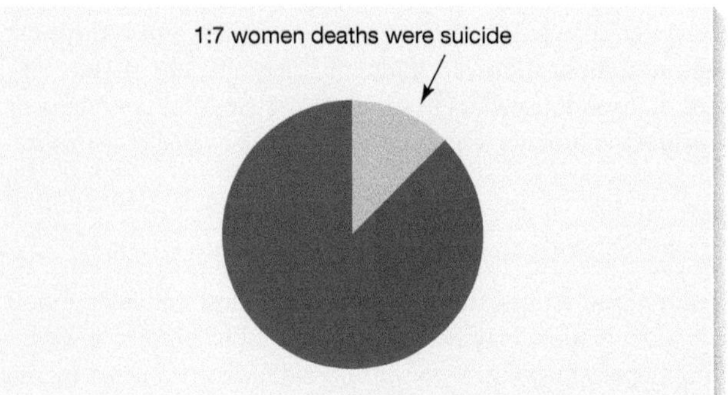

Box 21.1 Signs of severe maternal illness. Source: Data from Cantwell *et al.* (2015).

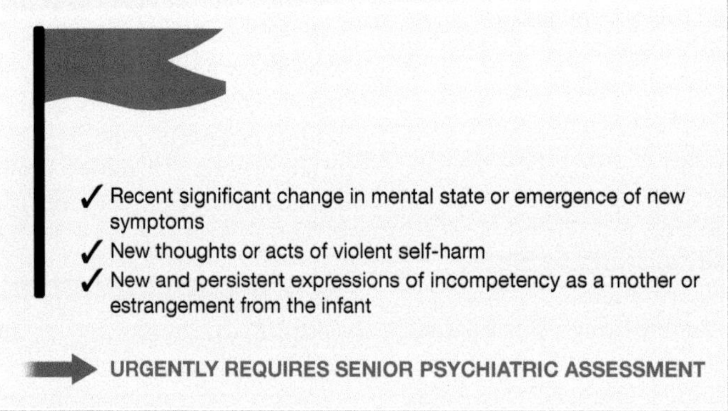

✓ Recent significant change in mental state or emergence of new symptoms
✓ New thoughts or acts of violent self-harm
✓ New and persistent expressions of incompetency as a mother or estrangement from the infant
URGENTLY REQUIRES SENIOR PSYCHIATRIC ASSESSMENT

Box 21.2 Consider admission to a mother and baby unit. Source: Data from Cantwell *et al.* (2015).

DOES THE MOTHER HAVE ANY OF THE FOLLOWING...

? Rapidly changing mental state
? Suicidal ideation (particularly of a violent nature)
? Pervasive guilt or hopelessness
? Significant estrangement from the infant
? Beliefs of inadequacy as a mother
? Evidence of psychosis

This is the most severe of the mood disorders that may affect the postnatal woman. It is rare (1–2:1000) and, whilst it can occasionally be unipolar, it is typically a bipolar disorder, with major depressive symptoms exhibited around psychotic episodes. Symptoms may develop as early as 3 days postpartum (particularly where there is a past history of mood disorder), but more commonly between 8 and 14 days postpartum with psychotic episodes lasting a median duration of 40 days (Bergink *et al.*, 2012).

Aetiology

The exact aetiology is unknown but various theories exist with varying degrees of evidence to support them. A selection of these are included here:

- Genetic link and chromosomal mutation – supported by familial trends and high incidence of occurrence with both monozygotic twins (Jones *et al.*, 2007).
- Frontal and temporal lobe developmental abnormalities alongside dopamine pathophysiology – supported by studies in neurobiology (Stone, 2008; Yonkers *et al.*, 2011).
- Sleep disruption and deprivation, particularly of total sleep time and rapid eye movement (REM) sleep -known to lead to psychotic symptoms such as hallucinations and feelings of persecution in the general population, and may also explain increased psychosis in primigravida (Haskett, 2010).

Predisposing factors (Essali *et al.*, 2013; Lewis *et al.*, 2016)

- Previous history or first degree relative with history of postpartum psychosis.
- Previous history or first degree relative with history of a bipolar disorder.
- Previous history or first degree relative with history of depressive disorder.
- Primigravida.
- Single parent.
- Older women.
- Major trauma experienced – particularly with sexual (e.g. rape or abuse) or pregnancy associations (e.g. traumatic birth history).
- Sleep deprivation.

Signs and symptoms (see Box 21.1) (Haskett, 2010; Bergink *et al.*, 2015; Lewis *et al.*, 2016)

- Sleep deprivation – unable to sleep or a feeling of not requiring sleep.
- Mood fluctuation with severe symptoms (e.g. mania, depression).
- Obsessive concerns regarding the newborn.
- Delusions.
- Hallucinations.
- Disorganised thoughts and behaviour.
- Loss of inhibitions.
- Restlessness and irritability.
- Confusion.
- Self or newborn neglect.

Risks to mother and newborn (Gutteridge and Lazarus, 2008)

- Inadequate or inappropriate care and diet.
- Self harm, including suicide (see Figures 21.1 and 21.2).
- Neglect or harm to the newborn, including infanticide.
- Harm to others – family, friends and carers.
- Relationship breakdown with infant.
- Relationship breakdown or depression in the partner.

Preventative management of known risk

Pregnant women who have a known risk are those with either a previous history of postpartum psychosis in an earlier pregnancy, or women with a known bipolar disorder (previously named manic-depressive disorder). Management of those with bipolar disorder should commence preconceptually with consideration of medications already being taken and a plan of preventative care. Bergink *et al.* (2015) advocates lithium treatment, alongside benzodiazepines and antipsychotics for those with bipolar disorders. Lithium during the first trimester may increase the risk of fetal heart malformations (Essali *et al.*, 2013) so the aim is to balance the time of commencement according to maternal condition and lowest risk.

Postpartum treatment with lithium is successful in preventing relapse for women who have experienced a previous postpartum psychosis (Bergink *et al.*, 2012; Bergink *et al.*, 2015; Wesseloo *et al.*, 2016). Lithium is passed on in breast milk and may cause toxicity (Essali *et al.*, 2013) so, when breastfeeding, alternative support options need to be planned to balance the risks and benefits.

Acute management in emergency (Haskett, 2010; Cantwell *et al.*, 2015)

Any unexpected acute episode of psychosis, including where planned management has failed, will require emergency management. This includes some or all of the following actions:

- Assess and minimise immediate risk of harm (to self, newborn or others).
- Consider duty of care and escalation of safeguarding responsibilities.
- Referral to mental health services – preferably a specialist perinatal team.
- Liaising with obstetrician, paediatrician and GP.
- Admission to psychiatric care – a specialist mother and baby unit where available (see Box 21.2).
- Prompt treatment of sleep deprivation – medication (e.g. benzodiazepines) and support with care of infant.
- Mood stabilisation – medication (e.g. antipsychotics).
- Long-term therapy – medication (including hormone replacement), psychotherapy, electroconvulsive therapy (ECT).
- Regular monitoring and coordinated on-going care with information and advice – intervention as required.
- Safe mother and newborn interaction and relationship building.
- Communications across midwife, health visitor, obstetrician, paediatrician, GP and psychiatry teams.

It is also imperative that all other pathophysiology is excluded through a full history and investigative screening process. This is because psychotic episodes can also occur secondary to numerous diseases including infection, eclampsia, thyroid disease, vitamin deficiency, cerebrovascular accident, medication, illicit drugs and metabolic disease (Bergink *et al.*, 2015; Cantwell *et al.*, 2015). Psychosis can also be secondary to major depression and require antidepressant treatment to counteract mood imbalance.

22 Pre-eclampsia

Box 22.1 Possible progression of pre-eclampsia symptoms.

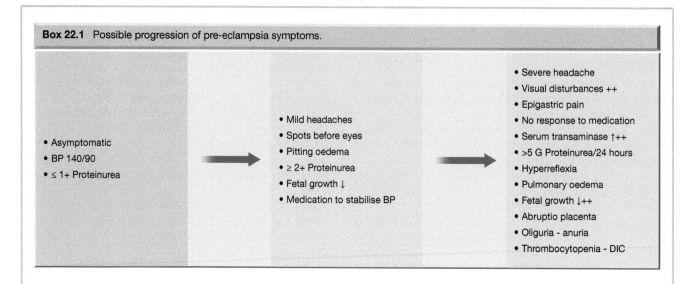

• Asymptomatic • BP 140/90 • ≤ 1+ Proteinurea	→	• Mild headaches • Spots before eyes • Pitting oedema • ≥ 2+ Proteinurea • Fetal growth ↓ • Medication to stabilise BP	→	• Severe headache • Visual disturbances ++ • Epigastric pain • No response to medication • Serum transaminase ↑++ • >5 G Proteinurea/24 hours • Hyperreflexia • Pulmonary oedema • Fetal growth ↓++ • Abruptio placenta • Oliguria - anuria • Thrombocytopenia - DIC

Box 22.2 Prophylactic anticonvulsant therapy.

Magnesium sulphate ($MgSO_4$):

- Loading dose of 4 g should be given intravenously over 5 minutes (Eclampsia trial collaborative group, 1995; NICE, 2010; NICE, 2012a)
- Followed by an infusion of 1 g / hour maintained for 24 hours (Eclampsia trial collaborative group, 1995; NICE, 2010; NICE, 2012a)
- Recurrent seizures should be treated with a further dose of 2–4 g given over 5 minutes
- Delivery typically within 24 hours. Avoid continuous administration beyond 7 days as can cause fetal harm

Box 22.3 Monitoring for magnesium toxicity.

$MgSO_4$ toxicity can cause respiratory arrest. To prevent this assess:

- Deep tendon reflexes – patellar reflex present
- Respiratory rate and oxygen saturation
- Level of consciousness – somnolence
- Visual changes
- Flushing
- Muscle paralysis
- Urine output (100 mL/s minimum over 4 hours)
- Measure serum magnesium level at 4–6 hours
- Adjust infusion to maintain 4–7 mEq/L(4.8–8.4 mg/dL)
- Measure serum magnesium level if serum creatinine ≥1.0 mg/dL
- Antidote ready – calcium gluconate 1g (10 mL/s of 10% solution) IV over 2 minutes

Hypertensive disorders of pregnancy

Pre-eclampsia is one of a number of gestational hypertensive disorders. Hypertensive disorders affect 14–20% of pregnancies and may exist prior to pregnancy (chronic hypertension), exacerbate due to the pregnancy (chronic hypertension compounded by gestational hypertension), or first develop during the pregnancy (pregnancy-induced or gestational hypertension – including pre-eclampsia or eclampsia) (Dekker, 2010). No longer a leading cause of maternal death, the improvements in management of hypertensive disorders now means only 1:400 000 women in the UK will die from a pregnancy-related, hypertensive disorder (Knight *et al.*, 2015).

Definitions

- **Hypertension** – a diastolic blood pressure (DBP) at or above 90 mmHg, or a systolic blood pressure (SBP) at or above 140 mmHg, on two occasions hours apart (Permezel, 2015b).
- **Chronic hypertension in pregnancy** – hypertension prior to pregnancy and present before 20 weeks' gestation (Permezel, 2015b).
- **Gestational hypertension** – newly developing hypertension after 20 weeks, with no systemic effects and resolving spontaneously postnatally (Permezel, 2015b).
- **Pre-eclampsia** (see Box 22.1)/**pre-eclamptic toxaemia (PET)** – new hypertension after 20 weeks; arising antenatally, intrapartum or postnatally with systemic involvement; proteinurea is a common, significant marker but one or more of the following systems may be affected (Permezel, 2015b, p. 130):
  - Renal – proteinurea, renal insufficiency, oliguria.
  - Haematological – thrombocytopenia, haemolysis, disseminated intravascular coagulation (DIC).
  - Hepatic – epigastric or right upper quadrant abdominal pain, elevated serum transaminase.
  - Neurological – visual disturbances, headache, hyperreflexia, stroke (sustained clonus and convulsions with eclampsia).
  - Pulmonary – oedema.
  - Placental – fetal growth restriction, abruption.
- **HELLP syndrome** – (haemolysis, elevated liver enzymes, low platelets) is a form of severe pre-eclampsia (Permezel, 2015b). In rare cases it will occur without true hypertension but the blood pressure (BP) will usually still have raised significantly (Cunningham *et al.*, 2014).
- **Eclampsia (see Chapter 23)** – the tonic–clonic seizure complication which follows PET when cerebral hypoxia has occurred (Permezel, 2015b). In rare cases it occurs without true hypertension, but the BP will usually have raised significantly (Cunningham *et al.*, 2014).

Pre-eclampsia

Pathophysiology

Permezel (2015b) suggests there are three possible causes for pre-eclampsia linked to placental ischaemia:

- Deficient placentation – abnormalities of the spiral arteries in the myometrium and a diminished utero-placental blood flow.
- Maternal vascular disease.
- Excessive placental size (multiple pregnancies, diabetes, hydatidiform mole).

Predisposing factors (Myatt *et al.*, 2012; Cunningham *et al.*, 2014; Permezel, 2015b)

- Maternal age – older mothers (complicating chronic hypertension).
- Nulliparous or previous pre-eclampsia.
- New partners.
- Multiple pregnancy (but not linked to zygosity).
- Race and ethnicity – 5% of White people, 11% of African-American people.
- Genetic predisposition – incidence is three to four times higher if a first degree relative experienced pre-eclampsia.
- Socio-economic factors – marital status, years of education.
- Body mass index (obesity) – increases progressively with weight.
- Raised SBP at booking.
- Raised mean platelet level at booking.
- First-trimester concentrations of ADAM-12, pregnancy-associated plasma protein-A and placental growth factor all raised.
- Diabetes mellitus.
- Hypercholesterolemia.
- Hydatidiform mole – when PET may occur before 20 weeks.

Management (Permezel, 2015b)

The aims of management of mild and moderate PET will be to prevent seizures, prevent cerebral haemorrhage, prolong the pregnancy to fetal maturity and expedite delivery. Severe PET requires intensive inpatient management with delivery within 24–48 hours, prioritising maternal health over the fetus.

- Monitor maternal condition and systemic damage – blood pressure, reflexes, oedema, visual disturbance, abdominal pain, proteinurea, platelet count, creatinine, hepatic transaminases, serum uric acid.
- Monitor fetal condition and development – heart rate activity, growth, weight.
- Monitor liquor volume and umbilical vessel flow.
- Convulsion prophylaxis (see Boxes 22.2 and 22.3) – routinely or linked to hyperreflexia (prior to antihypertensives due to vasodilatory effects).
- Antihypertensive medication to prevent abruptio and cerebral haemorrhage when SBP ≥ 160 mmHg; DBP ≥ 100 mmHg.
- Fluid balance – maximum 125 mL/hour (oral and intravenous) to counteract venous constriction and fall in central venous pressure (caused by antihypertensives and anticonvulsants). Avoid excessive transfusion (pulmonary oedema, ascites, cardiopulmonary overload) and insufficient transfusion (reduced cell volume and organ ischaemia, e.g. anuria – kidney failure).
- Assess urine output – 30 mL/hour minimum.
- Transfusion of platelets and/or plasma to include clotting factors.
- Corticosteroids if before 34 weeks.
- Delivery at 38 weeks – earlier if maternal or fetal compromise.

Complications

- Eclampsia.
- Abruptio placenta.
- Pulmonary oedema.
- Cerebral haemorrhage.
- Cerebrovascular accident (stroke).
- Premature birth.
- Intrauterine growth retardation.
- Death– fetus, woman or both.

23 Eclampsia

Figure 23.1 Significance of blood results. Source: Data from Raynor *et al.* (2012, p. 49).

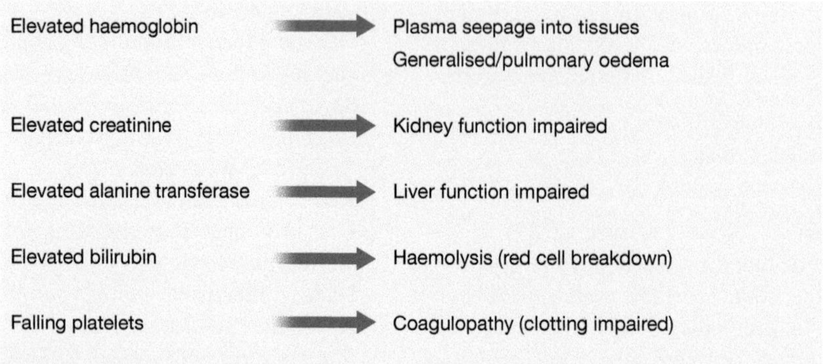

Box 23.1 $MgSO_4$ dosages during eclampsia. Source: Data from NICE (2010); NICE (2012a).

If already had a loading dose of $MgSO_4$ and now on continuous infusion

- Additional 2 g to be given IV

If not already receiving $MgSO_4$

- Requires 6 g IV over 15–20 minutes
- Followed by 2 g/hour infusion

$MgSO_4$ continues until 24 hours after last seizure. Monitor toxicity with calcium gluconate (antidote) and have resuscitation equipment available (see also Figure 29.3).

Box 23.2 Anaesthetic and surgery risks requiring increased monitoring and preventative management. Source: Data from Raynor *et al.* (2012, p. 50–51).

- Spinal/epidural anaesthesia risk of haematoma (due to coagulopathy)
- Haematoma at injection site could cause nerve/cord compression
- General anaesthetic intubation can cause further BP surge (pressor response)
- BP surge can cause cerebral haemorrhage
- BP surge can cause deterioration in placenta and/or placental abruption
- Deterioration in placenta can cause fetal compromise/hypoxia
- Surgical risk of haematoma or haemorrhage (due to coagulopathy)
- Preterm delivery may require classical incision
- Anaemia due to haemolysis makes any bleeding more significant

Eclampsia is one of a number of hypertensive disorders that occur in pregnancy (see Chapter 22) and is most often seen as a complication and worsening of pre-eclampsia. In cases where pre-eclampsia was not present the diagnosis may require exclusion of alternative causes of seizures, such as maternal hypotension, idiopathic epilepsy, intracranial neoplasia, cerebrovascular accident, local anaesthetic toxicity, alcohol withdrawal, or metabolic disturbances such as hyponatraemia or hypoglycaemia (Permezel, 2015b, p. 138).

Definition

Eclampsia is the tonic–clonic seizure complication when cerebral hypoxia has occurred (Permezel, 2015b). The hypoxia results from vasospasm, possibly further complicated by cerebral oedema, cerebral haemorrhage and/or cerebral thrombosis (Permezel, 2015b). In rare cases it can occur without true hypertension, but the blood pressure (BP) will usually have raised significantly (Cunningham *et al.*, 2014).

Incidence

Eclampsia occurs in 1:1500 deliveries presenting almost equally across both the antenatal and early postnatal periods but with a small number of first occurrences during labour (Premezel, 2015b).

Early warning signs

There may be no warning signs at all but on most occasions the woman will have pre-eclampsia, systemic symptoms and early features aligned to both cerebral hypoxia and severe pre-eclampsia:

- Rise in blood pressure.
- Increasing proteinurea.
- Severe headaches.
- Persistent visual disturbances.
- Drowsiness.
- Irritability.
- Restlessness.
- Twitching.
- Aura.

Convulsion progress

Most often a generalised tonic–clonic seizure occurs. Permezel (2015b) suggests that the pattern may include:

- An aura stage and dissociation with surroundings.
- Tonic stage – generalised spasm of skeletal muscles due to virtual cessation of respirations; cyanosis.
- Clonic stage – alternating muscle spasm and relaxation; lasts up to 2–3 minutes; high risk of self injury (tongue biting, knocking against an item, falling from a bed).
- Post-ictal stage – reduced level of consciousness; may last as long as a few hours particularly as numbers of fits increase linked to increasing cerebral hypoxia.
- Status eclampticus – continuous repeating seizures, which bring the dangers of suffocation and irreversible brain damage (caused by a combination of the initial hypoxia complicated by breath holding during seizures).

Management

Care during the convulsion (Permezel, 2015b)

- Prevent further injury or harm – remove objects nearby; add padding to objects that can't be removed (e.g. placing a pillow over a sharp corner); ensure there are no electrical, hot or sharp objects within reach; and protect against a fall (e.g. from a bed by using cot sides).
- Anticonvulsant medication – magnesium sulphate ($MgSO_4$) as soon as possible (see Boxes 23.1, 22.2 and 22.3). The use of diazepam is controversial due to the side effects of respiratory depression, aspiration and arrest (particularly when used with $MgSO_4$).
- Maintain airway and oxygen saturations – breath holding for the 60–90 seconds of the convulsion may cause cyanosis. Also, if diazepam is used, a significant drop in consciousness is likely. Insert an airway during the relaxed elements of the convulsion to protect the airway and limit the possibility of tongue biting. Give oxygen via a face mask as soon as possible.
- Prevent aspiration – lie the woman in the semi-prone, recovery position used for unconscious clients. This enables secretions to drain away – consider use of suction as required.
- Transfer to an obstetric unit (preferably with intensive care facilities), with 24-hour anaesthetic, paediatric, medical and obstetric cover.

Stabilisation of hypertensive condition

- Continue $MgSO_4$ therapy beyond the initial bolus (see Boxes 22.2 and 23.1).
- Monitor vital signs (maternal and fetal as required) including neurological observations, blood results (see Figure 23.1) and for early evidence of any $MgSO_4$ toxicity (see Box 22.3).
- Assess cerebral hypoxia damage as an indicator of further seizures.
- Antihypertensive medication – if BP remains severely elevated (after $MgSO_4$ effects stabilise). Labetalol therapy – 20 mg intravenously over 2 mins, doubled to 40 mg, then 80 mg at 10 minute intervals until BP responsive (total dose not to exceed 300 mg).

Delivery or termination of the pregnancy

This should happen as soon as the woman has stabilised and within a maximum of 24 hours. Corticosteroids should be administered to any woman $\leq$ 34 weeks pregnant whilst stabilising the BP (to help mature the fetal lungs) but the pregnancy should not be prolonged in the interest of the fetus – the health of the woman should be the priority. Caesarean section ensures the most expedited delivery.

Complications (Permezel, 2015b)

- Abruptio placenta.
- Pulmonary – oedema and/or aspiration pneumonia.
- Cerebral – haemorrhage or cerebrovascular accident.
- Renal failure.
- Cardiac failure.
- Disseminated intravascular coagulation.
- Corticol blindness.
- Premature delivery.
- Psychological problems.
- Anaesthetic complications (see Box 23.2).
- Maternal and/or fetal death.

24 Venous thromboembolism

Figure 24.1 Venous anatomy of the leg.

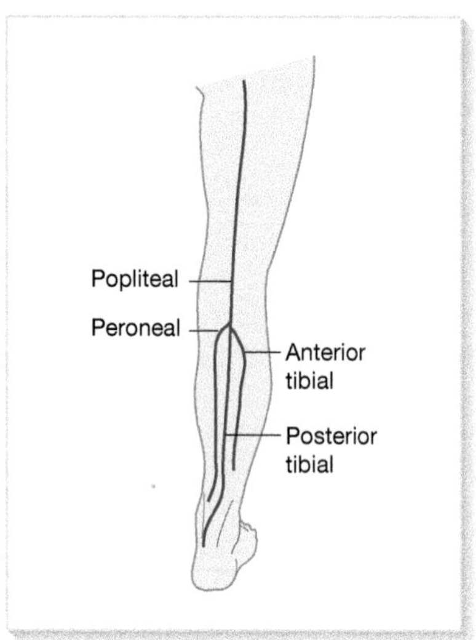

Figure 24.2 Thrombus and embolism formation.

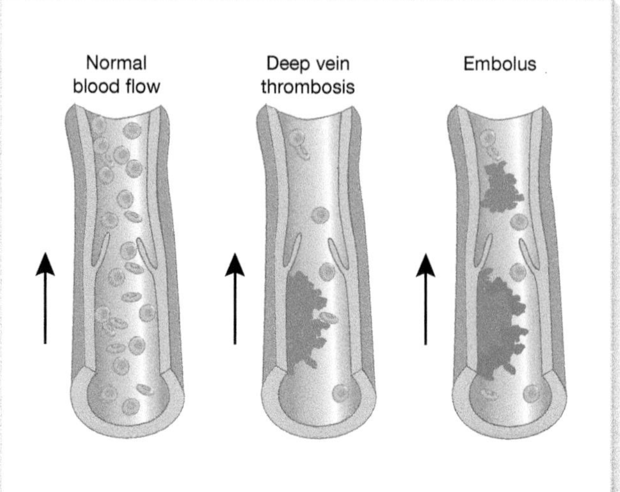

Figure 24.3 Pathophysiology.

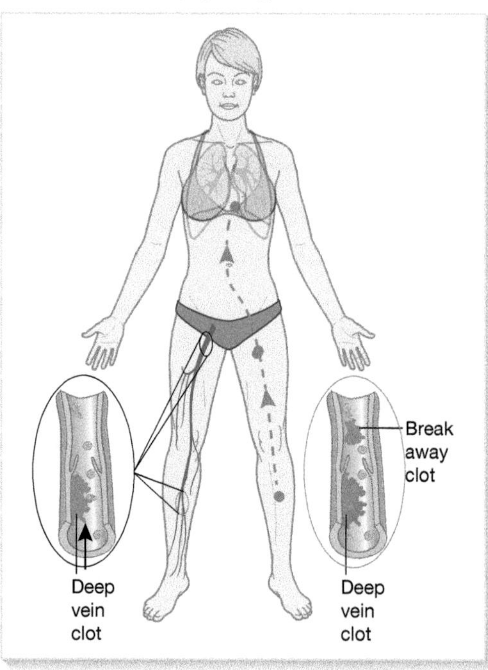

Figure 24.4 Antiembolism, graduated compression sock.

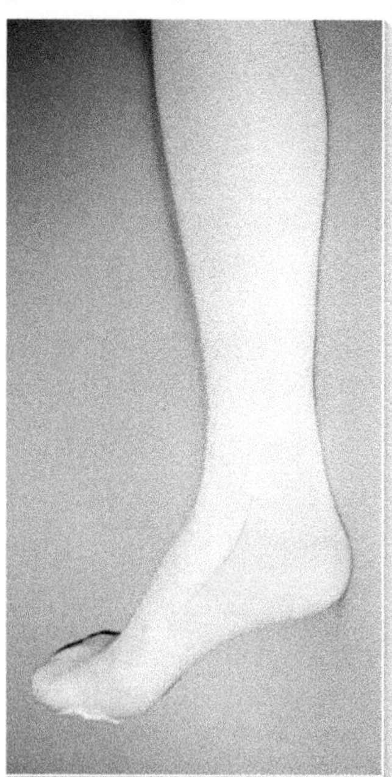

Venous thromboembolism (VTE) remains a leading cause of maternal mortality throughout pregnancy and the puerperium. VTE encompasses two main conditions – deep vein thrombosis (DVT) and pulmonary embolism (PE) – where a small piece of the DVT breaks off and travels through smaller veins until the vein becomes too small in the pulmonary circulation to allow the thromboembolus to pass. At this point, the blood supply to the area beyond the embolus is cut off (see Figures 24.1–24.3). The incidence of VTE remains relatively low with an estimated 1 in 1000 maternities complicated by VTE. Recent mortality rates indicate that although pregnant and postpartum women are four to six times more likely than non-pregnant women to suffer a venous thromboembolic episode, the mortality rate remains low at 1.01 per 100 000 maternities, equally shared between the antenatal and postnatal periods.

Risk factors

Pre-existing risk factors (Nelson-Piercy *et al.*, 2015)

- Previous VTE; family history in a first-degree relative.
- Known thrombophilia.
- Pre-existing medical condition (e.g. systemic lupus erythematosus [SLE], malignancy, liver disease).
- Age > 35 years.
- BMI > 35.
- Smoker.
- Varicosities in the lower leg(s).
- Previous history of postpartum haemorrhage, placenta praevia, Caesarean section.
- Parity > 3.
- Assisted conception.

Antenatal risk factors

- Pre-eclampsia (in current pregnancy).
- Hyperemesis.
- Multiple pregnancy.
- Caesarean section.
- Prolonged labour.
- Instrumental vaginal delivery.
- Haemorrhage.
- Severe infection.
- Preterm birth and stillbirth (in current pregnancy).
- Long haul flights.

Postpartum risk factors

- Immobility.
- Dehydration.
- Anaemia.
- Infection.
- Postpartum haemorrhage.

Signs and symptoms of acute VTE

The signs and symptoms of VTE in a pregnant or postnatal woman can be varied and on occasion, a woman may be asymptomatic. However, generally the following are demonstrated.

Deep vein thrombosis

- Redness, inflammation and swelling in the lower leg(s) with heat over the affected area.
- Pain in the calf which worsens on walking.
- Abdominal pain (if there is compression of the common iliac vein).
- Low-grade pyrexia.

Pulmonary embolism

- Sudden onset and collapse.
- Apprehension.
- Chest pain.
- Cough, haemoptysis, cyanosis, dyspnoea.

Diagnosis and management (Thomson & Greer, 2015; NICE, 2016a)

- Where there is a strong suspicion of VTE – start anticoagulation therapy before the diagnosis is confirmed (or excluded).

Confirm diagnosis

DVT

- History.
- Compression duplex ultrasound.
- Venography – 'gold standard'.

PE

- Chest X-ray.
- Electrocardiogram (ECG).
- Ventilation–perfusion (V/Q) lung scan or computerised tomography pulmonary angiogram (CTPA).

Note: D-dimer. The value of D-dimer is debatable and is not recommended by Royal College of Obstetricians and Gynaecologists (RCOG), because in an otherwise uncomplicated pregnancy, an increased level is not unusual.

Management (Thompson & Greer, 2015; NICE, 2016b)

DVT

- Blood tested for full blood count, coagulation screen, urea and electrolytes, liver function tests.
- Commence low molecular weight heparin therapy (LMWT). Dose titrated against the woman's booking or early pregnancy weight and clear guidelines should be available.
- Regular observations using the modified early obstetric warning system (MEOWS) chart.
- Antiembolism, graduated compression socks/stockings to improve circulation in veins of the lower limbs (see Figure 24.4).
- Maintain adequate hydration.

Acute PE

- Immediate assessment by experienced, multidisciplinary team.
- Intravenous unfractionated heparin therapy preferred first-line treatment with accompanying activated partial thromboplastin time (APTT) testing 4–6 hours after loading dose and at prescribed intervals thereafter.
- Manage in an appropriate location such as a high dependency unit or equivalent area on delivery suite.
- Surgical intervention (e.g. embolectomy – decided on individual basis).
- Resuscitation if cardiac arrest occurs, including perimortem Caesarean section within 5 minutes if resuscitation fails.

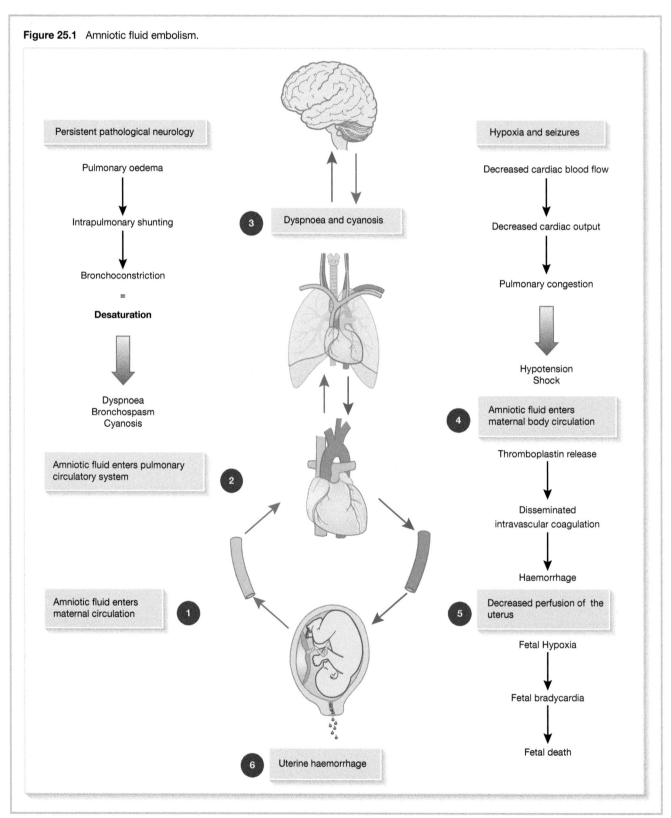

25 Amniotic fluid embolism

Figure 25.1 Amniotic fluid embolism.

Persistent pathological neurology

Pulmonary oedema

Intrapulmonary shunting

Bronchoconstriction

=

Desaturation

Dyspnoea
Bronchospasm
Cyanosis

3 Dyspnoea and cyanosis

Hypoxia and seizures

Decreased cardiac blood flow

Decreased cardiac output

Pulmonary congestion

Hypotension
Shock

4 Amniotic fluid enters maternal body circulation

Thromboplastin release

Disseminated intravascular coagulation

Haemorrhage

2 Amniotic fluid enters pulmonary circulatory system

1 Amniotic fluid enters maternal circulation

5 Decreased perfusion of the uterus

Fetal Hypoxia

Fetal bradycardia

Fetal death

6 Uterine haemorrhage

Amniotic fluid embolism – frequently referred to as AFE – is an often fatal obstetric emergency that is exclusive to labour and the immediate postpartum period. The onset is sudden, unpreventable and unpredictable. The condition occurs when amniotic fluid, fetal cells, hair, or other debris enters the mother's blood stream via the sinuses in the placental bed or small lacerations in the lower segment of the uterus or cervix. Initially it was supposed that the entry of amniotic fluid and/or fetal debris into the maternal circulation caused a mechanical blockage. However, more recent research seems to suggest that these invasive elements may in fact trigger an immune reaction (Dedhia & Mushambi, 2007).

Background

Although this condition was identified in the 1920s, it was not until Steiner and Lushbaugh (1941) identified that the histopathology of the pulmonary circulations of women who had died suddenly in or around the time of childbirth contained amniotic fluid and fetal debris such as hair, squamous cells etc. Initially maternal collapse was attributed to the embolisation of pulmonary blood vessels, but research undertaken in the 1990s suggested that immune/allergic responses were responsible (i.e. fetal antigens stimulating an outpouring of immune mediators as seen in anaphylactic reactions). Hence, AFE is now often referred to as 'anaphylactoid syndrome of pregnancy'.

Incidence

In the UK, the MBRRACE report (Knight *et al.*, 2014) states that AFE affects approximately 1:50 000 women giving birth and remains the fifth leading cause of maternal death. The percentage of fatalities ranges between 11 and 60%, although more recent estimates suggest 16–30% – this wide range may be due to early recognition of the condition, improved resuscitation techniques and improved intensive care facilities.

Predisposing factors

Although there are no proven predisposing/risk factors, certain conditions are thought to be related to the onset of AFE:

- Maternal age > 35 years.
- Multiparity.
- Multiple pregnancy.
- Intrauterine fetal death.
- Raised intra-amniotic pressure (e.g. termination of pregnancy).
- Polyhydramnios.
- Induction of labour.
- Strong, frequent or tetanic uterine contractions.
- Operative or instrumental delivery.
- Meconium-stained liquor.
- Maternal history of allergy.
- Chorioamnionitis.
- Uterine rupture.
- Placenta praevia/accreta.
- Eclampsia.

Pathophysiology (see Figure 25.1)

AFE occurs in the presence of ruptured membranes and demonstrates two main pathophysiological effects: haemodynamic collapse and coagulopathy (Ito et al., 2014).

Phase 1

The majority of fatalities occur during this phase.

- Amniotic fluid and fetal cells enter the maternal circulation.
- Production of biochemical mediators begins allergic response.
- Pulmonary artery vasospasm.
- Pulmonary hypertension leading to elevated right ventricular pressure and hypoxia.
- Myocardial and pulmonary capillary damage.
- Left heart failure.
- Acute respiratory distress syndrome.

Phase 2

May develop between 30 minutes and 4 hours after phase 1.

- Left ventricular failure and pulmonary oedema.
- Biochemical mediators trigger disseminated intravascular coagulation.
- Massive haemorrhage and uterine atony.

Signs and symptoms

It must be remembered that AFE begins suddenly and rapidly:

- Sudden dyspnoea and pulmonary oedema.
- Sudden drop in oxygen saturation.
- Cyanosis.
- Hypotension and cardiac collapse.
- Haemorrhage.
- Anxiety, nausea, vomiting.
- Chills and sweating.
- Tachycardia with possible arrhythmia.
- Seizure.
- Coma.

Management

This is best achieved via a multidisciplinary approach including obstetrician, anaesthetist, haematologist, neonatologist, midwife, porter.

- Early recognition – call for help.
- Rapid resuscitation:
  - oxygen and saturation monitor
  - monitor pulse, blood pressure, respirations
  - left lateral tilt or manual uterine displacement
  - two wide bore cannulae (one in each antecubital fossa)
  - blood sampling – full blood count, urea and electrolytes, liver function tests and urates, clotting studies, group and cross match
  - urinary catheterisation and fluid balance
  - rapid intravenous fluid replacement with crystalloids
  - manage uterine atony as per primary postpartum haemorrhage
  - disseminated intravascular coagulation therapy
  - plan for chest X-ray, electrocardiogram, VQ scan, echocardiogram.
- Delivery of the fetus within 5 minutes of decision to resuscitate the woman or as quickly as possible.
- Transfer to intensive care unit and maintain contemporaneous records throughout.

26 Disseminated intravascular coagulation

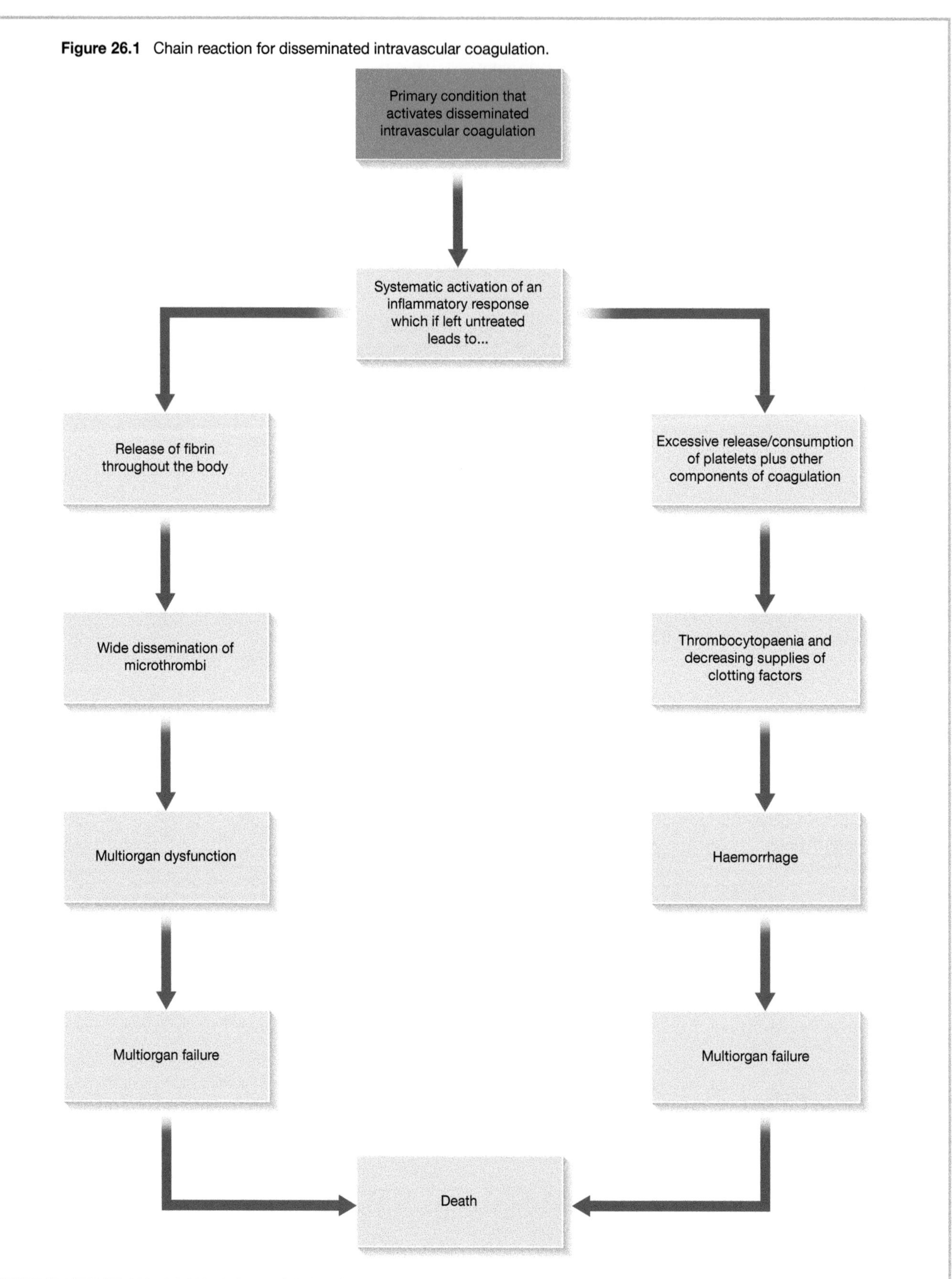

Figure 26.1 Chain reaction for disseminated intravascular coagulation.

Disseminated intravascular coagulation (DIC) (or coagulopathy) is an acute condition which affects approximately 13% of women. Abnormal coagulation takes place within the blood vessels, leading to over-consumption of the individual's clotting factors. This leads to a failure in the normal clotting mechanisms at the point of haemorrhage.

Aetiology

DIC is not an illness in itself, but rather a response to the development of another condition (Levi, 2015). It always occurs secondary to another event, for example pre-eclampsia, intrauterine fetal death, or postpartum haemorrhage, in which the body demonstrates a systemic inflammatory response and the eventual stimulation of a coagulation chain of events, culminating in the release of procoagulant material into the bloodstream.

Causes

In pregnant women, the causes of DIC includes (Moake, 2016):

- Amniotic fluid embolism.
- Sepsis.
- Acute fatty liver of pregnancy.
- Intrauterine infection.
- Pre-eclampsia and eclampsia.
- HELLP (haemolysis, elevated liver enzymes, low platelet count) syndrome.
- Abruptio placentae.
- Antepartum, intrapartum, postpartum haemorrhage.
- Retained intrauterine death of the fetus.
- Retained products of conception – with the release of placental tissue factor.
- Blood transfusion – haemolytic reaction.

Pathophysiology (see Figure 26.1) (Erez *et al.*, 2015)

Once the initiation of the systemic activation of coagulation has occurred, the resultant release of fibrin eventually leads to the formation of microthrombi throughout the organs of the body. This subsequently contributes towards multiorgan dysfunction and finally, failure. Massive haemorrhage may result from the consequent depletion of clotting factors. Thus, the morbidity and mortality of the woman will depend on the extent of intravascular thrombosis.

Occasionally DIC starts slowly, resulting in the development of thromboembolic events such as deep vein thrombosis. However, DIC generally develops rapidly leading to multiple microvascular thrombosis and haemorrhage, which if left unchecked will cause organ failure.

Increased clotting in the presence of diminishing fibrinolysis is a primary feature of DIC, which together with a reduction in anticoagulant features, results in a cascade of microthrombi production and consequent ischaemic damage to tissues and organs. This predisposes the woman to thrombocytopaenia as the microthrombi consume the woman's store of platelets and other coagulation factors.

Signs and symptoms of DIC

- The presence of a condition associated with DIC.
- Evidence of venous thromboembolic manifestations.
- Bruising.
- Petechial haemorrhages.
- Haemorrhage – persistent.
- Tachycardia.
- Hypotension.
- High fever – rapid onset.
- Chest pain.
- Dyspnoea.
- Dizziness.
- Haematuria (indicative of renal involvement).

Clinical diagnosis (Erez *et al.*, 2015)

- Increased levels of fibrinogen degradation products (FDPs) and D-dimer.
- Hypofibrinogenaemia.
- Thrombocytopaenia.
- Deranged clotting times.
- Presence of schistocytes – fragments of red blood cells typical of intravascular haemolysis.

Clinical care

- Monitor the woman's vital signs; maintain contemporaneous records.
- Care for her in a close-observation area/high dependency unit.
- Fluid replacement to correct hypovolaemia.
- Maintain accurate fluid balance; catheterise and attach a urometer.
- Oxygen therapy if bleeding.

Ongoing management

There is no specific 'cure' for DIC and thus accurate identification of the cause is essential. This may include treating sepsis with antibiotic therapy and evacuation of the uterus if retained products of conception are the suspected cause. Effective treatment of the cause is likely to bring about a rapid reversal of the woman's condition. However, if haemorrhage is present, the immediate transfusion replacement of platelets with platelet concentrate to reverse thrombocytopaenia, fresh frozen plasma to increase the body's natural anticoagulants and cryoprecipitate to restore levels of thrombin and factor VIII, is essential.

In cases where the development of DIC has been gradual, for example with the manifestation of deep vein thrombosis or pulmonary embolism, treatment involving the use of heparin can be helpful. However, where there is already evidence of bleeding or where the risk of haemorrhage is increased, heparin is not helpful – except in a woman with a retained dead fetus and whose blood results are showing deteriorating levels of coagulation factors as well as platelets and fibrinogen. In this case, the recommended treatment would be a course of heparin lasting several days to bring clotting factors levels, etc. under control before facilitating the delivery of the fetus or the evacuation of retained products of conception.

27 Prelabour rupture of membranes

Figure 27.1 Management of prelabour rupture of the membranes.

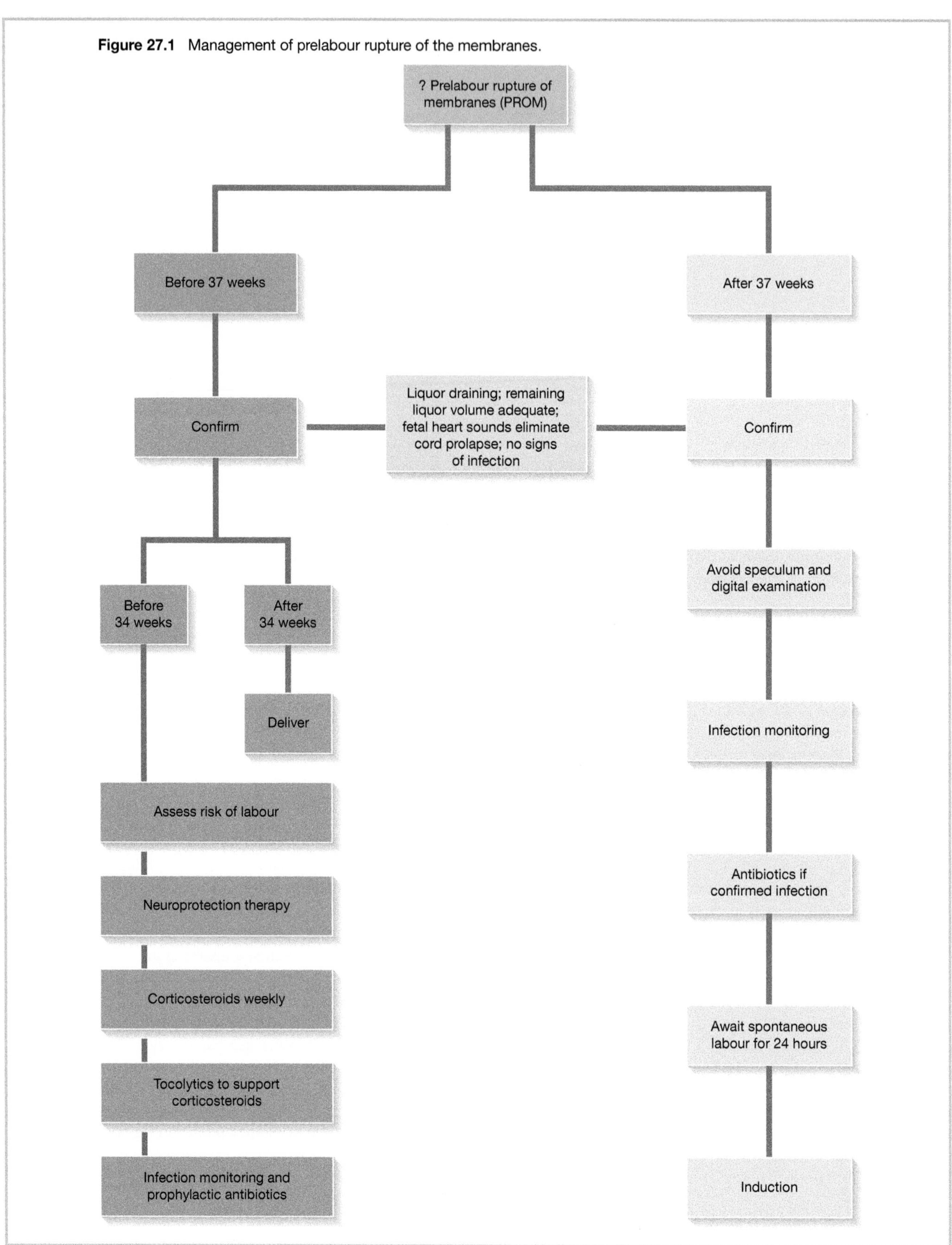

Physiology

Prelabour (premature) rupture of the membranes may be linked to: over-stretching of the membranes (e.g. polyhydramnios and twins); membrane defects (e.g. reduced collagen); or weakness (e.g. following uterine infection) (El Senoun *et al.*, 2014). It may also follow an increase in intrauterine pressure from trauma (e.g. external abdominal injury) or result from damage by the fetus (e.g. sharp nails).

Prelabour rupture of membranes (PROM)

This is the spontaneous breaking of the membranes at, or near, term without the onset of spontaneous contractions. It occurs in approximately 8% of pregnancies (Cunningham *et al.*, 2014). Spontaneous labour follows within 12 hours for 79%, rising to 95% by 24 hours (Permezel & Di Quinizio, 2015).

Risks associated with PROM

- Increased risk of infection for the woman, fetus and infant.
- Cerebral palsy associated with infection.
- Oligohydramnios.
- Abruptio placentae.
- Increased incidence of marginal cord insertion, battledore placentae and retained placentae (Svigos *et al.*, 2010).
- Increased operative delivery.

Predisposing factors for PROM

- Previous PROM.
- Smoking.
- Polyhydramnios.
- Multiple pregnancies.
- Poor diet/nutrition.
- Infection in the vagina, cervix or uterus.
- Previous cervical surgery or cerclage.

Management of PROM (see Figure 27.1)

- Confirm PROM and exclude cord prolapse via history and reassuring fetal heart sounds. Speculum examination only required with uncertain history (NICE, 2015a). No digital examination.
- Antibiotic therapy remains controversial. Whilst some evidence supports its use only when there is confirmed maternal infection and not as routine/prophylactic treatment (Wojcieszek *et al.*, 2014), more recently Saccone and Berghella (2015) identified significantly lower infection rates with prophylactic use when spontaneous labour had not occurred within 12 hours.
- Induce labour with prostaglandins or oxytocin at 24 hours post-PROM (NICE, 2013).
- Expectant management, when chosen by the mother, should include 4 hourly temperature and vaginal loss monitoring by woman (NICE, 2015a).

Preterm PROM

Spontaneous rupture of the membranes before 37 weeks occurs in 3% of pregnancies and is known as preterm PROM (P-PROM) (El Senoun *et al.*, 2014). It can be further classified into mid-trimester (<24 weeks), early (24–34 weeks) and near-term (34–37 weeks).

Risks associated with P-PROM

- Ascending infection – chorioamnionitis, endometritis and septicaemia (maternal or fetal) in one-third of cases (Fung, 2015).
- Cord prolapse/compression with fetal hypoxia/anoxia – associated with ill-fitting presenting part occurs in 1% of cases (Fung, 2015).
- Malpresentations and compound presentations.
- Anhydramnios and associated pulmonary hypoplasia (Fung, 2015).
- Fetal skeletal/postural deformities – limitation of movement *in utero.*
- Abruptio placenta – rapid decrease in uterine size.
- Fetal mortality – linked to degree of prematurity and infection.
- Premature labour – 50% labour within a week, and 75% within 2 weeks (El Senoun *et al.*, 2014).
- Neonatal morbidity (prematurity) – infection, jaundice, respiratory distress syndrome, feeding problems, cerebral palsy, hypothermia, intraventricular haemorrhage, necrotising enterocolitis (Fung, 2015).
- Increased operative delivery.
- Psychosocial and economic effects associated with hospitalisation and increased health concerns.

Predisposing factors for P-PROM (Mercer, 2007)

- History of premature birth.
- Black race.
- Genetic factors.
- Socioeconomic status.
- Smoking.
- Low maternal weight and nutritional deficiencies.
- Multiple pregnancy.
- Prior cervical conisation or cerclage.
- Amniocentesis.
- Vaginal bleeding in pregnancy.
- Infection.

Management of P-PROM

- Confirm P-PROM and exclude cord prolapse via history, speculum examination and vaginal fluid tests – without digital examination.
- Trans vaginal ultrasound of cervical length – to assess risk of labour.
- Magnesium sulphate therapy for neuroprotection.
- Conservative management to support maturing of fetus – unless infection risk is greater or fetal compromise evident.
- Monitor infection risk – C-reactive protein, white cell count and fetal heart monitoring (NICE 2015b).
- Fetal monitoring – may be omitted if fetus is on threshold of viability.
- Liquor, contraction and tenderness monitoring.
- Corticosteroid therapy before 34 weeks to increase surfactant development, then repeated weekly (Crowther *et al.*, 2015).
- Tocolytics (<34 weeks) support corticosteroid therapy (Fung, 2015). No benefit without corticosteroid therapy (Mackeen *et al.*, 2014).
- Delivery after 34 weeks – no greater risk (Buchanan *et al.*, 2010).
- Home vs hospital management – home before viability. Once viable – insufficient evidence to support home (El Senoun, *et al.*, 2014).
- Prophylactic antibiotics may prolong the pregnancy and reduce morbidities (but not mortality) (Kenyon *et al.*, 2013).

28 Preterm labour and delivery

Figure 28.1 Cervical cerclage.

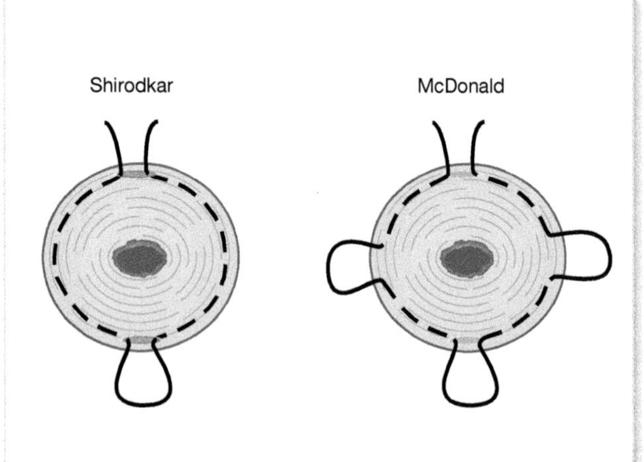

Figure 28.2 Cervical pessary.

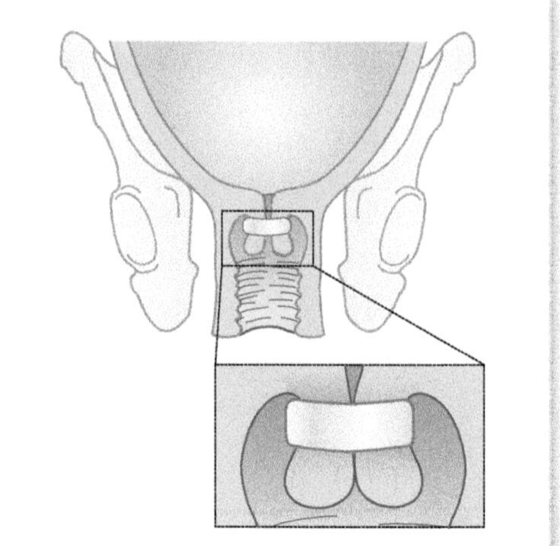

Box 28.1 Tocolysis dosage.
Source: Data from Fung (2015).

NIFEDIPINE

Loading dose (oral)

- either 4 × 10 mg @ 15 minute intervals
- or 3 × 20 mg @ 20 minute intervals

Maintenance dose (oral)

- 10–20 mg up to 4 times / day

Box 28.2 Corticosteroid dosage.
Source: Data from Fung (2015).

Either

BETAMETHASONE 11.4 mg IM
× 2 doses 24 hours apart

Or

DEXAMETHASONE 6 mg IM
x 4 doses 12 hours apart

Box 28.3 Contraindications to nifedepine.
Source: Data from Fung (2015).

Tocolysis contraindicated if:

- ≥ 34 weeks gestation
- Ruptured membranes
- Antepartum haemorrhage
- Suspected infection
- Fetal compromise

Box 28.4 $MgSo_4$ dosage for ≤30 weeks gestation. Source: Data from Fung (2015).

NEUROPROTECTIVE DOSAGE

(30% risk reduction of death/disability)

Loading dose (IV)

- 4 g over 20–30 minute

Maintenance dose (IV)

- 1 g / hour up to birth

Preterm or premature delivery is classified as before 37 weeks gestation, and may be elective (to support maternal or fetal health), or spontaneous (following an unexpected labour). The fetus is not considered legally viable until 24 weeks gestation. Whilst there have been rare reports of infants surviving from as early as 21^{+6} weeks, the general consensus remains that survival is rare before 22^{+6} weeks (RCOG, 2014). Additionally, prematurity is the leading cause of newborn death and disability worldwide with increased morbidity and mortality as the gestation reduces (Haas *et al.*, 2015). The most common morbidities are associated with long-term neurological or developmental disabilities. Active management and support for the viable fetus is normal practice but, for those infants on the edge of viability or earlier, there may be many ethical dilemmas to consider when making management decisions.

Incidence

Approximately 12% of births are preterm (Fung, 2015) with 66–75% of these occurring spontaneously and 25–33% linked to elective delivery for the health of the mother or fetus (Fung, 2015; NICE, 2016c).

Predisposing factors

There are no predictive risk scoring systems to identify those at greatest risk of preterm birth (Davey *et al.*, 2015). The main risk factor is a previous history of preterm birth (Fung, 2015). In the case of elective preterm birth, the most common maternal cause is pre-eclampsia and for the fetus it is growth restriction (Fung, 2015). Other significant factors include:

- Over distended uterus (e.g. multiple pregnancies, polyhydramnios [Fung, 2015]).
- Antepartum haemorrhage (e.g. persistent bleeding in first and second trimesters, placental abruption [Fung, 2015]).
- Smoking and significant passive smoking (UKTIS, 2011).
- Infection (e.g. urinary or genital tract infection [Sangkomkamhang *et al.*, 2015]).
- Preterm premature rupture of membranes (PPROM) (Fung, 2015).
- Uterine malformation (e.g. bicornuate, septate [Fung, 2015]).
- Placental damage (e.g. sickle cell crisis [Martí-Carvajal *et al.*, 2009]).
- Cervical incompetency/trauma including cone biopsy (Fung, 2015).
- Low socioeconomic status (Fung, 2015).

Prediction and diagnosis

The presence of regular contractions alongside the effacement and dilatation of the cervix before 37 weeks gestation will confirm preterm labour. When it is suspected but not yet confirmed, a vaginal swab test for fetal fibronectin (fFN) may be used between 24 and 36 weeks. Whilst it has a poor positive predictive value of imminent labour (15–30%), it has a high (97%) negative predictive value (Fung, 2015). It can therefore be very reassuring when a negative value is predicted that labour is not imminent in the next 7 days.

Prevention

- Smoking cessation.
- Cervical monitoring by ultrasound for early detection of changes.
- Infection screening and antibiotic therapy (Sangkomkamhang *et al.*, 2015).
- Inform women of signs of preterm labour and who to contact (NICE, 2016c).
- Prophylactic cervical cerclage (suturing) or vaginal progesterone should be considered for women with previous preterm birth, cervical incompetence or cervical shortening between 16 and 24 weeks gestation (Alfirevic *et al.*, 2012; NICE, 2016c) (see Figure 28.1).
- A silicone ring, known as a cervical pessary, may be used as a less invasive approach to closing the cervix instead of cervical cerclage (Abdel-Aleem, et al., 2013) (see Figure 28.2).

Management (RCOG, 2011; NICE, 2015b; NICE, 2016c)

- Coordinated multidisciplinary neonatal and obstetric team involving the woman and her partner in decision making.
- Confirm preterm labour – speculum examination plus digital examination if dilatation not determined (with intact membranes); transvaginal scan of cervical length or fFN swab.
- Preterm delivery risks and infant care needs explained to the woman – elective deliveries may allow time to tour facilities.
- Tocolysis and maternal corticosteroids between 26^{+0} and 29^{+6} weeks when preterm labour is suspected (see Box 28.1, 28.2 and 28.3 for dosage and contraindications) – to delay delivery and enable lung maturation.
- Corticosteroids only between 30^{+0} and 33^{+6} weeks when preterm labour confirmed, P-PROM has occurred, or elective delivery is planned – to promote fetal lung maturity.
- Repeat corticosteroid dose after 7 days if not yet delivered (Crowther *et al.*, 2015).
- Consider magnesium sulphate when delivery is expected within 24 hours if between 24 and 29^{+6} weeks gestation – to reduce neurological morbidities (see Box 28.4 for dosage).
- Infection screening – clinical assessment and checking for raised C-reactive protein, raised white cell count and fetal tachycardia. Antibiotics if infection detected or if P-PROM proven
- Decide re fetal heart monitoring – typically electrocardiogram after 26 weeks.
- Decide if vaginal delivery contraindicated.
- Delayed cord clamping (30 seconds – 3 minutes) if infant healthy; or milk cord before clamping if resuscitation required.

Possible outcomes and complications

- Benefits outweigh disadvantages, but prenatal corticosteroids are associated with a small reduction in size at birth (Crowther *et al.*, 2015).
- Caesarean section is more likely in women who have had a cervical suture inserted during pregnancy (Alfirevic *et al.*, 2012).
- Premature delivery is associated with increased neonatal risk of:
  - death
  - respiratory distress syndrome
  - intraventricular haemorrhage
  - necrotising enterocolitis
  - jaundice
  - long-term neurological or developmental disabilities.

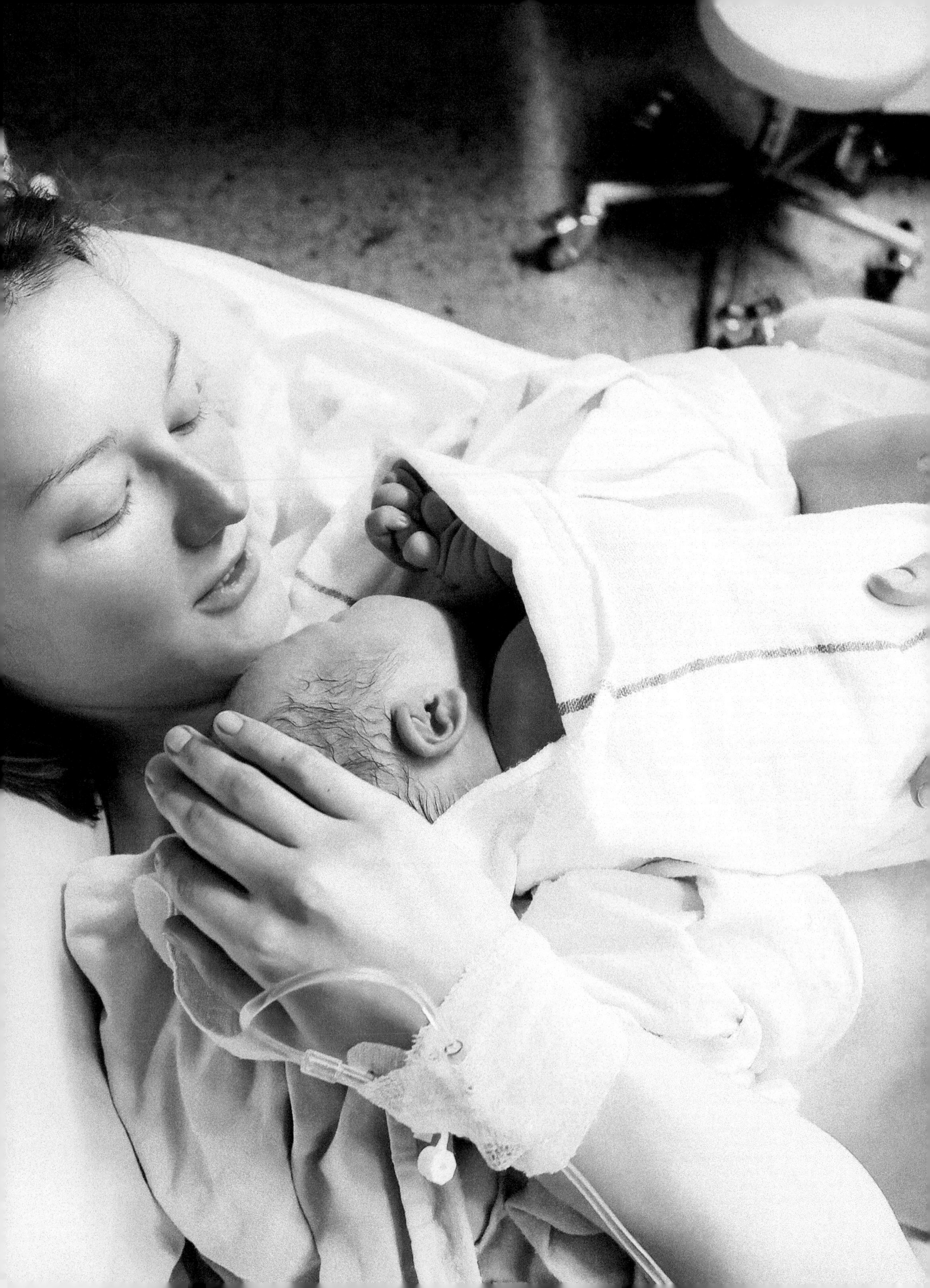

Associated skills

Chapters

Section 12 Instrumental and Operative deliveries

29 Instrumental vaginal delivery 66
30 Preparation and transfer to the operating theatre 68
31 Role of the scrub midwife or nurse 70
32 Receiving the baby in the operating theatre 72
33 Immediate care following surgery 74

Section 13 Fetal surveillance

34 Electronic fetal monitoring – actions following a suspicious or pathological trace 76
35 Fetal scalp electrode 78
36 Fetal blood sampling 80

Section 14 Maternal monitoring

37 Recognising the deteriorating woman 82
38 Examination *per vaginam* 84
39 Speculum examination 86
40 Urinary catheterisation 88

Section 15 Venous skills

41 Venepuncture 90
42 Intravenous cannulation 92
43 Blood transfusion therapy 94

Section 16 Augmentation

44 Artificial rupture of membranes 96
45 Oxytocic augmentation 98

Section 17 Perineal Trauma

46 Third- and fourth-degree tears 100
47 Perineal suturing 102

Section 18 Infection awareness

48 Maternal sepsis 104
49 Source isolation nursing 106
50 Group B streptococcus 108
51 Infection control 110

29 Instrumental vaginal delivery

Figure 29.1 Image of forceps.

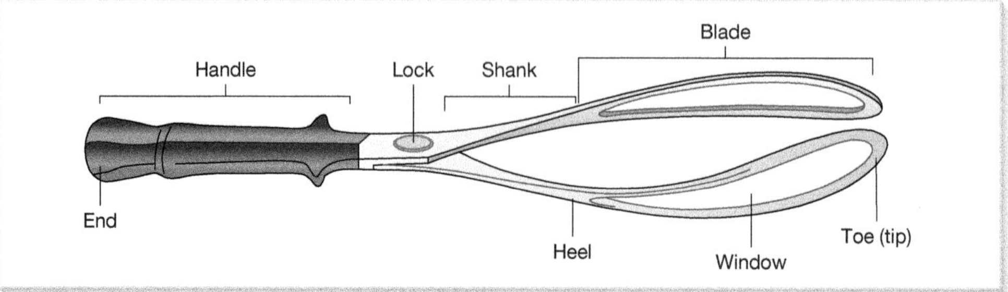

Box 29.1 Exceptions to full cervical dilatation (vacuum only).

- Second twin
- Small baby
- Urgent delivery required
  - maternal haemorrhage
  - maternal collapse
  - severe fetal hypoxia
  - fetal anoxia

Box 29.2 STOP attempts when …

- No contractions
- Ineffective anaesthesia
- Vacuum disengages three times (pop offs)
- No descent or rotation progress over 3 consecutive episodes of traction
- 15 minutes of vacuum

Box 29.3 Beware possible complications.

Neonatal

- Intracranial haemorrhage/subgaleal haematoma (more common with a vacuum delivery than forceps)
- Facial nerve palsy
- Brachial plexus injury secondary to shoulder dystocia
- Forceps marks on the face
- Facial or scalp lacerations
- Neonatal jaundice
- Retinal haemorrhages

Maternal

- Postpartum haemorrhage
- Increased trauma – cervical, vaginal and third or fourth degree tears
- Urinary retention and bladder problems
- Psychological trauma

Table 29.1 Station prior to instrumental birth. Source: Data from Permezel & Paulsen (2015).

Station	Descriptors (PP= presenting part)
Outlet	Head has reached pelvic floor – visible without parting introitus. Anterior position.
Low	Maximum cephalic diameter passed ischial spines. PP at least 3 cm below ischial spines without caput or moulding.
Mid cavity	Head engaged – maximum diameter has passed through pelvic inlet. No head palpable abdominally. PP at ischial spines. No caput or moulding. Maximum cephalic diameter has not yet passed through smallest pelvic diameter – Caesarean section may be required.
High	Head not engaged. PP above ischial spines. Instrumental delivery not recommended.

The instruments that are available to assist vaginal delivery are either vacuum extraction devices or more than 70 types of obstetric forceps. These instruments provide a means of applying traction to the fetus to facilitate a vaginal delivery.

Vacuum extraction involves placement of a correctly sized cup (metal or plastic) to the flexion point (3 cm anterior of the posterior fontanelle), with the cup edge over the posterior fontanelle. A safe level of vacuum is created using a hand or electrical pump and traction is applied during a contraction alongside maternal effort. The traction encourages flexion, follows the birth canal, shadows normal physiological manoeuvres and allows natural rotation to occipito anterior (when required), appropriate for outlet and low pelvic deliveries. Vacuum is self-limiting in the degree of traction that can be used.

Forceps delivery (see Figure 29.1) involves two blunt blades being individually inserted posteriorly between contractions following the curve of the pelvis, then slid around to each side of the fetal head, before being interlocked at the shank end of the handle. When in place, the sagittal suture will be midline, the posterior fontanelle one finger's breadth above the shanks, with a fingertip between the heel of the blade and the fetal head. Their cephalic curve both fits around the fetal head and enables them to follow the sacral curve during delivery (this is minimised for rotational forceps). The handles have a projection (shoulder) to help with grip and traction is applied during a contraction alongside maternal effort.

Incidence

The incidence of instrumental deliveries varies across Europe, from 0.5% in Romania to 16.4% in Ireland, with an average of 7.5% (Rather *et al.*, 2016). In the UK, incidence remains stable at between 10 and 13% (Bahl *et al.*, 2011). Vacuum methods have gained in popularity with the use of forceps decreasing. This has had an impact on Caesarean section rates as forceps delivery is not a second option for those obstetricians now deskilled in the use of forceps (Rather *et al.*, 2016).

Indications (Bahl *et al.*, 2011; Nikpoor and Bain, 2013; Permezel and Paulsen, 2015; NICE, 2016d)

An instrumental delivery is only possible when there are no contraindications. It may become necessary when the second stage fails to progress to delivery or when an expedited delivery is required for either fetal or maternal reasons such as:

- Lack of progress – suspect delay and actively manage after 1 hour of second stage for nulliparous and 30 minutes for multiparous women; refer for instrumental/operative delivery at 2 or 1 hours respectively.
- Fetal compromise – evidence of fetal hypoxia, non-reassuring electrocardiogram.
- Maternal medical or obstetric conditions – e.g. heart weakness, severe hypertension, tumour, psychological trauma, haemorrhage.
- Maternal exhaustion – e.g. prolonged first and second stage of labour.
- Inability to perform maternal effort effectively – e.g. due to disability, epidural anaesthesia.
- Aftercoming head following a breech delivery.

Contraindications

- Lack of maternal consent.
- Incomplete dilatation of cervix (see Box 29.1 for exceptions).
- Inadequate pelvis – cephalo-pelvic disproportion.
- Excessive caput and/or moulding.
- No uterine contractions.
- Non-cephalic presentation (except for aftercoming head of breech).
- Fetal bleeding conditions.
- High presenting part – the biparietal diameter is still above the ischial spines (see Table 29.1).
- Preterm – forceps possible as they protect the head, but no ventouse before 34 weeks.
- Inability to determine position of head and correctly place equipment.

Choice of instrument

This is influenced by numerous factors including availability of equipment, obstetric factors and training of operator (this is essential to positive outcomes). The literature supports that both the forceps and metal vacuum cups make vaginal birth more likely than the soft or hand held vacuum cups. However, maternal trauma, incontinence and Caesarean rates increase following forceps, and the metal cup increases risk of neonatal trauma, scalp injury and cephalhaematoma (O'Mahony *et al.*, 2010). Therefore, the plastic cup is a common choice for non-complicated deliveries.

Management (Bahl *et al.*, 2011; Suwannachat *et al.*, 2012; Permezel and Paulsen, 2015; NICE, 2016d)

- Multiprofessional team – fully staffed theatre; equipment checked.
- Ensure adequate contractions present.
- Signed informed consent – prepared for chignon/forceps marks.
- Psychological support from same midwife throughout procedure.
- Anaesthesia – regional (pudendal plus perineal if low cavity only).
- Well lit, lithotomy position (edge of bed and at operator height).
- Aseptic procedure followed.
- Empty bladder required – remove any indwelling catheter.
- Confirm station (see Table 29.1), presentation, position and no caput or moulding – use vaginal examination/ultrasound as needed.
- Membranes ruptured.
- Lubricate chosen instrument and insert.
- Check no maternal tissue caught and correct application.
- Monitor contractions – inform obstetrician and coach maternal effort.
- Apply forceps or vacuum (rapid negative pressure; maximum 15 minutes).
- Maintain flexion; traction with contraction and maternal effort; follow pelvic 'J' curve.
- Stop procedure if no descent/progress after three pulls; or three pop offs (ventouse); or 15 minutes have elapsed (see Box 29.2).
- Perineal infiltration and mediolateral episiotomy at crowning only if indicated – guard perineum against laceration/extension.
- Remove instrument once jaw delivered; normal delivery from here.
- Mange third stage – ensure haemostasis (oxytocics as required).
- Examine cervix, vagina, perineum and anus – suture as required.
- Contemporaneous record keeping.
- Reassess for risk of thromboembolism and analgesia needs.
- Monitor first void/bladder – indwelling catheter for at least 12 hours.
- Review by obstetrician to discuss indications for delivery and assess for psychological trauma.
- Monitor for any possible complications throughout (see Box 29.3).

30 Preparation and transfer to the operating theatre

Figure 30.1 Preoperative checklist.

Preoperative checklist

Surname:
Forename:
Hospital number:
Date of birth:
Consultant:
Ward: Date:

Tick as appropriate

Checklist	**Yes**	**No**
Emergency procedure		
Next of kin informed		
Identification bracelet correct		
All notes including initial assessment		
All X-rays		
Consent form signed		
English first language? (If not, specify ……………………………….)		
All jewellery removed; rings taped		
Make up/nail varnish removed		
Dentures removed		
Hearing aid *in situ*		
Prosthesis/hip/knee/replacement/metalwork		
Pacemaker		
Operation site shaved/marked		
Catheter in bladder		
Passed urine/catheter released		
Antiembolus stockings		
Infection risk		
MRSA		
Other		

Bloods	**Date taken**	**Baseline observations**	**Sickle cell screen**
Hb	INR	BP	Positive
FBC	APPT	Pulse	Negative
WBC	Glucose	Temperature	N/A
Platelets	Blood gases	Respirations	
Na	Blood group	Existing skin/pressure damage	**Other**
K	Cross match?		
Urea	Yes /No		
Creatinine			

Diabetic: Yes/No	BM Stick	Time	Sliding scale running at

Allergies/sensitivities
Time last ate/drank
Premedication given (specify)

Print name:	Designation:
Signature:	Dare:

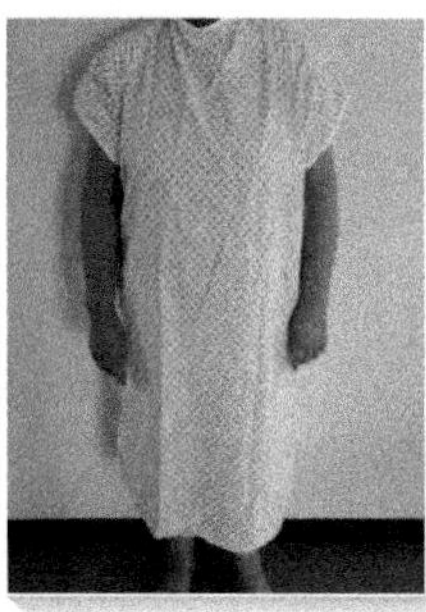

Figure 30.2 Theatre gown.

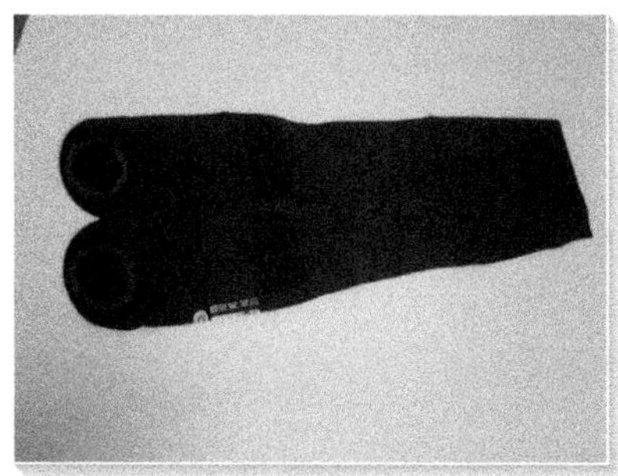

Figure 30.3 Graduated compression socks (thromboembolus deterrent socks - TEDS).

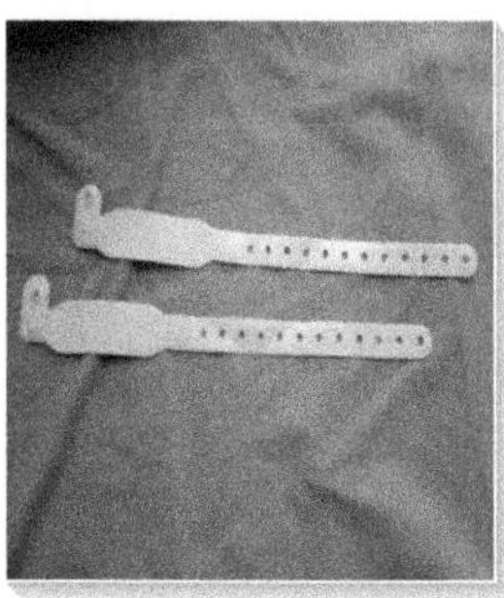

Figure 30.4 Identity bands.

Midwifery Emergencies at a Glance, First Edition. Denise (Dee) Campbell and Susan M. Carr. © 2018 John Wiley & Sons, Ltd. Published 2018 by John Wiley & Sons, Ltd.
Companion website: www.ataglanceseries.com/midwiferyemergencies

The preparation of a woman for transfer to the operating theatre will depend on the reason for the operative procedure. This will determine whether or not this is an elective or an emergency procedure and therefore the approach to the required preparations. The midwife has a pivotal role in supporting the woman and her birth partner(s). and where possible should remain with the woman from admission, or decision to operate, until she is transferred to the operating theatre. The most common operative procedure undertaken in the maternity unit is a lower segment Caesarean section (LSCS) in order to deliver the baby through an incision in the woman's abdomen. Throughout, the woman should be offered evidence-based information to assist with her decision-making related to the treatment and care being recommended. Similarly, good communication between the woman, her family and the carers must be fostered, taking into account any psychosocial and learning needs or disabilities that she may have (Dougherty *et al.*, 2015).

Antepartum preparations (see Figure 30.1)

In the event of a planned/elective LSCS, the woman should be welcomed to the maternity unit on arrival. It is common practice for Trusts to advise against eating from midnight the previous evening, but to permit sips of water up to 2 hours before the procedure. Prior to admission to the maternity unit, blood tests will be performed to include:

- Full blood count (FBC) – haemoglobin to identify women who may be anaemic (NICE, 2011).
- Group and save serum/cross-match – especially if the woman is at an increased risk of bleeding during the operation, for example, placenta praevia (NICE, 2011).

On admission

On admission, the woman will have routine observations taken including:

- Temperature.
- Pulse.
- Blood pressure.

She will also be asked to remove all her clothes and put on a hospital gown and a pair of graduated compression socks (thrombembolus deterrent socks [TEDS]) (see Figures 30.2 and 30.3). An identity band will be attached to her wrist stating her full name, date of birth and hospital or NHS number (see Figure 30.4). All jewellery should be removed and where this is not possible (e.g. a wedding band), the item should be covered with tape to prevent loss. Should the woman have any prosthetic items such as teeth, it will be necessary to discuss this with the anaesthetist as their removal may be preferred.

If this is an elective procedure, the mode of anaesthesia to be used will have been discussed with the woman prior to admission. Nonetheless, it is likely that the woman will be visited by an anaesthetist to ensure that she remains comfortable with her earlier decisions. Regional anaesthesia in the form of a spinal block is generally recommended as this is safer and reduces the risk of maternal and neonatal morbidity when compared with a general anaesthetic (NICE, 2011). The anaesthetist may cannulate the woman on arrival in the operating theatre.

Consent

The obstetrician will visit the woman to elicit her consent to the procedure. This should only be requested once the woman has received a full explanation which takes into consideration her views and her cultural concerns, gives the reasons for the procedure and the possible accompanying risks (NICE, 2011). It must be remembered that the woman may refuse the procedure. Should this be the case, the midwife must support the woman in her decision in a non-judgmental manner.

Preparation for theatre

The midwife will support the woman by answering any questions related to what will happen when she arrives in the operating theatre suite. This may include:

- Explaining how many people will be present:
  - the surgeon – consultant or registrar obstetrician
  - the anaesthetist to ensure that the anaesthetic is functioning adequately
  - the operating department practitioner (or similar) to assist the anaesthetist
  - the scrub nurse or midwife who will assist with the instruments
  - the health care assistant to assist the scrub nurse/midwife
  - the midwife who will assist the baby at delivery
  - a neonatologist to assist the baby if required
  - the woman's birth partner(s) – if the anaesthesia is regional
  - possibly any student midwives or medical students with permission from the woman.
- The midwife will catheterise the woman's bladder using an aseptic technique in order to prevent damage by ensuring that it is empty throughout the operation.
- The woman will be informed that the operating table will be tilted initially to offset maternal hypotension when laying in a supine position.
- Pubic shaving may have been carried out by the woman prior to admission or this may be performed immediately prior to surgery.
- Should the reason for the LSCS be for a breech presentation, the woman's abdomen may be palpated by the obstetrician and the fetus examined using ultrasound to confirm its presentation and position. External cephalic version may be offered and attempted immediately prior to surgery in a last effort to rotate the fetus to a cephalic presentation.
- Preoperative medication may have been given to the woman to take prior to admission. However, this may be prescribed and administered prior to transfer to theatre. This may include preoperative antibiotics or gastric acid reduction medication (e.g. 150 mg ranitidine given orally the night before surgery and in the morning before surgery). In an emergency, 50 mg can be given intravenously, 30 minutes before surgery.

If an emergency LSCS is advised, all the above will be undertaken, but without the luxury of time to prepare the woman in a relaxed and leisurely manner. The time from decision to deliver and the delivery itself will be critical and thus the event is likely to be psychologically more stressful for the woman, her birth partner and the staff caring for her.

31 Role of the scrub midwife or nurse

Figure 31.1 Sterile surgical gown pack. Source: From Thomas (2015). Reproduced with permission of John Wiley & Sons.

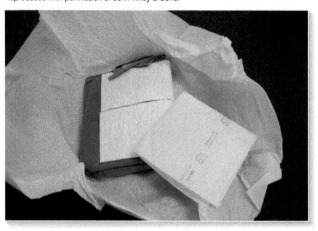

Figure 31.2 (a, b) Donning sterile gloves. Source: From Thomas (2015). Reproduced with permission of John Wiley & Sons.

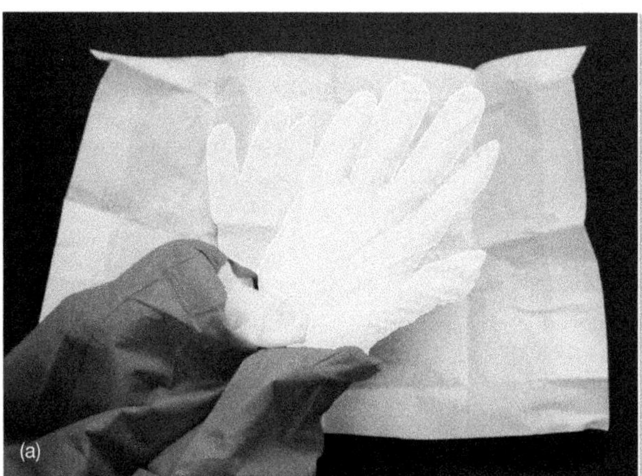

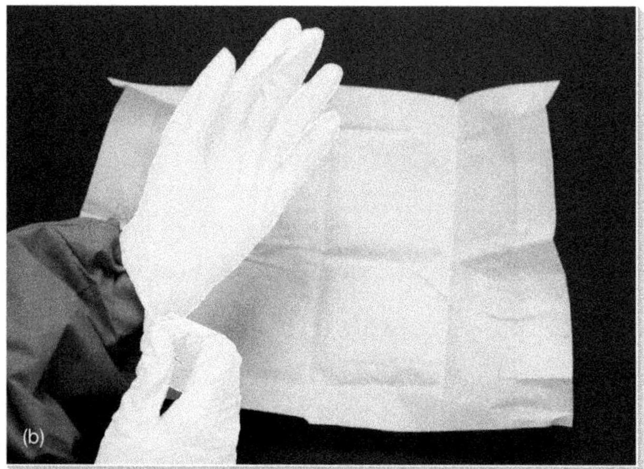

Figure 31.3 Ready for theatre. Source: From Thomas (2015). Reproduced with permission of John Wiley & Sons.

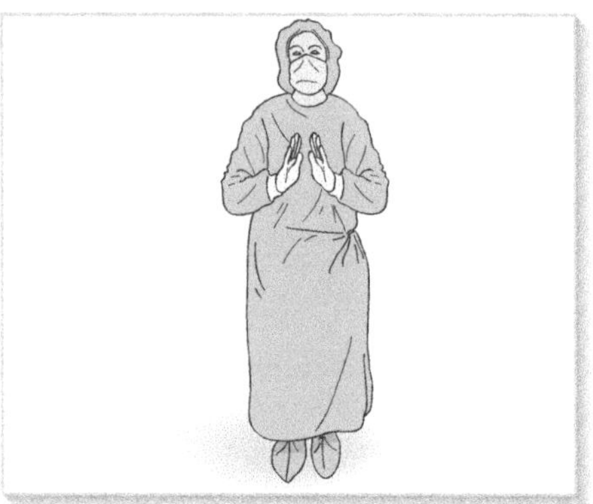

Figure 31.4 Setting out the sterile equipment.

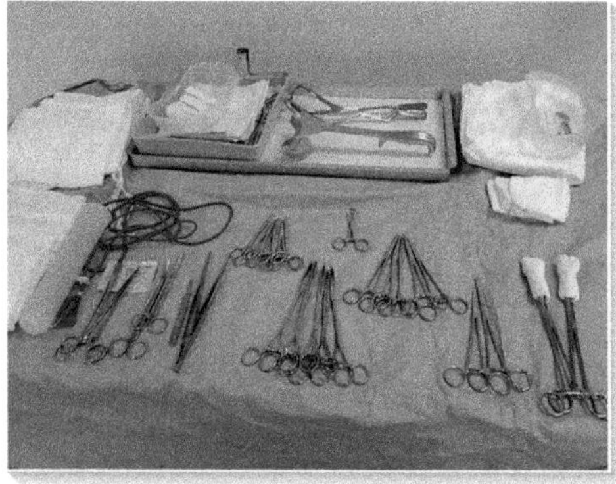

Figure 31.5 Umbilical cord clamp, scissors and sterile towel.

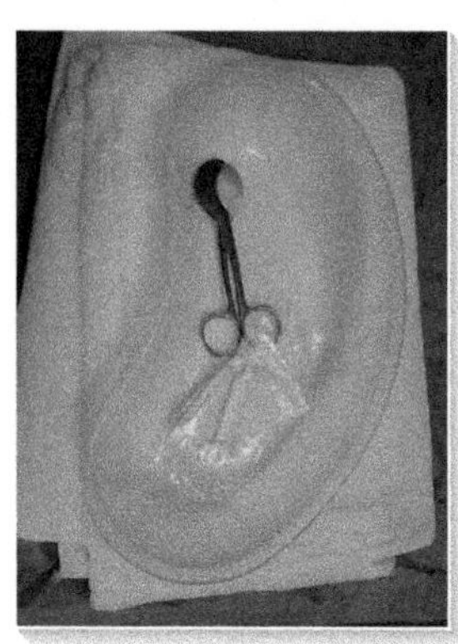

In recent years there has been an ongoing debate about the staffing of the operating theatre in an obstetric unit and the appropriateness of the midwife taking on the role of the instrument or scrub assistant, especially where shortages of midwifery staff exist. Many argue that the midwife's prime area of responsibility is to the woman, and subsequently the infant, and that it is not the midwife's role to offer scrub/instrument assistance. However, others espouse the belief that being 'with woman' also incorporates the competence and ability to assume the role of scrub midwife, thereby supporting the woman by being the advocate for her body during the birth (Pusey, 2011). Competence is essential and must be demonstrated before the midwife, nurse or on occasion, operating department practitioner, can assume this role and assist as the instrument/scrub assistant (CODP, RCM, AfPP, 2009).

Preoperative preparations

- Whenever possible, it is helpful for the parents to meet the midwife who will be assisting the obstetrician during the forthcoming surgical procedure. The midwife should introduce him/herself and explain their role. It is important to explain that a theatre gown and possibly a cap will be worn and that they will not be immediately recognisable to the parents.
- The scrub midwife/nurse will enter the theatre wearing a cap to cover the hair, plus a face mask (with integral visor to protect the eyes if available) and/or a pair of goggles. Any special items or equipment that may be required will be discussed with the circulating assistant, who may be a midwife, a nurse or a member of support staff trained in perioperative skills.
- The scrub midwife/nurse will 'scrub up' and don a sterile gown followed by double-gloving with sterile latex surgical gloves, according to local policy (see Figures 31.1, 31.2 and 31.3).
- Once the scrub assistant has completed the previous steps they will proceed to the preparation room and, with the assistance of the circulating assistant, will begin to set up the equipment and instruments in an orderly manner (see Figure 31.4).
- All instruments are counted and verified by the scrub assistant and circulating assistant and subsequently documented on a Trust-specific pro forma.
- All swabs are counted, verified and documented as above.
- Any needles (hypodermic or attached to suture material) are counted, verified and documented on the relevant Trust-specific pro forma.
- Any lotions to be used are poured into the appropriate receiver after the name and the expiry date of the liquid are checked and verified as above.

Once the woman has been prepared to the satisfaction of the anaesthetist and obstetrician, the scrub assistant will enter the theatre and position themselves in close proximity to the operating table and the obstetricians.

Intrapartum responsibilities

- It is the prime responsibility of the scrub assistant to ensure that the whereabouts of all instruments, swabs, 'sharps' and other equipment are known throughout the procedure, including items which, once used, are removed from the sterile field of operation and are stored away from the scrub assistant's trolley (e.g. cord scissors used to tidy the umbilical cord following the application of the cord clamp by the midwife receiving the baby).
- The scrub assistant must maintain sterility throughout the procedure.
- The initial preparations, including the cleansing and draping of the woman's abdomen with sterile sheets, will be undertaken by the obstetrician and their assistant.
- Throughout the procedure the scrub assistant will remain alert to and anticipate the needs of the obstetrician, passing instruments and swabs, blades and sutures as required.
- As a rule, the 'scrub' midwife or nurse will pass a sterile towel to the midwife waiting to receive the baby (see Figure 31.5).
- The scrub midwife will pass the placenta and membranes, contained in a suitable receptacle, to the midwife who has care of the infant at birth, to be checked for completeness. The result of this examination is then relayed to the scrub assistant, who will then inform the obstetrician.
- A first instrument, blade, suture and swab count will be conducted typically prior to the closure of the peritoneum. Then before the obstetrician closes the woman's abdomen, the scrub and circulating assistants will re-count all instruments, swabs, blades and needles and confirm to the surgeon that all equipment has been accounted for. This will be entered onto the Trust-specific documentation.

Postoperative responsibilities

- The scrub assistant will remove all equipment to the sluice area for collation and packing before transfer to the central sterile supplies department to be cleaned, autoclaved and re-packed. Trust protocol may require the scrub assistant to complete and sign specific documentation prior to the equipment leaving the delivery suite, confirming that all instruments are present.
- The postoperative documentation will include the completion of the woman's notes to indicate the presence of all instruments, swabs, blades and needles following the completion of the surgery.
- As soon as is practicable, the scrub assistant may return to the woman and her support person to reassure them that the procedure has been completed successfully, to demonstrate care and concern for the newly-delivered woman and to share the enjoyment of welcoming the new baby.
- In some Trusts it is the duty of the scrub midwife/assistant to complete certain sections of the woman's notes. Therefore, it is their responsibility to become familiar with Trust protocol for postoperative care.

32 Receiving the baby in the operating theatre

Figure 32.1 Umbilical cord clamp, scissors and sterile towel.

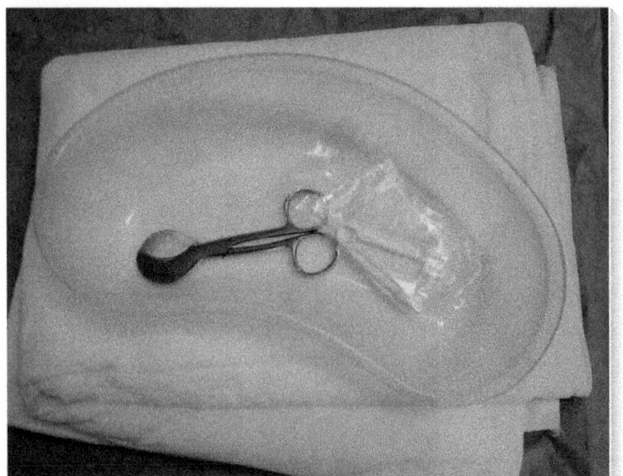

Figure 32.2 Identity wrist bands, cards and hat.

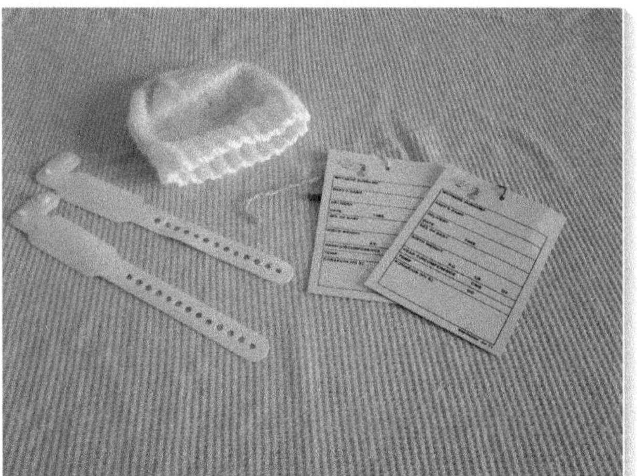

Figure 32.3 Resuscitaire.

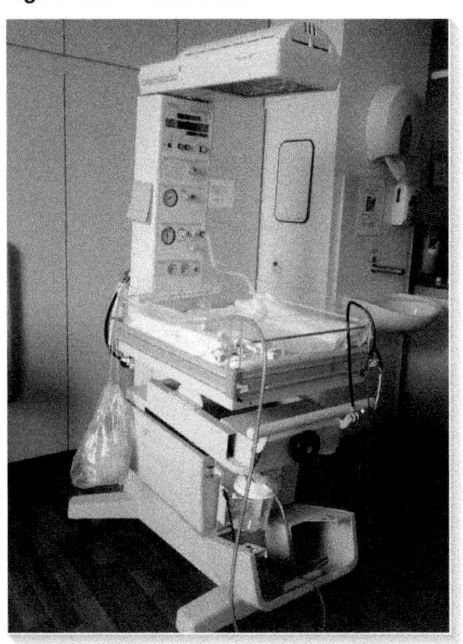

Figure 32.4 Weighing scales.

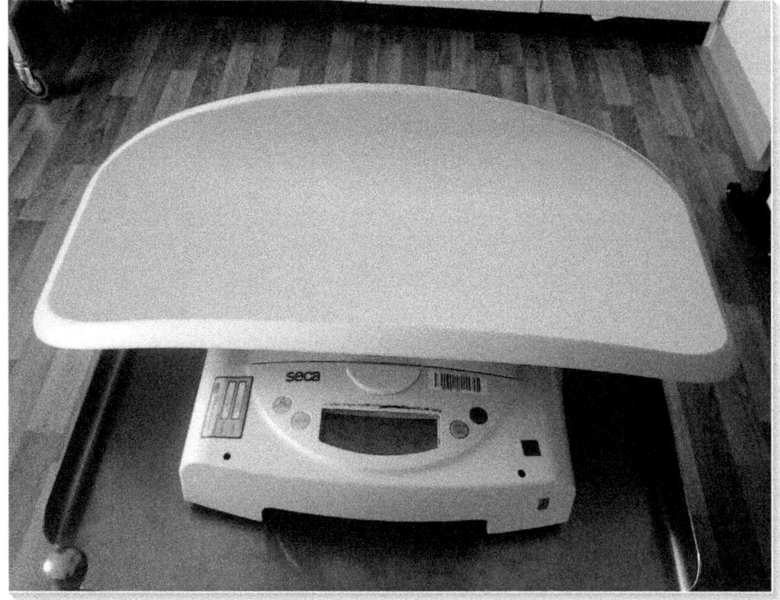

The infant born in the operating theatre, by elective or emergency Caesarean section or instrumental delivery, is generally received by a midwife. The midwife's sole responsibility in this birth situation is to support, monitor and care for the baby in the initial minutes after birth (Macdonald & Johnson, 2017).

Antepartum preparations

- Whenever possible, it is helpful for the parents to meet the midwife who will receive their baby during the forthcoming surgical procedure. The midwife should introduce him/herself and explain the likely course of events in the theatre related to the moments immediately after the birth of the baby. It is important to explain a theatre gown and possibly a cap will be worn and therefore they will not be immediately recognisable to the parents. At this point it is appropriate to enquire how the woman has decided to feed her baby.
- Review the mother's history to assess for potential risks to the baby.
- The midwife checks that any equipment that may be needed is present in the theatre, including the Resuscitaire. This should be switched on before the birth to enable good visualisation for the midwife and provide a warm surface on which to place the baby.
- The documentation to be completed following the birth should be available, together with two ID labels for the baby.
- If it is expected that fetal blood sampling (sampling from the placenta) may be necessary, especially if the procedure is being undertaken due to a deterioration in the fetal condition, the appropriate syringe(s), needles and sample bottles should be made ready but not labelled until the mother's notes are available in the theatre and her identity has been confirmed.
- A cot for the baby should be prepared outside the theatre in the recovery area together with a nappy and clothes. The environment should be kept warm.
- The neonatologist may be alerted at this point, if the condition of the baby has been called into question (NICE, 2011).
- Once the midwife has confirmed that everything is ready to receive the infant, they may put on a theatre hat to cover their hair – this will be determined by the local Trust policy. They should then wash and dry their hands and don a sterile gown and gloves before entering the theatre.

Intrapartum responsibilities

- It is imperative that the midwife remains vigilant throughout the procedure and is ready to receive the baby.
- As a rule, the 'scrub' midwife or nurse will pass a sterile towel to the midwife waiting to receive the baby together with an umbilical cord clamp and scissors to trim the umbilical cord as necessary (see Figure 32.1).
- As the baby emerges from the woman's abdomen the time of birth and the sex of the baby are noted, and the umbilical cord will be clamped and divided. The baby will then be passed to the waiting midwife.
- If the baby is in good condition, the midwife will take the baby to the mother (if alert and comfortable) and offer skin-to-skin contact via her upper abdomen and chest, covering the baby with blankets and a hat to maintain its body temperature (NICE, 2011).
- Two ID bands will be secured to the baby – usually one around each ankle, having been verified against the mother's notes and by the mother herself (see Figure 32.2).
- In general, the placenta and membranes are passed to the midwife receiving the baby in a suitable receptacle to be examined for their completeness. The result of this examination is then relayed to the scrub assistant.
- If the baby requires support or assistance after birth, the neonatologist will be called and the midwife will remove the baby to the Resuscitaire, ensuring where possible that the mother has uninterrupted visual contact with her baby (see Figure 32.3). On arrival, the neonatologist will be informed about the gestation of the infant, the nature of the problem and the reason for the operative procedure. The midwife will also ensure that the special care baby unit (SCBU) or neonatal intensive care unit (NICU) has been informed.
- The midwife will commence systematic resuscitation, ensuring that the woman and her partner are kept informed of what is being done for their baby (see Chapter 4).
- Blood may be taken from the umbilical vessels in the placenta to assess the baby's blood gases.

Criteria preventing the baby from moving to the recovery room with its mother

- The mother's condition is unstable.
- The neonate's condition requires attention.
- If the midwife receiving the baby is unable to remain with the mother and the baby.
- If the baby is to be removed from the woman for known social reasons, such as adoption at birth.

Postpartum responsibilities (Macdonald & Johnson, 2017)

- On completion of the surgery, if the baby is to be transferred to the SCBU or NICU, it generally travels the short distance either on the Resuscitaire or in a cot accompanied by the receiving midwife and the partner/support person.
- If the baby is in good condition, the woman may continue with skin-to-skin contact until such time as she is transferred to the recovery area. At this point the baby should be wrapped and handed to the woman's partner/support person (seated), while the woman is moved onto her ward bed. The baby can then be returned to its mother and together they are removed from the theatre to the recovery area.
- Skin-to-skin contact can be resumed once in the recovery area and while the baby's documentation is being completed. This may include the birth notification in addition to the baby's birth/postnatal observations.
- The midwife will perform the initial newborn examination and the cord will be trimmed and a cord clamp applied.
- At an appropriate time agreed with the parents, the baby can be weighed and measured and receive vitamin K if the parents consent (see Figure 32.4).
- The midwife can assist with breastfeeding as and when the infant and the woman show a readiness to do so (NICE, 2011).
- The midwife may be required to return to the operating theatre to clean and stock the Resuscitaire if used.
- Once the woman's condition is stable, the midwife may be called upon to accompany the woman and the baby to the postnatal ward where she will hand over their care to the ward staff using an SBAR (situation; background; assessment; recommendation) chart to aid good communication between staff.

33 Immediate care following surgery

Figure 33.1 Fluid balance chart.

FLUID BALANCE CHART

HOSPITAL NUMBER:
SURNAME:
FIRST NAME:

DATE	INDICATE NATURE AND VOLUME IN MILLILITRES OF ALL FLUID							
	INTAKE			OUTPUT				
						Drainage		
TIME	Oral	Intravenous/ subcutaneous	Other	Urine	Vomit aspirate	Specify	Specify	Other
01.00								
02.00								
03.00								
04.00								
05.00								
06.00								
08.00								
09.00								
10.00								
11.00								
12.00								
13.00								
14.00								
15.00								
16.00								
17.00								
18.00								
19.00								
20.00								
21.00								
22.00								
23.00								
24.00								
TOTAL INTAKE:		mL.		TOTAL OUTPUT:				mL.

FLUID BALANCE (Intake minus output): mL.

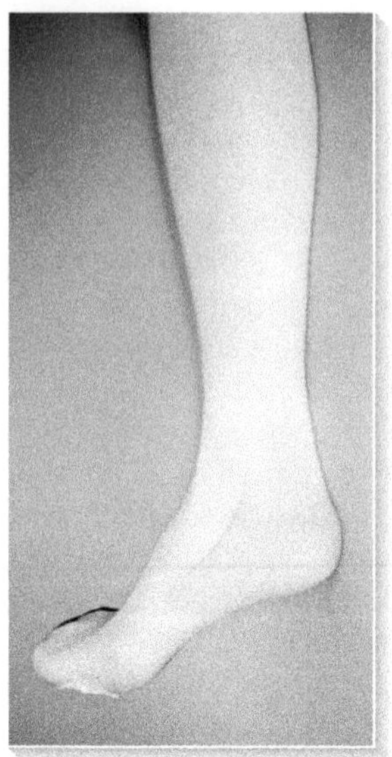

Figure 33.2 Graduated compression socks.

Figure 33.3 Catheter insertion form.

Urinary Catheter Insertion Form and Ongoing Care Plan
NB. One sheet per catheter. If catheter is resited start a new assessment and monitoring form

SURNAME:
FIRST NAME:
DATE OF BIRTH:
ID NUMBER:

		Insertion checklist	
Area/Dept.: ……………………………… Date/time of insertion: ………………….. Inserted by: ………………………………. (Print name and designation) Urethral: Suprapubic: Other: Catheter size: Anticipated date of removal: Actual removal date: Allergies:	**Reason for catheterisation** Retention of urine Measurement of urine output Preoperative drainage Bladder irrigation **Type of catheter** Latex short term max 4 weeks PTFE-coated short term max 4 weeks Silicone-coated long term max 12 weeks Hydrogel-coated long term max 12 weeks Other	**Insertion checklist** **Verbal/written consent:** **Chaperone present:** Hand hygiene and apply apron Prepare equipment (sterile technique) Apply FIRST sterile gloves Clean urethral orifice with 0.9% NaCl Apply sterile lubrication gel Apply SECOND sterile gloves Insert catheter – non-touch technique Inflate balloon with H_2O ……… mL Attach and label urine bag (start date) Residual	**First urinalysis result after catheter insertion** **Traceability label**

Please write in boxes YES or NO and where actions are indicated document in medical notes

Ward ____	Is catheter still required? **(Daily review)**	Catheter entry site cleaned with soap and water? **(Daily catheter site hygiene)**	Ensure drainage bag is positioned below bladder and off the floor **(At all times)**	Is drainage bag due to be changed today? **(Bag to be changed within 7 days)**	Is there any sign of infection (offensive cloudy urine, pyrexia, positive urinalysis)? **(If YES send CSU)**	Urine sample (CSU) taken and sent to lab. **(From designated closed needle-free port)**	**Print name and signature**
Date							
Date							
Date							
Date							
Date							
Date							
Date							

The prime concern for the midwife or nurse assigned to caring for a woman following surgery is to receive her into an environment that is safe and which enables individualised management. The woman and her baby will be moved from the operating theatre to the recovery room thereby beginning the transition from surgery to continuing her recuperation on the ward. The woman will be transferred on her bed and if she is well enough, the baby may be cradled in her arms or held close to her for skin-to-skin contact. However, if the woman is unwell or does not feel confident in holding her baby, the baby may be moved in a cot to the recovery area.

It is essential that all equipment and documentation that may be required during the recovery of a postoperative woman is available, including items that may be needed for emergency resuscitation. The time spent in the recovery area will depend on the type of anaesthesia used during the operation. This will determine the woman's ability to control her own airway postoperatively and communicate with her carers (Dougherty *et al.*, 2015).

Postoperative care

- The woman will be received into the recovery area and the midwife/nurse will introduce themselves to her.
- The midwife or nurse caring for the woman in the operating theatre should give a comprehensive handover to the individual who will continue her care in the recovery area. The use of a tool similar to an SBAR chart (Situation; Background; Assessment; Recommendation) should be used to ensure that the receiving member of staff is given a full picture of what has been carried out, why the procedure was necessary, what the current situation regarding the woman's recovery might be and what is required in the immediate future (see Chapter 37, Figure 37.2). This should include:
  - the woman's name
  - her relevant medical/surgical history
  - the procedure that has been undertaken, including any unforeseen events during or around the time of the surgery
  - any history of allergies, especially to medicines
  - any drugs (including fluids) administered during surgery or that may need to be infused post-operatively
  - any postoperative instructions related to her care.
- On admission to the recovery area a full set of observations should be carried out and documented on a Modified Early Obstetric Warning System (MEOWS) chart, including:
  - respiratory rate
  - blood pressure
  - heart rate
  - pain score
  - level of consciousness/neurological score in relation to sedation following anaesthesia (if appropriate) or pain relief
  - oxygen saturations if required (i.e. woman using oxygen postoperatively).
- Observations will continue at regular intervals throughout the woman's stay in the recovery area according to Trust policy and recommendations (Liddle, 2013). Generally, observations will be carried out every 15 minutes initially, gradually increasing the interval between recordings as the woman's condition improves. Should there be any deviation from the norm as noted on the MEOWS chart, either through abnormal observations or high numbers of items noted in the 'red' zone, referral to the obstetric team will be initiated (see Chapter 37, Figure 37.1).
- The midwife/nurse will monitor the woman's urine output, documenting this on a fluid balance chart (see Figure 33.1). She will also ensure that the urinary catheter remains *in situ* and is draining freely into a catheter bag mounted on a stand to prevent unnecessary tugging on the catheter.
- Any drainage devices will also be checked regularly and amounts of exudate entered onto the fluid balance chart.
- The woman's wound should be inspected for leakage and also the integrity of the dressing should be checked. This will be entered on the MEOWS chart.
- The woman's lochia will be examined for quantity, colour and consistency (e.g. the presence/absence of clots). The findings will be included on the MEOWS chart. In conjunction with the observation of the lochia, the fundus of the woman's uterus will be palpated gently, to confirm that it remains well-contracted.
- It is essential that the risk assessment for venous thromboembolism has been read and that the woman is wearing a pair of graduated compression socks/stockings (thromboembolus deterrent socks/stockings – TEDS) (NICE, 2011) (see Figure 33.2). Similarly, the instructions for the commencement and continuing administration of prophylactic anticoagulant therapy using a preparation of low molecular weight heparin (e.g. Clexane) should be available and actioned.
- As long as the woman is well, she may commence eating and drinking as soon as she feels hungry and thirsty (NICE, 2011).
- Contemporaneous documentation should be maintained throughout, including:
  - MEOWS chart
  - fluid balance chart
  - prescription chart to include all medication and intravenous therapy.
  - care bundles (e.g. intravenous cannula, urinary catheter) (see Figures 33.3)
  - the client's hand-held notes, which must be kept up-to-date throughout the time spent in the recovery area.
- Following a regional anaesthetic for an operative procedure, the woman should be settled in her bed in a sitting position, ensuring her comfort.
- Early skin-to-skin contact should be recommended and initiated as soon as possible after the birth. The midwife/nurse caring for the mother (and baby) should support and encourage the woman to feed her baby within the first hour after birth by her chosen method as soon as she is ready and happy to do so.
- Analgesia should be offered when the woman identifies that she is in pain. This may be administered by a patient-controlled pump or, initially, intramuscularly. Similarly, all prescribed medication should be given in a timely manner as detailed on the prescription chart (NICE, 2011).
- An opportunity to discuss and ask questions (about previous and ongoing management) should be facilitated as soon as practicable after the birth.

Electronic fetal monitoring – actions following a suspicious or pathological trace

Table 34.1 Cardiotocography interpretation. Source: Data from NICE (2017b).

	Salient features		
Description	**Baseline rate**	**Baseline variability**	**Decelerations**
Normal (reassuring) trace All three features reassuring	110–160 beats per minute (bpm)	5–25 bpm	• None or early decelerations • Variable decelerations with no concerning features such as lasting more than 60 seconds ▪ no 'shouldering' ▪ reduced variability during the contraction
Suspicious (non-reassuring) trace One non-reassuring feature **AND** two reassuring features	100–109 bpm **OR** 161–180 bpm	Less than 5 bpm for 30–50 minutes **OR** More than 25 bpm for 15–25 minutes	• Variable decelerations with no concerning features for 90 minutes or more **OR** Variable decelerations with any concerning feature in up to 50% of contractions for 30 minutes or more **OR** Variable decelerations with any concerning features in over 50% of contractions for less than 30 minutes **OR** Late decelerations in over 50% of contractions for less than 30 minutes, with no maternal or fetal risk factors such as vaginal bleeding or significant meconium
Pathological (abnormal) trace One abnormal **OR** Two non-reassuring features	Less than 100 bpm **OR** More than 160 bpm **OR** Sinusoidal pattern for more than 10 minutes	Less than 5 bpm for 90 minutes	Variable decelerations with any concerning features in over 50% of contractions for 30 minutes (or less if any maternal or clinical risk factors [see above]) **OR** Late decelerations for 30 minutes (or less if any maternal or fetal clinical risk factors) **OR** Acute bradycardia, or a single prolonged deceleration lasting 3 minutes or more

The presence of accelerations in the fetal heart rate, even in the presence of reduced baseline variability, is generally a sign that the fetus is healthy. Similarly, the absence of accelerations in the presence of an otherwise normal CTG trace, does not indicate fetal acidosis (NICE, 2017b).

Companion website: www.ataglanceseries.com/midwiferyemergencies

Continuous electronic fetal monitoring is achieved by cardiotocography (CTG) during which the fetal heart rate is auscultated either via a transducer attached to the maternal abdomen or via an electrode clipped to the fetal scalp. In addition, a separate transducer is attached to the maternal abdomen to record the uterine contractions. Thus, the fetal heart rate and the uterine contractions are both assessed simultaneously and plotted graphically enabling the midwife/medical practitioner to interpret the fetal reaction to the uterine contractions via the changes in the heart rate and pattern.

Reasons for continuous CTG monitoring

Continuous cardiotocography is recommended for the following (NICE, 2014):

- Meconium stained liquor defined as dark green amniotic fluid containing particulate meconium.
- Abnormality in fetal heart rate.
- Maternal pyrexia.
- Maternal tachycardia.
- Maternal hypertension.
- Fresh vaginal bleeding.
- Hypertonic contractions.
- Confirmed delay in the first or second stage of labour.
- Suspected amnionitis.
- Multiple pregnancy.
- Breech presentation.
- Oxytocin induction or augmentation of labour.
- Intrauterine growth restriction.
- Previous Caesarean section.

Risks impacting CTG monitoring

- Misinterpretation of the monitoring. This may lead to a delay in responding to the situation, taking inappropriate action or the misuse of oxytocic therapy.
- Failure of the CTG equipment.
- Poor positioning of the transducers.
- Poor documentation and record keeping.
- Inadequate staffing levels.
- Inadequate training and updating of staff.

Definition of a suspicious or pathological CTG trace (NICE, 2017b)

The diagnosis of a suspicious (non-reassuring) trace and a pathological (abnormal) trace is determined by the presence of reassuring, non-reassuring and abnormal salient features. These are the baseline heart rate, the baseline variability and the presence and character of decelerations in the fetal heart rate (see Table 34.1).

When reviewing a CTG trace, a systematic approach is recommended and thus the use of a mnemonic is favoured by some as an aide memoire to ensure that all aspects of the trace are reviewed and assessed.

- **CTG suspicious (non-reassuring):** a suspicious (non-reassuring) heart rate would demonstrate one non-reassuring feature **and** two reassuring feature.
- **CTG pathological (abnormal):** a pathologica l (abnormal) heart rate would consist of one abnormal **or** two non-reassuring features.

Management

Suspicious (non-reassuring) CTG trace

- Inform the senior midwife and obstetrician.
- Inform the woman and her birth companion about what is happening.
- Correct any underlying hypotension by commencing intravenous infusion.
- For uterine hyperstimulation, consider reducing or stopping oxytocin or offer tocolysis (e.g. terbutaline infusion).
- Undertake a set of maternal observations.
- Consider offering conservative measures (NICE, 2014) as determined by the most likely cause (e.g. encourage the woman to change her position – not supine).
- Document a plan for reviewing the CTG findings in the context of the entire clinical picture.

Pathological (abnormal) CTG trace

- Seek immediate review by senior obstetrician and senior midwife.
- Inform the woman and her birth companion about what is happening.
- Commence conservative measures (e.g. correct underlying hypotension and or hyperstimulation of the uterus) (NICE, 2017b).
- Exclude acute events (e.g. placental abruption, cord prolapse).
- Consider digital fetal scalp stimulation as an adjunct to CTG (NICE, 2014). If fetal scalp stimulation does not elicit and increase the fetal heart rate, fetal blood sampling should be considered.
- Consider expediting delivery of the fetus.

Acute bradycardia (or prolonged deceleration of more than 3 minutes)

- Urgent obstetric assistance is needed.
- Inform the woman and her birth companion about what is happening.
- Plans for an emergency birth should be made, especially if a sudden, acute event is suspected.
- Correct any underlying hypotension and or hyperstimulation of the uterus (NICE, 2017b).
- Instigate one or more conservative measures such as changing the woman's position; rehydrate the woman if necessary.
- Should the fetal heart rate increase any time up to 9 minutes after the acute episode, the decision to expedite the birth should be reviewed in consultation with the woman.

Decisions related to the care of a woman in labour should not be made on the evidence from CTG monitoring alone. The wellbeing of the woman, fetal movement, maternal observations, any vaginal bleeding, meconium staining of the liquor amnii, uterine contractions, maternal medication, etc. should also be taken into account.

35 Fetal scalp electrode

Figure 35.1 Images of a fetal scalp electrode and its parts.

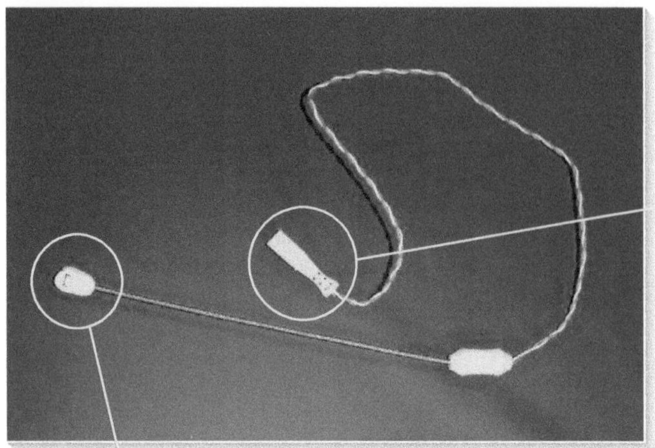

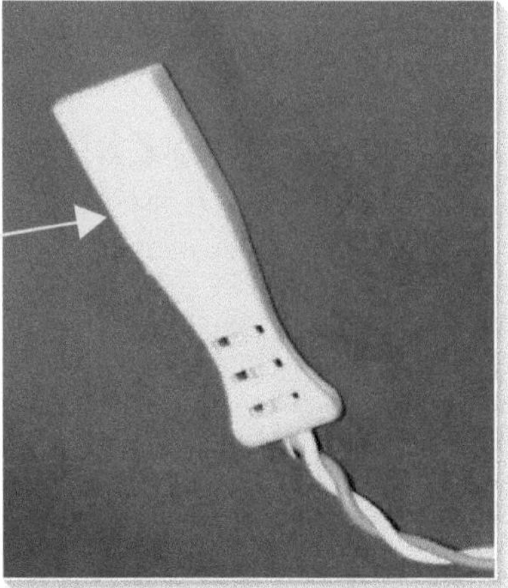

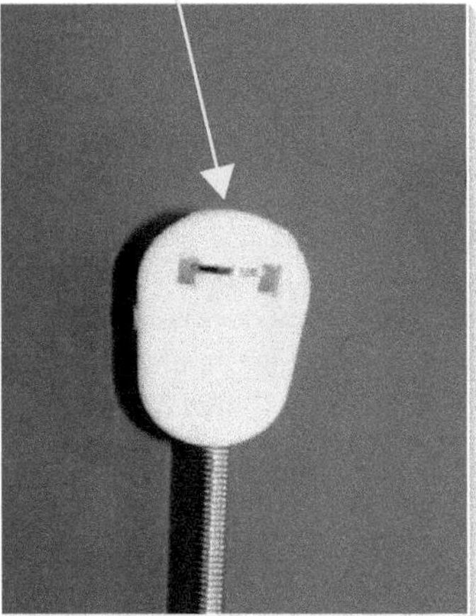

Figure 35.2 FSE slides along fingers with electrode facing fingers.

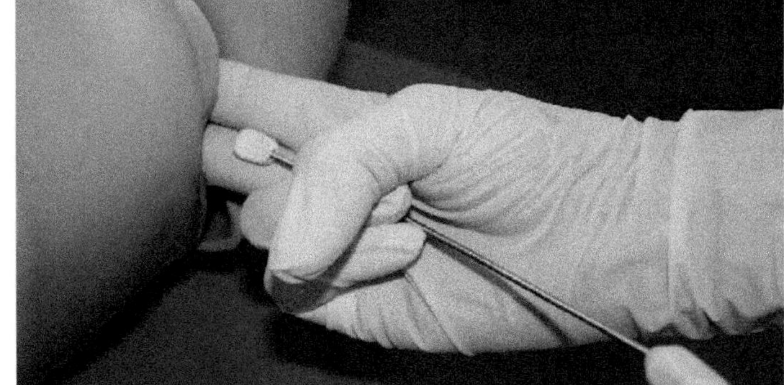

Figure 35.3 Head fully closed.

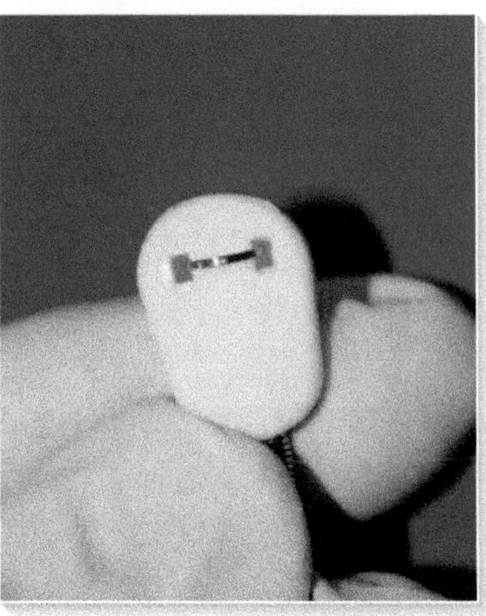

Figure 35.4 Head partially open.

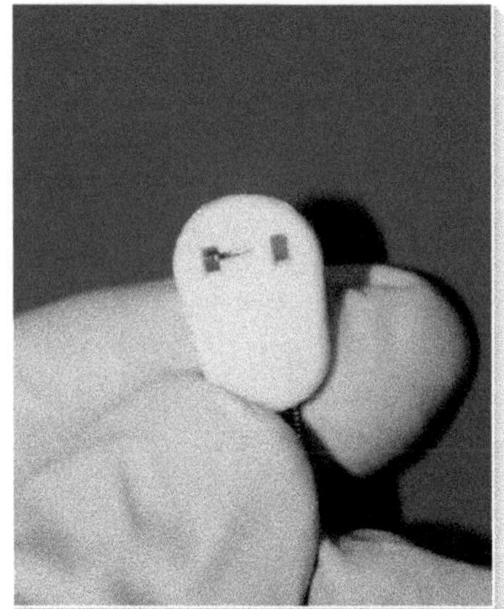

Figure 35.5 Head fully open.

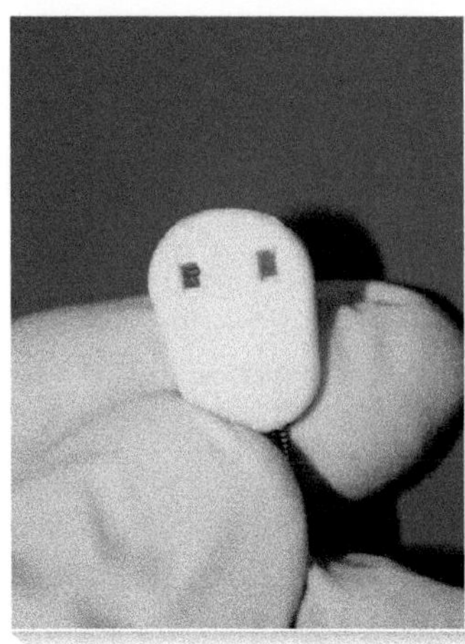

Most commonly, the fetal heart will be intermittently auscultated during labour using a pinard stethoscope or a Doppler system. When continuous monitoring is required, invasive procedures can be avoided through the use of an external transducer optimally positioned on the maternal abdomen over the site of the fetal heart. This is electrocardiotocography (ECTG) and it records an average of the beats it detects. The alternative is the application of an electrode to the scalp of the fetus during a vaginal examination, which occur in as many as 22% of deliveries (Kawakita *et al.*, 2016).

The fetal scalp electrode (FSE) (see Figure 35.1) enables monitoring of the actual fetal heart beats and electrical activity using single lead electrocardiography (ECG). The electrode is attached to the fetal scalp using either a clip or a screw technique. It can also be attached to a breech presentation. Interpretation of the recordings can prove challenging where traces are neither clearly normal nor clearly abnormal. False diagnosis of hypoxia can lead to unnecessary operative deliveries and the non-identification of hypoxia is associated with increased fetal morbidity. It is essential that each trace is considered individually alongside the woman's full history and by an experienced professional.

Predisposing factors

The women more likely to require continuous monitoring are those with a high-risk pregnancy and an associated greater risk of fetal hypoxia. An American study (Kawakita *et al.*, 2016) identified that FSEs were more commonly associated with:

- First pregnancies after 34 weeks.
- Younger women.
- Ethnicity.
- Raised body mass index.
- Smokers.
- Medical complications – diabetes, hypertension, heart/renal disease.
- Operative vaginal or Caesarean deliveries.

Indications

An FSE is indicated when continuous monitoring is required (a fetus at greater risk of hypoxia) but abdominal auscultation proves challenging through loss of contact or intermittent contact only from the ECTG. This is more likely with:

- Fetal arrhythmia.
- Increased fetal movement.
- Multiple pregnancy.
- Long labour.
- Trial of labour.
- Obese women.

Contraindications

The application of a FSE is an invasive procedure which can only take place when there is a full commitment to delivery. It is contraindicated when:

- Maternal consent is withheld.
- Labour has not been confirmed.
- Attempts are being made to stop labour.
- Vaginal examination is contraindicated.
- Artificial rupture of membranes is contraindicated.
- A high presenting part is identified.
- The cervix is closed or minimally dilated.
- Elective Caesarean section is planned.
- Cross-infection risk is increased (haemolytic strep B, herpes, hepatitis, HIV).
- Fetal coagulation problems exist.
- Prematurity < 34 weeks.
- Fetal death is suspected.

Note: HIV cross-infection is unlikely if there is an undetectable viral load (British HIV Association, 2014).

Management

- Explain indications and procedure (including difference in sound of heart beats); ensure no contraindications; gain informed consent.
- Check equipment and position the woman before starting.
- Secure transducer onto internal aspect of thigh with conductive gel.
- Aseptic procedure throughout and manage between contractions.
- Perform vaginal examination – to confirm cervix sufficiently dilated, normal cephalic or breech presentation, and at (or below) ischial spines.
- Amniotomy if membranes intact.
- Protect electrode from catching vaginal wall – clip towards fingers or spiral conector covered (see Figure 35.2).
- Hold electrode against fetal scalp (ensure not over face, suture line or fontanelle) – use index finger against clip.
- Either rotate clip back into head and allow it to spring back or rotate in direction of spiral (clockwise) until firmly held (see Figures 35.3, 35.4 and 35.5).
- Ensure fetal attachment – no cervical or vaginal tissue caught.
- Gently pull to check attachment.
- Assistant attaches wires to transducer to ensure it is working before removing fingers from vagina.
- Make the woman comfortable.
- Document indications, procedure and equipment used in records and start time of FSE on ECG recording.

Removal

This must be done at or just before birth, or on transfer to theatre if Caesarean required. The procedure is as above with the clip head held firmly whilst rotating the pin back into the head – to ensure it does not break off or tear the scalp. Check it is complete after removal. Examine the scalp of the neonate for puncture marks, clean the area and apply antiseptic cream if needed. Dispose of electrode in sharps box and document procedure.

Possible outcomes and complications

- Electrode may dislodge, need replacement or record maternal heart.
- Scalp bruising (contributing to jaundice), abscess, scarring or necrosis.
- Accidental needle stick injury to practitioner.
- Maternal infection – not due to FSE alone (Harper *et al.*, 2013).
- Reduced fetal blood sampling and operative deliveries (Neilson, 2015).
- Electrode may break, leaving a part in the scalp.
- Increased trauma with vacuum extraction (Kawakita *et al.*, 2016).
- Routine use of FSEs, even including ECG waveform analysis, is not evidenced as improving fetal outcomes (Neilson, 2015).

36 Fetal blood sampling

Figure 36.1 Equipment required for FBS.

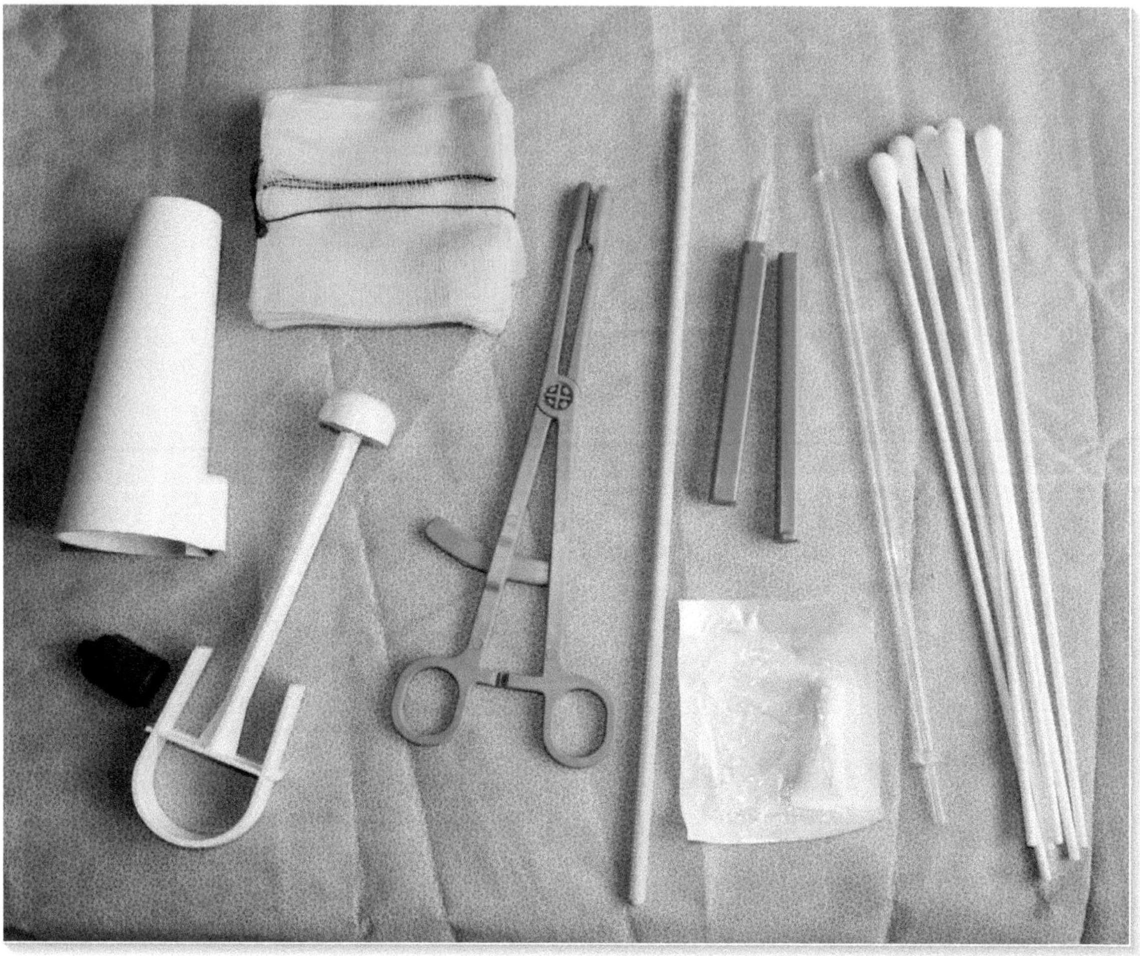

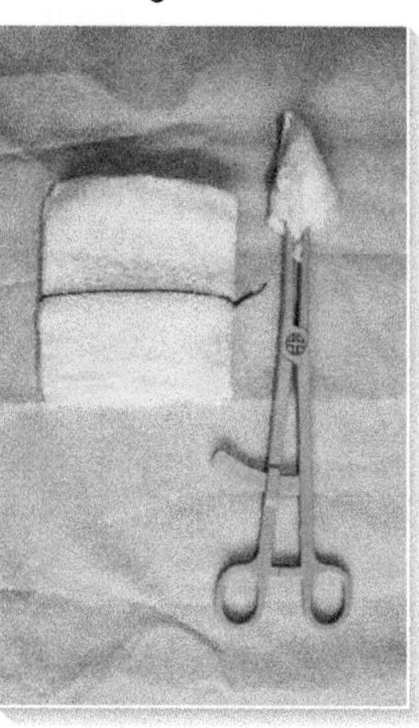
Figure 36.2 Prepared swab for cleaning.

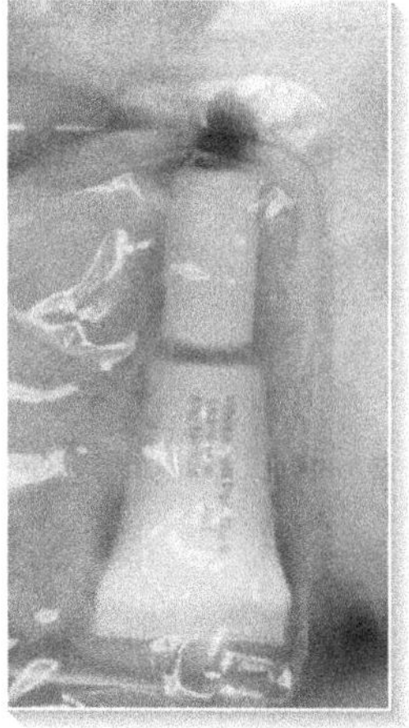
Figure 36.3 White soft paraffin – helps blood pool.

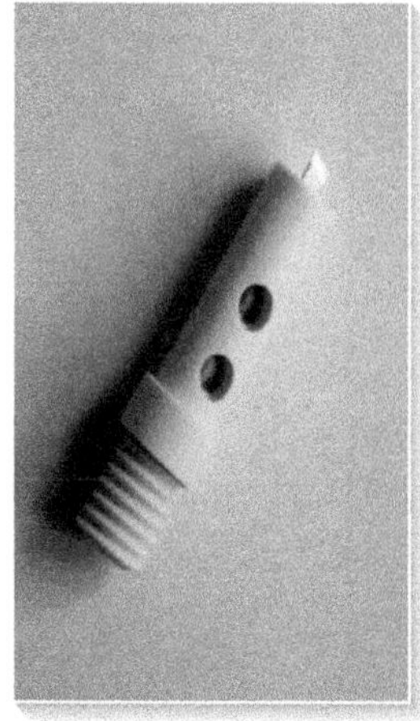
Figure 36.4 FBS blade.

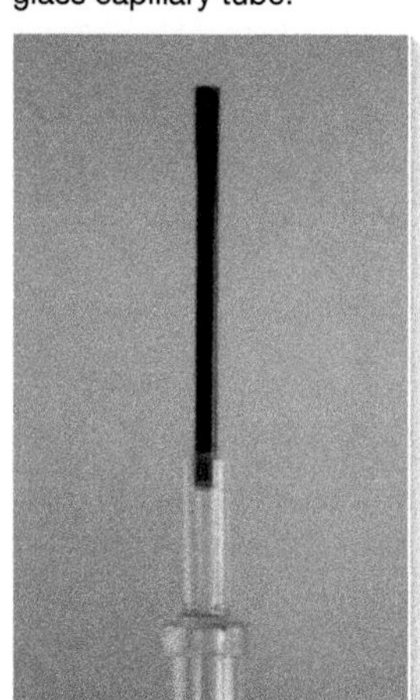
Figure 36.5 Blood-filled glass capillary tube.

It is a normal process to monitor the fetal heart through labour as an indicator of how the fetus is coping with the reduced oxygenation that occurs during contractions. It should be remembered though that a mild hypoxia and slight metabolic acidosis (in the presence of no other concerns) is a normal adaptive process by the fetus. When intermittent auscultation of the fetal heart indicates concerns, or when the pregnancy is of identified high risk, the primary screening process typically involves continuous heart monitoring using the electrocardiotocograph (ECTG). Recording the fetal heart alongside contractions is a useful screening tool – reassuring in the presence of accelerations; non-reassuring in the presence of late decelerations, reduced variability, falling baseline or a sinus rhythm. Whilst it is reliable for predicting a healthy fetus, it is less reliable in predicting morbidity. It has a high false positive rate, associated with increased rates of unnecessary operative deliveries (East *et al.*, 2015a, 2015b).

When the fetal heart pattern raises concern, management may escalate to include the screening of fetal capillary blood pH or lactate levels. This is because fetal acidosis is indicated by reduced pH and increased lactate levels also occur when oxygenation reduces. Despite this, fetal blood sampling (FBS) is not a reliable diagnostic test for fetal hypoxia – it does not reduce Caesarean section rates and misclassification of non-hypoxia is still common (Mahendru & Lees, 2011). It is not a gold standard test but will continue to be used until a better diagnostic test replaces it.

Indications

The indications for FBS relate to obtaining more information about how the fetus is coping with the challenges of labour. This screening tool can inform decision making on either allowing labour to continue, escalating management or expediting the delivery. Typically, it will be used:

- In the presence of a non-reassuring/suspicious ECTG.
- To support a decision to delay operative delivery.
- To support a decision to expedite delivery.
- Prior to Caesarean section to confirm necessity.

Note: A FBS may also be obtained from a placental sample at a Caesarean section to precisely inform about the fetal condition.

Contraindications

The most significant contraindication is the presence of fetal compromise – if the fetus is already known to be compromised then immediate delivery is indicated and there is no time for FBS. Other contraindications include:

- Cross-infection risk to fetus (HIV, hepatitis, herpes simplex) – HIV unlikely if viral load is undetectable (British HIV Association, 2014).
- Fetal coagulation disorders – thrombocytopenia.
- Prematurity < 34 weeks.
- Face presentation.
- Inability to perform FBS – cervical dilatation < 3 cm.
- Intact membranes – if membrane rupture is contraindicated.

Choosing which test to use

Capillary blood samples can be used to test for pH or lactate levels. In the UK capillary samples are most commonly tested for their pH level – screening for lactate levels is uncommon. Testing lactate levels will necessitate availability of different equipment, but a recent Cochrane review (East *et al.*, 2015b) strongly supports lactate screening as:

- A better indicator of fetal morbidity than pH and/or base deficit.
- Quicker and easier to obtain – smaller sample required.
- More sensitive in predicting hypoxic ischaemic encephalopathy.
- More accurate in predicting Apgar scores.
- Routinely used in Sweden, France and Australia.

Ongoing research within the Flamingo Trial (East *et al.*, 2015a) is expected to contribute further to the debate about which test to use.

Management

- Maintain ECTG monitoring throughout the procedure.
- Informed consent – to include details of the procedure, advantages and limitations, and that it may cause discomfort for the woman and leave a small scar on the fetal scalp.
- Ensure no known contraindications.
- Adequate analgesia.
- Gather and check all equipment in advance (see Figure 36.1).
- Ensure blood gas analyser machine is ready for use.
- Aseptic procedure throughout.
- Position for vaginal examination – left lateral recommended but lithotomy position may be used.
- Cleanse as for vaginal examination.
- Perform amniotomy if required.
- Insert amnioscope with obturator through the cervix.
- Remove the obturator and attach light source/illuminator.
- Visualise the scalp.
- Wipe scalp clean with swabs (see Figure 36.2).
- Spray scalp with ethyl chloride to numb area for fetus and increase capillary blood flow.
- Apply silicone gel or soft white paraffin to cause blood globules to form (see Figure 36.3).
- Attach blade to the blade holder and capillary tube to its holder.
- Pierce scalp with small disposable, long-handled blade to a controlled, maximum depth of 2 mm (see Figure 36.4).
- If a second cut is needed, do this at 90 degrees to the first incision.
- Collect 30–50 μl of blood (approximately 3 cm) in the heparinised tube supplied, avoiding air bubbles and contaminants (see Figure 36.5).
- If required, insert a mixing wire and end caps and gently shake the tube.
- Test the sample immediately to achieve greater accuracy of results.
- Document the indications, procedure and results in addition to noting the event on the ECTG trace.

Possible outcomes and complications

General (repeat sample required)

- Insufficient blood sample to test.
- Scalp oedema or caput succedaneum affects test results.
- Sample contaminated with air or amniotic fluid.

Maternal

- Infection – vaginal or uterine (e.g. endometriosis).
- Reduced necessity for operative delivery.

Fetal/neonatal

- Persistent scalp bleeding (coagulopathy problem).
- Scalp infection.

Recognising the deteriorating woman

Figure 37.1 Obstetric early warning chart.

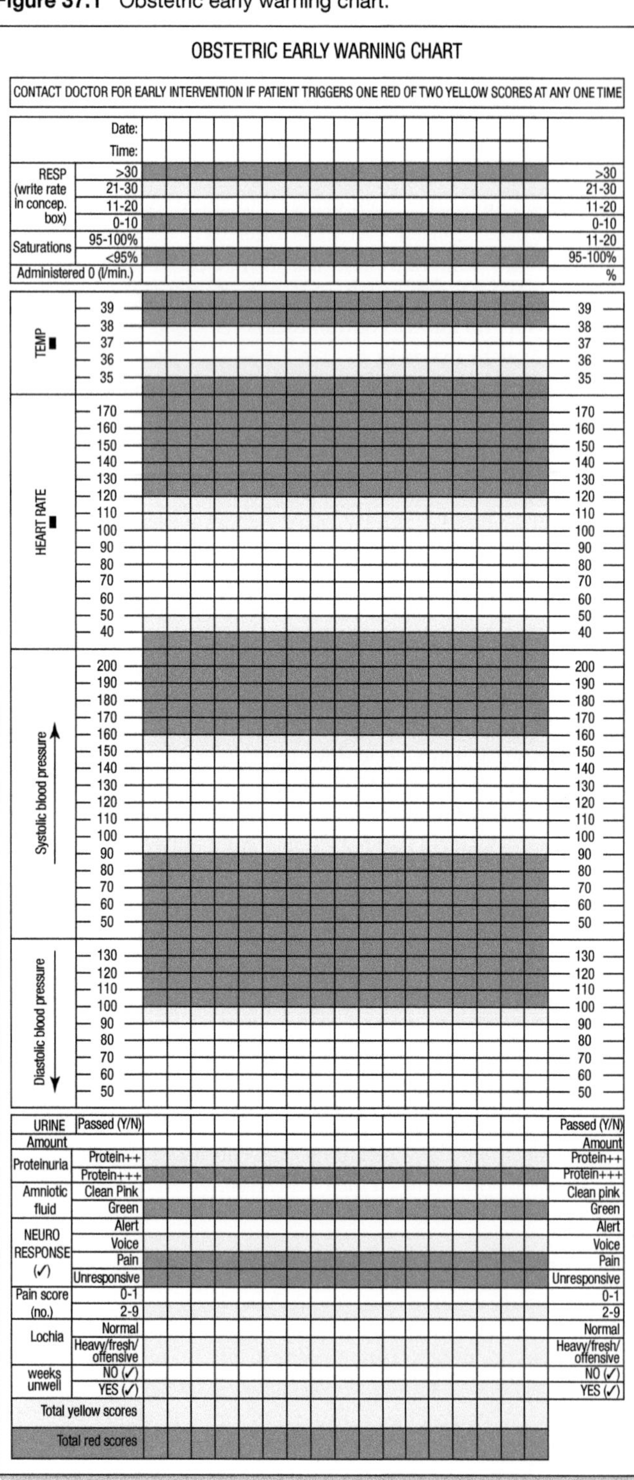

OBSTETRIC EARLY WARNING CHART

CONTACT DOCTOR FOR EARLY INTERVENTION IF PATIENT TRIGGERS ONE RED OF TWO YELLOW SCORES AT ANY ONE TIME

Date:
Time:

RESP (write rate in concep. box): >30; 21-30; 11-20; 0-10 | >30; 21-30; 11-20; 0-10

Saturations: 95-100%; <95% | 11-20; 95-100%

Administered 0 (l/min.) | %

TEMP: 39; 38; 37; 36; 35

HEART RATE: 170; 160; 150; 140; 130; 120; 110; 100; 90; 80; 70; 60; 50; 40

Systolic blood pressure: 200; 190; 180; 170; 160; 150; 140; 130; 120; 110; 100; 90; 80; 70; 60; 50

Diastolic blood pressure: 130; 120; 110; 100; 90; 80; 70; 60; 50

URINE: Passed (Y/N); Amount

Proteinuria: Protein++; Protein+++

Amniotic fluid: Clean Pink; Green

NEURO RESPONSE (✓): Alert; Voice; Pain; Unresponsive

Pain score (no.): 0-1; 2-9

Lochia: Normal; Heavy/fresh/offensive

weeks unwell: NO (✓); YES (✓)

Total yellow scores

Total red scores

Box 37.1 SBAR – handover tool.

SBAR–handover tool

Situation

- Client name and age:
- Hospital ID number:
- Consultant:
- Date and time of admission:
- Current situation

Background

- Client history – medical; surgical; obstetric
- Comorbidities
- Medication
- Recent/current treatment
- Investigations
- Any allergies

Assessment

- Reason for handover
- Clinical overview
- Any concerns
- Vital signs
- IV requirement
- Pain management
- MEOWS score

Recommendations

- Confirm plan of care
- Confirm actions required
- Any tests/investigations needed
- Any change in treatment required

The deterioration of a woman's condition can happen at any point in their care journey, but especially during an acute illness and after operative procedures have been performed (Luettel *et al.*, 2007). This is no less true for a woman undergoing childbirth; the recognition that a woman's wellbeing is being compromised can mean the difference between life and death. It has been demonstrated in recent years that women who fall victim to cardiac and/or pulmonary arrest demonstrate signs of deterioration in the 24 hours prior to the arrest. It is, therefore, essential that all midwives, nurses and doctors remain familiar with the physiological signs that herald a catastrophic deterioration in a woman's condition. The early intervention of senior clinical staff, alerted by the midwife caring for the woman in an obstetric setting, will enhance the woman's chances of survival.

Track and trigger

The use of early warning systems is now commonplace in the UK, with the National Early Warning System (NEWS) having been adapted to capture the unique characteristics of a woman during childbirth – the Modified Early Obstetric Warning System (MEOWS) (see Figure 37.1) (Banfield & Roberts, 2015). This system uses a colour-coded chart which should trigger an urgent response when one **red** or two **yellow** scores are demonstrated. The rationales behind the use of such observation charts are:

- To assess the woman presenting with an acute or exacerbating illness.
- To ensure an amelioration in the recognition of the deteriorating condition of a woman.
- To ensure timely recognition and response, with appropriate referral to clinical expertise.

These charts are no substitute for close observation by an appropriately trained midwife/nurse, but act as an aid to assessing the physiological wellbeing of the individual woman by the monitoring of her clinical responses. By observing the scores achieved during the regular monitoring process, the condition of the woman will be plotted and thus a visible representation of her clinical status will become available, triggering an escalation in her care should this be necessary.

Monitoring

Monitoring of the critically ill woman forms the foundation of her care upon which all subsequent interventions are based. It is thus essential that:

- Base-line readings of the woman's clinical status are recorded on admission. The following physiological observations are recommended:
  - blood pressure
  - temperature
  - heart rate
  - respiratory rate
  - oxygen saturations
  - level of consciousness.
- In certain situations, the evaluation of urinary output and pain assessment may be included together with biochemical analyses (e.g. lactate levels, arterial pH, etc).
- A written plan should be in place outlining which observations should be made and at what interval. This will take into consideration the woman's diagnosis (if known on admission) and any co-morbidities that may be known to clinical staff. The frequency of monitoring may change once a plan of treatment has been finalised and should therefore be reviewed regularly, but at all times the measurement of physiological observations represents a holistic assessment of the woman's wellbeing and not just a 'set of obs'.
- The monitoring of an acutely ill woman should be undertaken by an appropriately trained midwife/nurse, competent in the measurement and interpretation of observations.

Escalation

It is recommended that an escalation policy should be in place in all acute hospital settings, with the degree of escalation matching the level of response and staff competence required to meet the woman's changing needs (Banfield & Roberts, 2015). The policy may include a graded response system determined by the degree of deterioration as per locally agreed parameters, for example:

- Minimal deterioration – the midwife/nurse in charge of the area should be informed and the frequency of observations increased.
- Moderate deterioration – an urgent referral to the medical team caring for the woman and members of the multidisciplinary team (MDT) with the relevant competencies required for this level of care
- High level of deterioration – an emergency referral to a consultant with critical care capabilities including airway management and diagnostic skills. This referral should generate an immediate response regardless of the time of day.

Teamwork and communication

It has been identified that poor team working and inadequate communication between clinical staff can cause a delay in the recognition and assessment of a deterioration in a critically ill woman and the subsequent response to the acute situation. The following are recommended:

- Clearly defined roles for members of the MDT.
- Structured handovers by the MDT using recognised tools such as SBAR (Situation; Background; Assessment; Recommendations) (see Box 37.1) (Banfield & Roberts, 2015).
- MDTs in the ward area and in the critical care facility have a shared responsibility for the woman's care.
- The decision to transfer the woman to or from a critical care area and ward should be a joint decision involving the MDT. Careful planning of the transfer will ensure continuity of care and a safe, effective transfer.
- Education and training should be ongoing to ensure that staff possess the appropriate competencies. Assessment in practice should be implemented to enable staff to demonstrate their competence.

38 Examination *per vaginam*

Figure 38.1 Insertion of fingers.

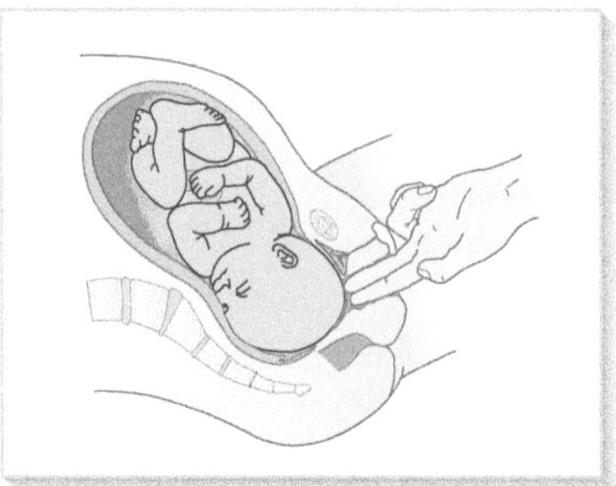

Figure 38.2 (a–h) Logical identification of the findings.

Clitoris
Urethra
Labia minora
Labia majora
Vaginal orifice
Anus

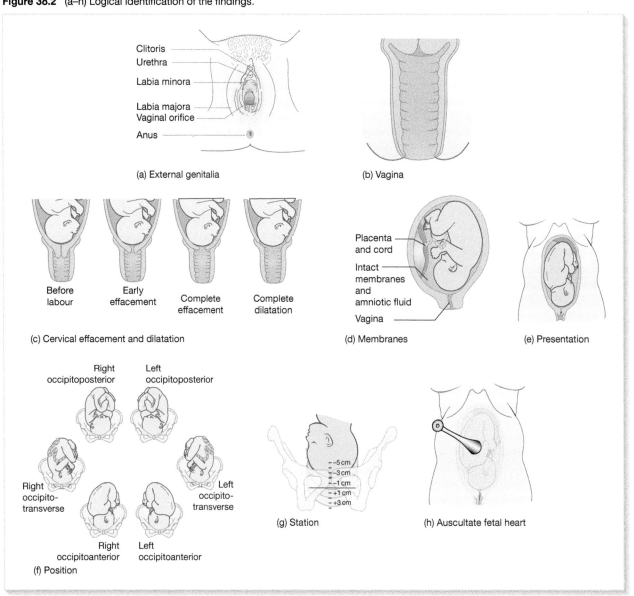

(a) External genitalia

(b) Vagina

Before labour
Early effacement
Complete effacement
Complete dilatation

(c) Cervical effacement and dilatation

Placenta and cord
Intact membranes and amniotic fluid
Vagina

(d) Membranes

(e) Presentation

Right occipitoposterior
Left occipitoposterior
Right occipito-transverse
Left occipito-transverse
Right occipitoanterior
Left occipitoanterior

(f) Position

–5 cm
–3 cm
–1 cm
+1 cm
+3 cm

(g) Station

(h) Auscultate fetal heart

Midwifery Emergencies at a Glance, First Edition. Denise (Dee) Campbell and Susan M. Carr. © 2018 John Wiley & Sons, Ltd. Published 2018 by John Wiley & Sons, Ltd.
Companion website: www.ataglanceseries.com/midwiferyemergencies

This internal procedure may be carried out antenatally, during the intrapartum period and postnatally. The procedure should be carried out in an efficient manner, taking into consideration the woman's sensitivity related to such an intimate procedure – her privacy and dignity are of paramount importance throughout. Vital information can be elicited from this vaginal examination (VE), which together with external findings, will contribute to the decisions made concerning the ongoing care of the woman.

Indications for performing a VE (Harris, 2011)

Antenatal

Examination *per vaginam* is seldom performed antenatally. However, the following circumstances may require a VE:

- To confirm presentation of the fetus *in utero* (e.g. breech, brow).
- Induction of labour (e.g. by artificial rupture of the membranes, insertion of a prostaglandin pessary or similar equivalent).
- To confirm abdominal findings where there is doubt.

Intrapartum

- To confirm the onset of labour.
- To assess the progress of labour – or lack of it.
- To identify the presentation and position of the fetus.
- To assess the degree of flexion of the fetal head.
- To perform artificial rupture of the membranes.
- To undertake fetal blood sampling.
- To attach a fetal scalp electrode to monitor the wellbeing of the fetus using electronic surveillance via a cardiotocograph machine.
- To exclude cord prolapse in the presence of confirmed spontaneous rupture of the membranes.
- To confirm full dilatation of the cervix.
- To confirm the lie, presentation and position of a second fetus in a multiple pregnancy.
- To undertake the manual removal of adherent placenta and membranes in the third stage of labour.
- Occasionally – maternal request.

Postpartum

Examination *per vaginam* is seldom performed postnatally. However, it may be performed in such circumstances as secondary postpartum haemorrhage due to an atonic uterus caused by retained products of conception such as a cotyledon of placenta or fragments of membrane.

Contraindications

Vaginal examination should not be undertaken if:

- There is lack of maternal consent.
- There is any history of antepartum haemorrhage.
- Placenta praevia is known to exist.
- Vasa praevia is suspected.
- Preterm and/or prelabour rupture of membranes is suspected.

Risk factors

Risk factors associated with a vaginal examination include:

- The introduction of infection especially in the presence of ruptured membranes.
- Unplanned digital rupture of the membranes.
- Haemorrhage if the location of the placenta has not been confirmed.
- Exacerbation of psychological trauma.

Procedure (Johnson & Taylor, 2016)

Preparation

- Confirm a valid reason for performing the vaginal examination.
- Secure verbal, informed consent from the woman.
- Gather equipment as required.
- Undertake an abdominal examination and palpation to ascertain the current lie, presentation, position, attitude and station/engagement of the fetus.
- Auscultate the fetal heart following the abdominal examination.
- Prepare the woman in a semi-recumbent position:
  - ensure an empty bladder
  - position the woman appropriately with her undergarments removed and her legs abducted.
- Don a pair of sterile gloves.

Examination in labour (Macdonald & Johnson, 2017)

- The woman's vulva should be visualised for any abnormality and then cleaned using warm water. In order to reduce the possibility of introducing an ascending infection, the midwife or doctor should use the hand which will not subsequently be inserted into the vagina to perform the examination.
- The examining fingers (index and middle fingers) should be lubricated and inserted gently into the vagina with the cooperation of the woman and the examination is performed between contractions (see Figure 38.1).
- On completion, the fingers are withdrawn carefully noting any discharge that may be present.
- The fetal heart should be auscultated (see Figure 38.2h).
- The woman should be made comfortable and her dignity restored.
- The appropriate disposal of all used items should be completed.
- The findings should be communicated to the woman and a plan of care explained, to include the possibility of a blood-stained 'show' following the procedure.
- The woman's notes and partogram (if appropriate) should be updated with the information.
- Appropriate referral should be made where necessary.

Findings (see Figure 38.2)

- **External genitalia** – while separating the labia any abnormalities should be noted, including perineal scarring, vulval varicosities and abnormal discharge.
- **Vagina** – it should be warm and moist. The vaginal walls should be soft and distensible and the sub-pubic arch should be equal or greater than 90 degrees.
- **Cervix** – it should be assessed for its position, effacement, dilatation and application to the presenting fetal part.
- **Membranes** – confirmation of intact or ruptured membranes should be made and colour of liquor amnii should be noted if membranes have ruptured.
- **Presentation and position of the fetal head** – using the landmarks on the presenting part (e.g. sagittal suture and fontanelles, ischial tuberosities and anus), an assessment of the position of the fetus in relation to the woman's pelvic landmarks should be made. At this point the degree of flexion and any moulding may also be determined.
- **Station of the fetal head** – descent of the fetal head is noted in terms of the relationship of the presenting part to the maternal ischial spines.

Speculum examination

Figure 39.1 Cusco speculum – various sizes.

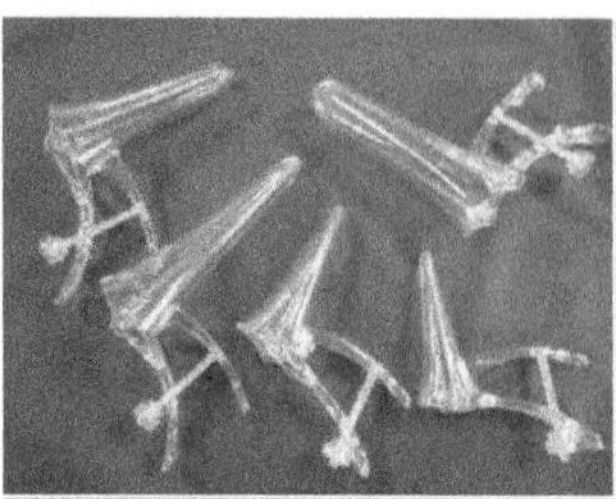

Cusco speculum – various sizes

Figure 39.2 Sims speculum.

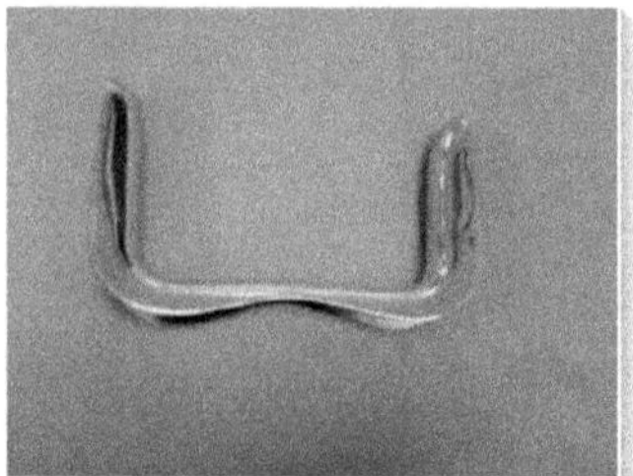

Sims speculum

Figure 39.3 (a–f) Speculum examination.

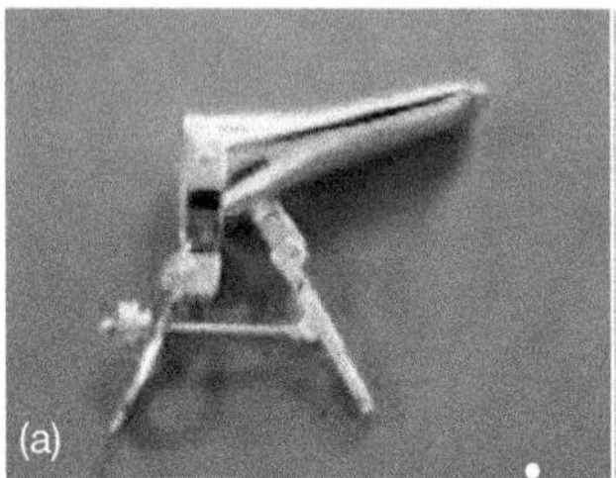

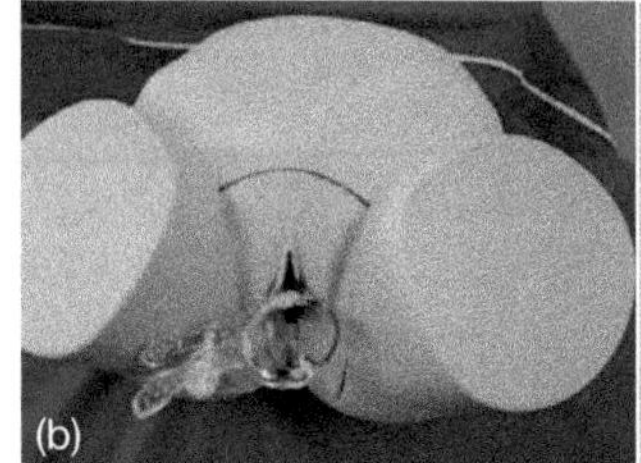

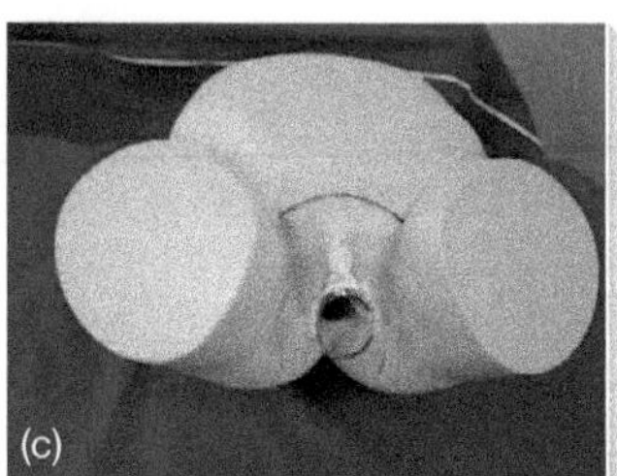

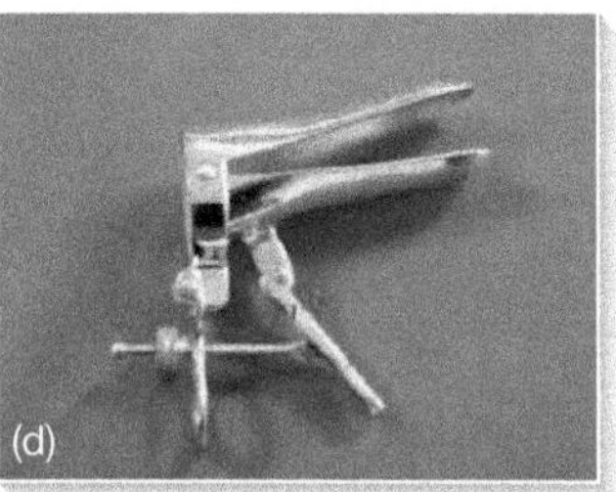

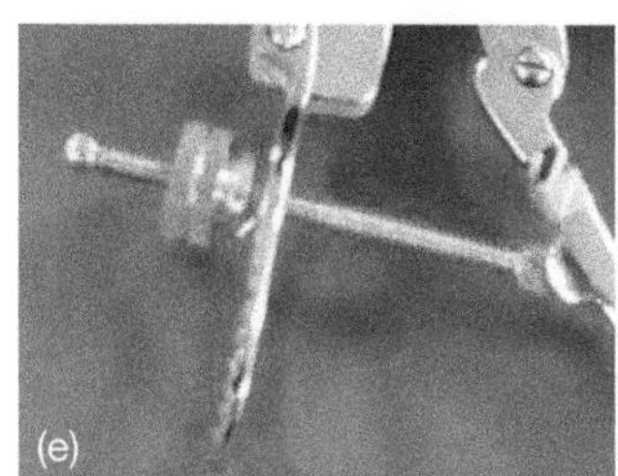

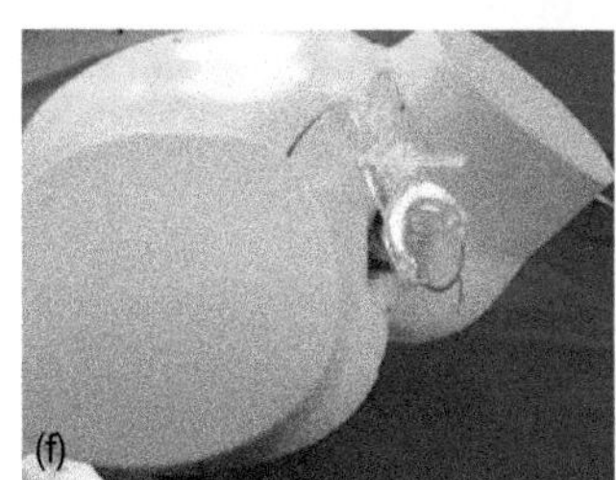

A speculum is an instrument used to open the vagina. The two most commonly used types of speculum are:

1 Bi-valve or Cusco speculum (see Figure 39.1).
2 Sims' speculum (see Figure 39.2).

Indications for use

Antenatal/intrapartum indications

- To obtain a high vaginal swab.
- To assess the state of the cervix in preterm labour.
- To inspect the fornices in the upper vagina around the cervix for the presence of amniotic fluid, in cases of suspected prelabour spontaneous rupture of membranes (NICE, 2014).
- To obtain a cervical sample for screening purposes.

Postnatal indications

- To obtain a cervical sample for screening purposes.
- To obtain a high vaginal swab.
- To inspect the upper vagina around the cervix for presence of trauma.

Contraindications for use

- Lack of consent from the woman.
- If it is certain that the membranes have ruptured.

Preparation for a speculum examination

Prior to commencing the speculum examination

- The midwife/health care practitioner should introduce themselves to the woman and aim to establish a rapport with her before commencing the examination.
- Informed, verbal consent must be secured before commencing the procedure and therefore the woman must understand the reason(s) why the procedure is required as well as how it is to be performed.
- It is important to explain to the woman that although the procedure may be uncomfortable, it should not be painful.
- Ensure that the woman's bladder is empty by asking her to visit the toilet if appropriate, or by inserting an intermittent urinary catheter.
- Ensure that the woman is in a semirecumbent position with her knees bent, heels together and her legs apart.
- Maintain her dignity by covering her with a sheet, having removed any underwear, sanitary pad, etc.
- Identify a suitable light source.

Performing a speculum examination

(Johnson & Taylor, 2016)

- This examination should be performed using an aseptic technique and standard precautions to minimise the risk of introducing an infection into the genital tract during the antenatal, intrapartum or postnatal period.
- The trolley should be cleaned using an appropriate technique.
- Gather the appropriate sterile equipment and any additional items, such as a swab used for taking a high vaginal specimen, and place on the bottom shelf of the clean dressing trolley.
- Return to the woman with the trolley.
- The midwife/health care practitioner should wash their hands and prepare the equipment on the upper shelf of the trolley before removing the cover from the woman.
- The midwife/health care practitioner may put on a pair of protective goggles to protect their eyes from a splash injury.
- Don a disposable apron and a pair of sterile gloves.
- Clean the external genitalia from front to back using a non-touch/clean hand, dirty hand technique, using each swab only once before discarding.
- Ensure that the blades of the Cusco speculum are closed.
- Lubricate with sterile gel if necessary.
- Place the speculum in the dominant hand and separate the labia with the non-dominant hand, exposing the introitus.
- Inform the woman that the speculum is about to be introduced and gently insert the closed blades of the speculum in the antero-posterior position, in a downward manner at an angle of 45 degrees to the floor (see Figures 39.3a and 39.3b).
- Once in place the speculum is rotated through 90 degrees into the transverse position with handles uppermost (i.e. towards the woman's abdomen) and the anterior blade against the anterior vaginal wall and the posterior blade against the posterior vaginal wall) (see Figure 39.3c).
- The blades can then be opened gently by bringing the handles together – pressure may be felt as the blades open and stretch the vagina.
- The screw securing the blades in the open position can be tightened to prevent unexpected closure of the blades (see Figures 39.3d, 39.3e and 39.3f).
- Using the light source, the vagina, cervix and state of the membranes can be visualised and any swabs taken at this point.
- Note any discharge, bleeding or evidence of ruptured membranes $\pm$ amniotic fluid.

Completing the speculum examination

Once the examination has been completed:

- The screw should be released before attempting to close the blades.
- The blades are closed gently ensuring that maternal vaginal tissue does not become trapped between the blades.
- At this point the speculum may be rotated back through 90 degrees into the antero posterior position.
- The speculum can now be withdrawn from the vagina.
- Take note of any vaginal discharge, bleeding, amniotic fluid and cover the introitus with a sterile sanitary pad.
- Restore the woman to a comfortable position and cover her with a suitable sheet.
- Auscultate the fetal heart if performing the examination in the antenatal or intrapartum period.
- Dispose of all equipment.
- Label any swabs and complete investigation request documentation and arrange for their transport to the appropriate laboratory.
- Return to the woman and assess her wellbeing following the procedure and explain to her the findings of the procedure, outlining the immediate plan of care.
- Ensure that a contemporaneous record of the examination is maintained in the woman's case notes, including the following:
  - the date and time of the procedure
  - the rationale for the examination
  - the confirmation of informed, verbal consent to the procedure by the woman
  - the details of the procedure
  - any investigations undertaken (e.g. high vaginal swab)
  - the state of the vagina, cervix and membranes (if appropriate)
  - the condition of the woman on completion of the procedure
  - the fetal heart rate – if appropriate
  - the immediate and future plan of care
  - the signature of the midwife/ health care professional who undertook the procedure and the name printed in full.

40 Urinary catheterisation

Figure 40.1 Anatomy of the perineum showing the urethral meatus.

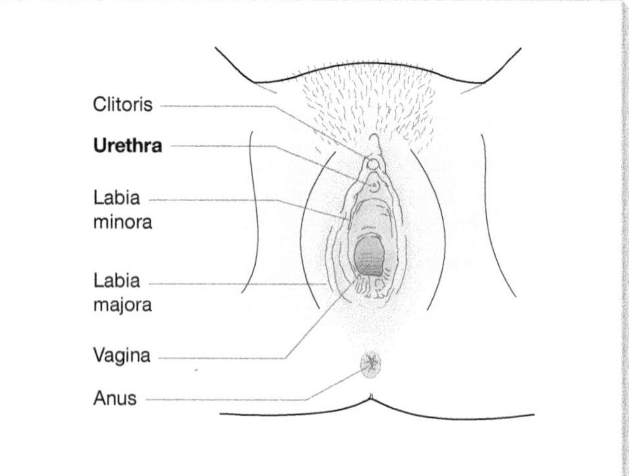

Figure 40.2 Anatomy of the pelvis showing the urethra and bladder.

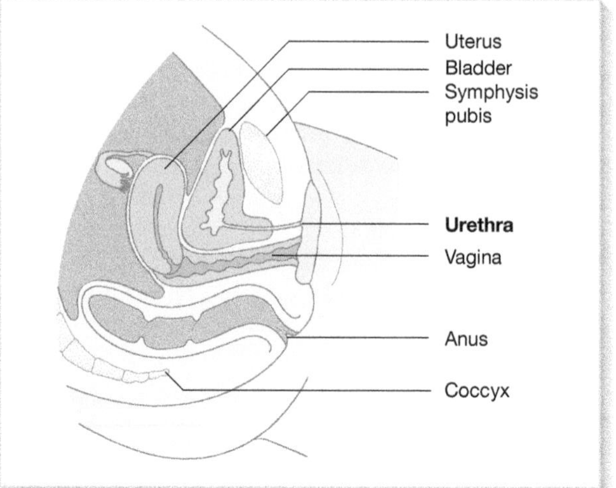

Figure 40.3 Single-use catheters.

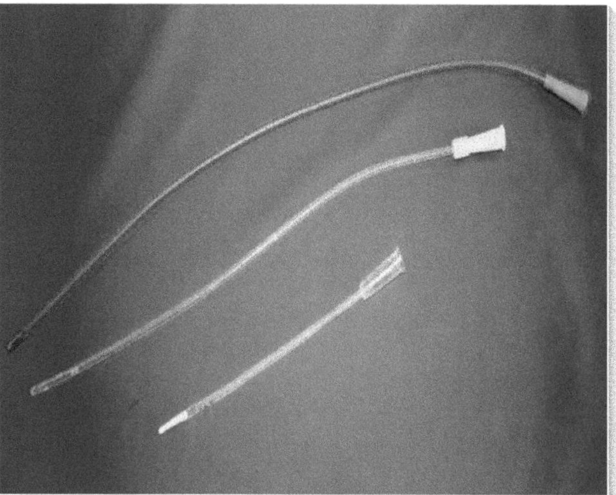

Figure 40.4 Indwelling catheters.

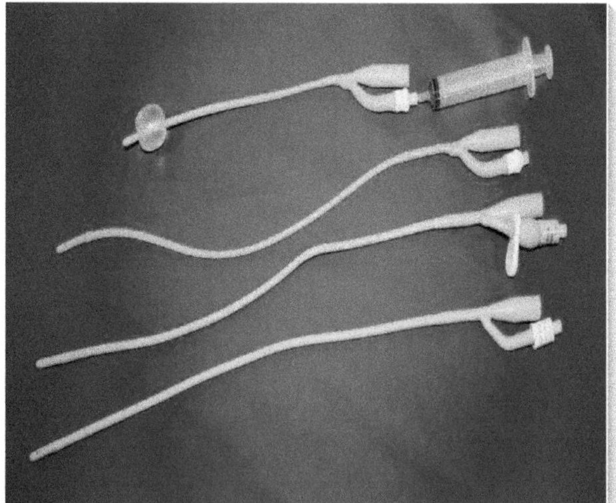

Box 40.1 Considerations when choosing your catheter.

- Ensure that any allergies are known and avoided – many catheters are made from latex and allergy is possible
- Have you chosen a 'Female' length catheter (25 cm long) – a longer one might allow pooling of urine?
- Is the service user obese and better suited to the 'Male' length catheter (40 cm long) – too short and any balloon may inflate in the urethra?
- Have you chosen a 12–14 Fr catheter diameter – larger bore are only appropriate for special procedures?
- Have you inflated the catheter balloon to manufacturers instructions (10–30 mL) as under inflation may cause pressure

Box 40.2 Indwelling catheter care.

- Daily shower or bath for general hygiene
- Standard precautions should be used at all times
- Ensure that the catheter bag and tubing are never above the height of the bladder
- Ensure that the bag and tubing is supported and does not pull on the catheter
- Never allow the catheter drainage valve to touch the floor
- Regularly empty the collection bag to encourage free drainage and no backflow of urine
- Ensure jug used to empty bag is clean, used once only (before cleaning) and does not touch drainage valve
- Catheter bags should be aseptically changed weekly

Definition

Urinary catheterisation is the insertion of a sterile, purpose-designed tube via the urethral canal to release urine from the bladder.

Possible indications

In all cases other than when an indwelling catheter is required, natural micturition is preferred to catheterisation and particularly for non-emergency situations (such as inability to void urine, screening and diagnostic care, or postoperatively to maintain an empty bladder). Emergency catheterisation can enable screening/diagnosis, uterine involution, access to the pelvis and/or abdomen, and prevent bladder trauma before or during:

- Caesarean delivery.
- Instrumental vaginal delivery (e.g. forceps delivery).
- Manoeuvres to assist delivery (e.g. shoulder dystocia).
- Malpositions with wider diameters (e.g. occipito posterior).
- Malpresentations (e.g. breech).
- Prevention or management of postpartum haemorrhage.
- Screening or diagnostic testing before emergency management.
- Manual removal of a retained placenta.
- Continuous monitoring of an accurate fluid balance.
- Treatment of urinary retention.

Catheterisation during emergency care

Single use (intermittent)

This is the acute use of catheterisation to empty the bladder immediately but not continuously. The catheter is inserted and then removed as soon as there is no further urinary drainage. This is the technique most commonly used in emergency obstetric care, ensuring maximum pelvic space and no bladder trauma.

Indwelling

This is a longer term catheterisation which empties the bladder immediately, then ensures the bladder continues to drain. Most commonly, indwelling catheters are left in place during a particular procedure (e.g. Caesarean section). Longer periods may be associated with postoperative recovery, bladder trauma or when management includes strict fluid balance.

Risks associated with catheterisation

Urinary catheterisation associated with an emergency procedure may be complicated by difficult access and constriction of the urethra due to fetal descent through the pelvis and distention of the pelvic floor and perineum. These aspects and the procedure itself increase the risk of:

- Urinary tract infection (UTI) – affecting the urethra, bladder or kidneys. This may occur when commensal bacteria from the perineum are introduced to the urinary tract by a contaminated catheter. The close proximity of the urethra, vagina and anus and the physical changes to these during labour (dilation of the vaginal introitus and anus, alongside relaxation and compression of the urethra) increase the likelihood of bacterial cross-infection. Additionally, bacteria can enter an indwelling catheter via drainage ports or from a backflow of urine.
- Urethral or bladder trauma – hormones relax the urethral tube and the fetal presenting part distorts and constricts it. Even the most careful insertion of a catheter can damage the lining of the urethra and bladder.
- Urinary retention – following removal of the catheter, there may be a delay in the return of normal physiological micturition.

Risk reduction

A number of key aspects will reduce morbidity including:

- Bladder care throughout labour and natural emptying of the bladder.
- Full consent and cooperation of the woman to be catheterised.
- A skilled professional performing the procedure.
- Choice of the correct size and type of equipment.
- Perineal hygiene.
- Sterile equipment and closed system.
- Aseptic technique – insertion, indwelling and removal.
- Any drainage bag must be kept below the height of the bladder.
- Remove catheter promptly when no longer required.

Method of catheterisation

- **Informed consent** is required.
- **Gather equipment** – sterile gloves, aseptic pack, catheter (see Box 40.1) and bag (if indwelling), torch, sterile water, lubricant, anaesthetic gel, receiver, disposable sheet.
- **Standard precautions** must be applied throughout including hand hygiene, aseptic technique, perineal cleansing and, for an indwelling catheter, use of a closed drainage system (preconnected).
- **Position** the woman semi-recumbent, ankles together, knees apart (if not already in a lithotomy position), on a disposable pad, with underwear and sanitary protection removed. The sheet covering her should only be removed at the last moment.
- **Cleanse** the vulva from front to back with the non-dominant hand using sterile water, then establish your sterile field.
- **Locate the urethra** by separating the labia with the non-dominant hand, using a good light source (see Figures 40.1 and 40.2).
- **Insert the catheter** gently, using the dominant hand and a backwards and upwards direction. The plastic wrapper is slid back along the catheter as the catheter progresses further into the urethra. Stop if there is a contraction, severe pain or resistance.
- **Urine voiding** occurs once the catheter reaches the bladder.
- **Single use catheters** (see Figure 40.3) allow drainage of the urine into a receiver. When drainage stops the catheter is gently removed.
- **Indwelling catheters** (see Figure 40.4) require that the catheter is inserted a further 5 cm once urine begins to drain to ensure that the retaining balloon is within the bladder. Sterile water is inserted into the port to inflate the retaining balloon. The catheter bag is secured to a stand below bladder height to allow continuous drainage. Increased fluid intake, regular drainage and measurement of urine, the need for ongoing catheterisation and catheter care (see Box 40.2) are reviewed regularly and recorded accordingly.

41 Venepuncture

Figure 41.1 Select a vein.
Source: Thomas (2015). Reproduced with permission of John Wiley & Sons.

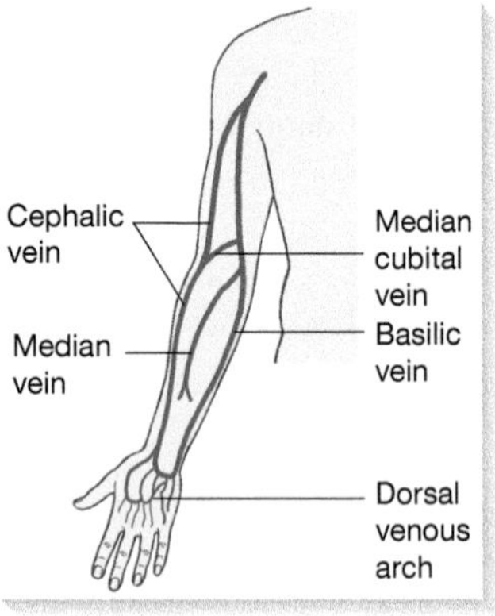

Figure 41.2 Equipment for venepuncture.
Source (a-d): Thomas (2015). Reproduced with permission of John Wiley & Sons.

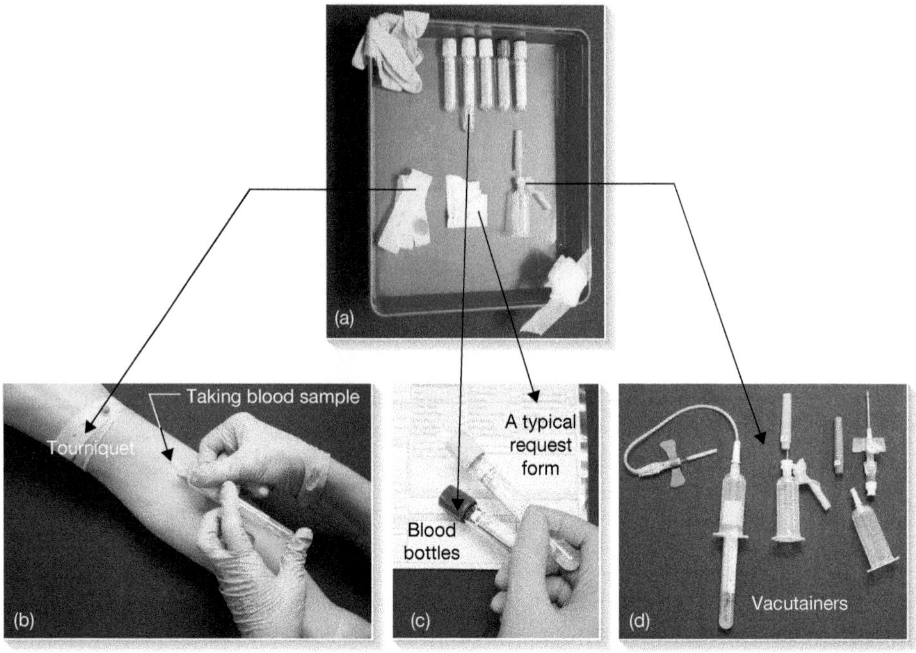

Table 41.1 Risks to client and the health worker.

Risks to the client	Reducing the risks
• Allergic reaction, e.g. to latex, adhesive tape, antiseptic products	• Question the patient before commencing the procedure • Check the patient's notes
• Pain at the site of venepuncture	• Ensure staff are well trained in venepuncture • Careful selection of needle size in relation to vein size
• Haematoma formation at puncture site	• Pierce the skin at 30° angle or less • With the arm straight, apply pressure to the puncture site for 3–5 minutes
• Infection at the site of venepuncture	• Use standard safety precautions throughout procedure • Wash hands before and after the procedure • Cleanse the proposed puncture site with 70% alcohol swab and allow to air-dry completely • Use only sterile equipment
• Prolonged or extensive bleeding	• Read patient's notes to identify use of anticoagulant therapy or a history of bleeding
• Patient anxiety, e.g. fainting	• Use a semirecumbent position for the procedure • Talk to the patient throughout to distract them
Risks to the health care worker	**Reducing the risks**
• Needle-stick injury	• Only use safety devices such as retractable needles • Never re-cap needles • Dispose of equipment appropriately and immediately following procedure
• Exposure to blood	• Wear non-sterile gloves • Wear goggles where appropriate • Use vacuum extraction devices when taking several samples from one patient • Cover injuries with waterproof dressing • If exposed to blood via a splash or needle-stick injury, follow local protocols including reporting the incident • Ensure hepatitis B vaccination is up to date

Venepuncture is the most common invasive procedure carried out on patients, but it should always be remembered that it carries with it a measure of fear for many patients and also the increased risk of needle-stick injury to the health care worker. Venepuncture can be defined as the insertion of a sterile, hollow needle into a vein, usually for the purpose of drawing blood (Scales, 2008).

Purpose of venepuncture (Harris, 2008)

- To draw blood for diagnostic investigations.
- For routine assessment of blood components such as haemoglobin.
- To assess the levels of drugs in the blood.
- To establish the body's response to differing forms of treatment.
- To harvest blood for assessment of its group and Rhesus factor prior to cross-matching blood for transfusion.
- To screen for infection.

Anatomy of the vein

Veins carry oxygen depleted blood back to the heart for reoxygenation. They have three distinct layers:

- Tunica adventitia/externa or outermost layer composed of connective tissue which surrounds and supports the vein.
- Tunica media: the middle, muscular layer which enables the vein to contract, relax or spasm when stimulated for example, by venepuncture, changes in temperature, hypotension and dehydration. Because the muscles are poorly developed, the vein can collapse or distend in response to an increase or fall in blood pressure.
- Tunica intima or innermost layer composed of smooth endothelial cells to ensure the free-flow of the blood in the vein. Semilunar valves in the larger vessels generally at the junctions of veins prevent the backflow of blood ensuring that the blood continually moves towards the heart. The valves can be seen as a bulge in a vein and can be palpated by an experienced practitioner.

Issues associated with venepuncture

There are issues attached to venepuncture which can affect both health care personnel and patients, but which can be minimised by appropriate training. Every step in the process of securing an adequate blood sample will affect the quality of the sample and by consequence the speed at which results are returned and treatment initiated. The three main issues affecting patient care are incorrect labelling of samples, haemolysis of a sample and contamination of a sample.

Preparation

- Secure consent from the patient, ensuring their dignity and privacy.
- Make the patient comfortable in a sitting or semirecumbent position.
- Position the arm with an absorbent towel beneath.
- Ensure adequate lighting and a warm environment – if it is too cold, vasodilatation will be inhibited.
- Select a vein (see Figure 41.1). A vein in the patient's non-dominant arm is generally preferred; either the median cubital vein or basilic vein would be the vein of choice. The median cubital vein is often the easiest vessel to puncture as it lies between muscles, whereas the basilic vein overlies an artery and a nerve and thus has the accompanying risk of damage to these structures.
- Gather equipment onto a cleaned trolley (see Figure 41.2).
  - vacuum extraction chamber, needles and appropriate sample tubes, winged collection tubes or whatever is agreed with the laboratory. These should be placed on a carrying tray
  - disposable tourniquet
  - goggles and non-sterile gloves are recommended to protect from accidental splash injury
  - sharps container
  - transport bags
  - dressing.

Procedure

Be aware of risks to client and self (Johnson & Taylor, 2016) (see Table 41.1):

- Extend the patient's arm and visualise the antecubital fossa – a vein should be visible without the application of the tourniquet.
- Label the blood bottles in front of the patient.
- Wash hands and don non-sterile gloves.
- Apply the tourniquet approximately 7–8 cm above the proposed puncture site. Tapping, stroking and asking the patient to open and close their hand repeatedly may also assist venous filling.
- Clean the skin using a circular, rubbing motion for 30–60 seconds with an antiseptic solution such as 70% alcohol swab. Allow this to air-dry completely to ensure the disinfection of the skin and prevent discomfort during cannulation. Once dry the vein should not be re-palpated, tapped or touched.
- Assemble the needle and vacuum extraction tube holder.
- Draw the skin tight below the venepuncture site towards the patient's hand and insert the needle into the vein at an angle of approximately 30 degrees with the bevel side uppermost.
- Insert the collection bottle into the vacuum chamber and commence collection, replacing the tube with others until all sampling has been completed. Ensure this is done in the correct order to avoid contamination.
- Tubes containing an additive should be inverted 8–10 times – they should **not** be shaken.
- Release the tourniquet and apply a dry gauze pad over the puncture site.
- Gently press down on the gauze pad over the puncture site while removing the needle.
- Apply pressure to the straightened arm for 3–5 minutes or until the bleeding has stopped and then cover with an adhesive dressing.
- Dispose of the equipment immediately in a sharps container which should be within arm's reach. Do not separate the needle from the vacuum extraction device or syringe – whichever method has been used – as this increases the risk of needle-stick injury.
- Check the labels for accuracy and also the accompanying request forms.
- Place bottle(s) into the transport bag and seal, and the request form(s) into the outer section, and arrange for dispatch.

42 Intravenous cannulation

Figure 42.1 Suitable sites for cannulation.

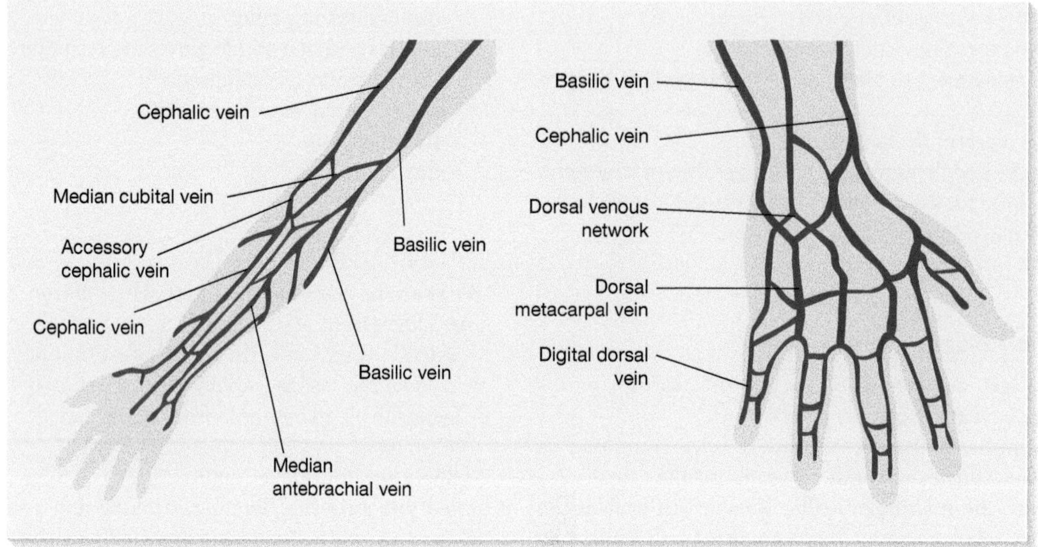

Figure 42.2 Equipment required for cannula insertion. Source: Thomas (2015). Reproduced with permission of John Wiley & Sons.

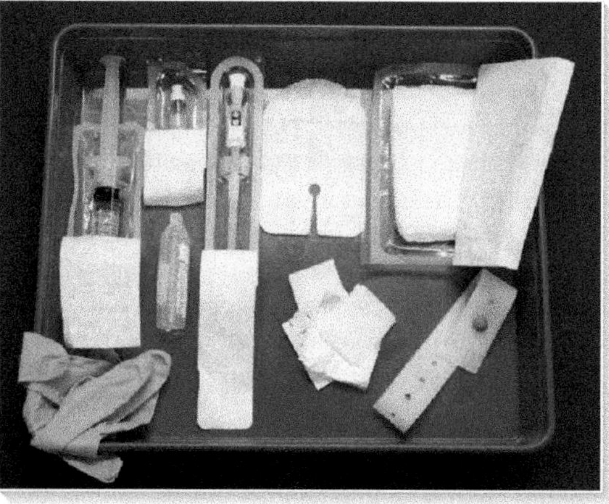

Figure 42.3 Intravenous cannula sizes. Source: Thomas (2015). Reproduced with permission of John Wiley & Sons.

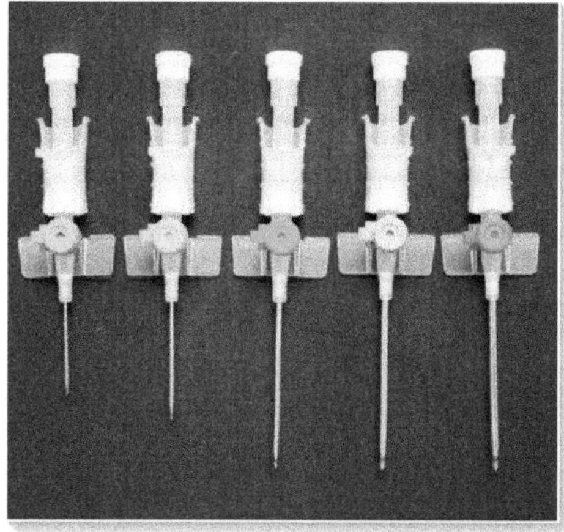

Figure 42.4 Angle of cannula insertion. Source: Thomas (2015). Reproduced with permission of John Wiley & Sons.

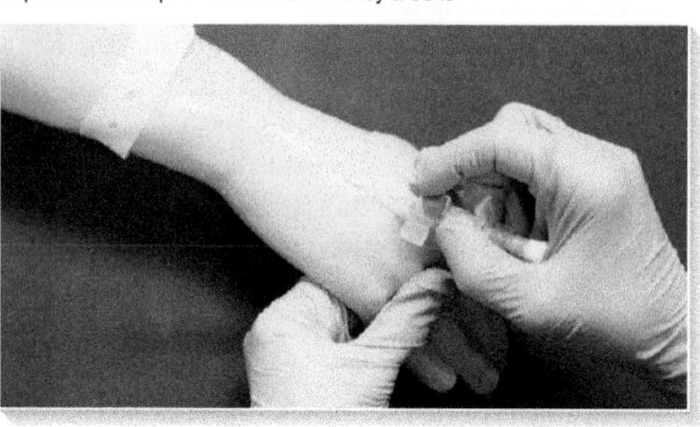

Figure 42.5 Taking a blood sample. Source: Thomas (2015). Reproduced with permission of John Wiley & Sons.

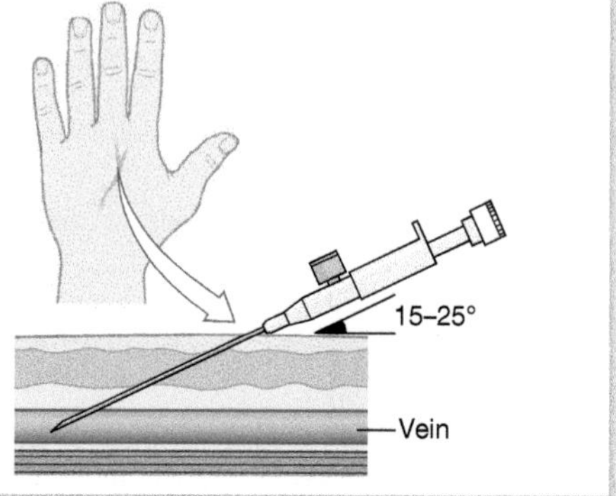

The purpose of inserting a cannula into a vein is to provide venous access to allow blood to be drawn for testing and for the administration of medications, intravenous fluids, blood products and parenteral nutrition (Shlamovitz, 2017).

Contraindications

There are no contraindications. However, there may be situations which would prevent a health care professional from proceeding with the procedure:

- Failure to secure consent from a conscious, competent patient (NMC, 2015).
- The presence of an infected and/or injured limb or extremity.

The success of the procedure will be judged on the cooperation of the patient and their informed consent together with the skill of the operator in maintaining patency of the portal and the maintenance of a 'closed' system, thereby reducing the risk of infection.

Structure of the vein (Martini *et al.*, 2014)

The veins return oxygen-depleted blood to the right side of the heart. There are exceptions to this rule, but these will not be discussed here. The vein has three layers (tunicae):

- Tunica externa or adventitia.
- Tunica media.
- Tunica intima.

The presence of valves in the veins ensures that backflow of the blood returning to the heart is prevented because the pressure within the vein is much lower than that in the arteries, as the lumen of the vein is significantly larger. The contraction and relaxation of muscles surrounding the veins also ensure the onward flow of the blood back to the heart.

Preparation

- Secure consent from the patient, ensuring their dignity and privacy.
- Position the arm (or extremity).
- Ensure adequate lighting.
- Ensure that the environment is warm – if it is too chilly, vasodilatation will be inhibited.
- Gather equipment (see Figure 42.2):
  - suitably sized cannula (see Figure 42.3)
  - tourniquet
  - goggles and non-sterile gloves to protect from accidental splash injury
  - 0.9% sodium chloride flush (occasionally heparin flush)
  - local anaesthetic if required – subcutaneous injection or topical gel
  - blood bottles if required
  - dressing.

Procedure (Harty, 2017)

The selection of an appropriate vein is related to the intended purpose of the intravenous cannulation. A vein in the patient's non-dominant arm is generally preferred – either the cephalic or basilic vein would be the vein of choice in the antecubital fossa, especially if rapid infusion of fluids or blood products is anticipated (see Figure 42.1). A 'good' vein is one which is large and visible and which refills after being compressed. The application of a disposable tourniquet approximately 7–8 cm above the proposed puncture site will assist the identification of a suitable vein as this encourages venous filling. Tapping, stroking and asking the patient to open and close their hand repeatedly may also assist venous filling. Asking the patient to allow their arm to hang and the application of a warm compress may also help. Ultrasound guidance can also be used to good effect. A vein on the dorsal aspect of the wrist or hand may also be adequate depending on the reason for cannulation.

- Wash hands and don non-sterile gloves.
- Clean the skin using a rubbing motion for 30–60 seconds with an antiseptic solution such as 70% alcohol swab. Allow this to air-dry completely to ensure the disinfection of the skin and prevent discomfort during cannulation. Once dry the vein should not be re-palpated, tapped or touched.
- Separate the needle (trochar) and the cannula and then replace them gently to ensure the smooth insertion of the needle and its subsequent removal during the advancing of the cannula into the vein.
- Stabilise the vein throughout by applying the non-dominant thumb distal to the expected puncture site and stretching the skin in a downward fashion.
- The access device is inserted with the needle bevel uppermost as this ensures that the sharpest part of the device pierces the skin, entering at an angle appropriate for the size of the cannula and the depth of the selected vein (i.e. 10–20 degrees for a superficial vein using a 20–22 G cannula or 30–40 degrees for a deeper vein and using a larger device such as 16–18 G (see Figure 42.4).
- A 'flashback' of blood will be seen in the chamber on successful insertion of the needle into the vein. The angle of entry can then be reduced to avoid piercing the posterior wall of the vessel. If there is no flashback, withdraw the device until just beneath the skin and then attempt cannulation again. If extravasation occurs and a swelling develops, remove the device and tourniquet, applying pressure to the puncture site for 5 minutes to avoid a significant haematoma. Do not return the needle/trochar to that cannula as this may damage the cannula and increase the risk of embolism.
- Once cannulation has been achieved the device is lowered to the skin and advanced a little further (maintaining the traction on the skin), then the cannula is eased into the vein over the needle.
- Apply pressure over the cannula to avoid bleeding and while supporting the cannula with the non-dominant hand, remove the needle with the dominant hand, disposing of it in a sharps container.
- Blood can be withdrawn at this point if required, following which the tourniquet is released and the 0.9% sodium chloride flush (or heparin) may be attached as the external wings of the cannula are secured using clear tape (See Figure 42.5).
- Withdraw a small amount of blood to ensure patency then flush the cannula.
- Ensure that the cannula is secure and then apply a label to the dressing, indicating the date and time of insertion, as the cannula should be reviewed in 72 hours.
- Complete the patient's written records and care bundle forms as Trust protocols require, identifying the type and size of the cannula.

43 Blood transfusion therapy

Figure 43.1 Blood groups.

Group	Antigen	Antibody
A	A	B
B	B	A
AB	AB	None
O	None	AB

Figure 43.2 Blood group compatability.

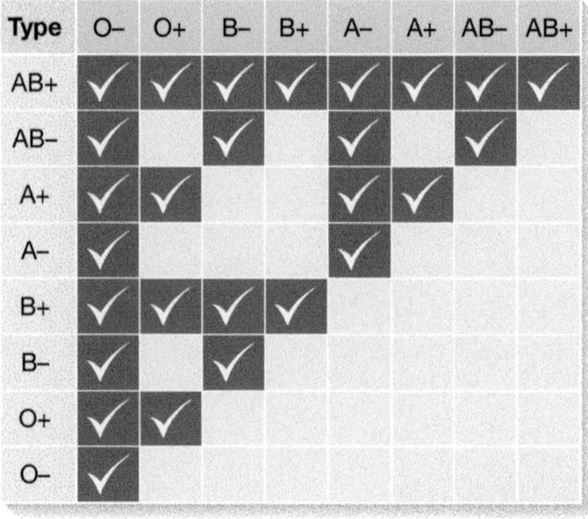

Type	O–	O+	B–	B+	A–	A+	AB–	AB+
AB+	✓	✓	✓	✓	✓	✓	✓	✓
AB–	✓		✓		✓		✓	
A+	✓	✓			✓	✓		
A–	✓				✓			
B+	✓	✓	✓	✓				
B–	✓		✓					
O+	✓	✓						
O–	✓							

Figure 43.3 Blood sample.

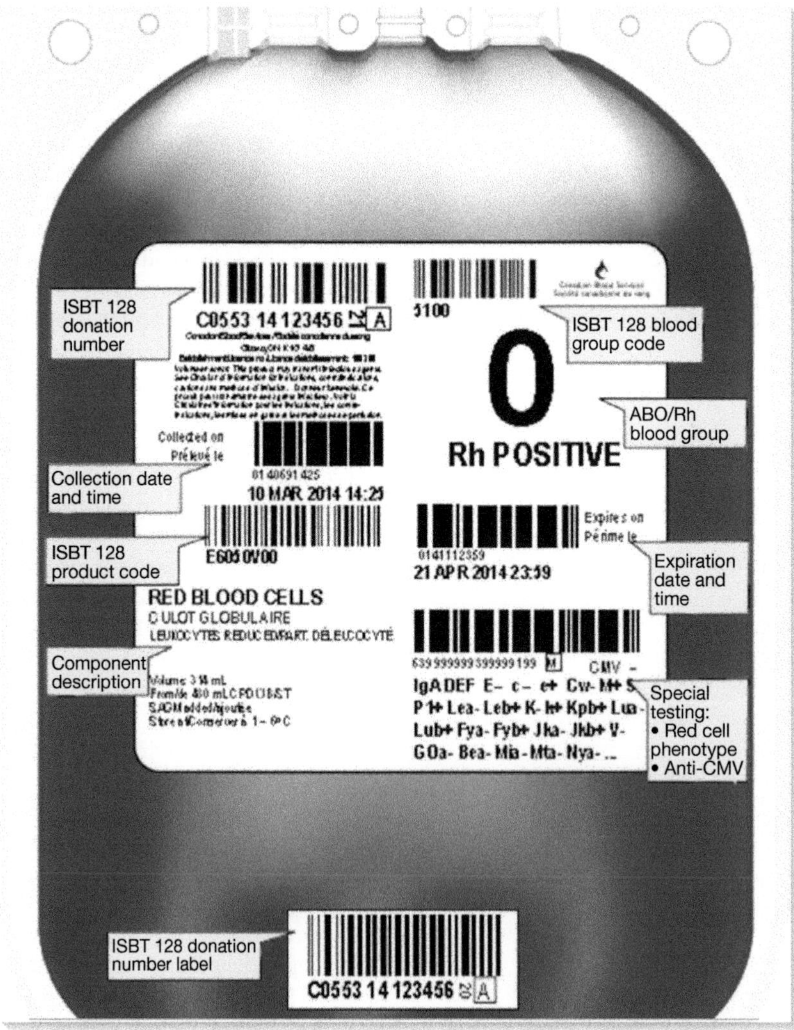

Midwifery Emergencies at a Glance, First Edition. Denise (Dee) Campbell and Susan M. Carr. Published 2018 by John Wiley & Sons, Ltd.
Companion website: www.ataglanceseries.com/midwiferyemergencies

Blood transfusion therapy is the intravenous administration of red blood cells or other blood products following informed, verbal consent from the woman (where possible) having identified an appropriate reason for transfusion. Written consent may be required under local policy but is not mandatory nationally. Transfusion should only be used when the benefits outweigh the risks of transfusion and there are no appropriate alternatives. The decision to transfuse a woman should be based on sound clinical assessment which has been underpinned by evidence-based guidelines and haematological sampling.

Reasons for blood administration

Women may require a transfusion at any stage of their antenatal, intrapartum or postnatal journey:

- For the correction of hypovolaemia (e.g. following haemorrhage).
- When the woman has a low haemoglobin and is anaemic.
- In the presence of a clotting disorder.
- In the presence of blood disorders and diseases (e.g. sickle cell).
- When an exchange transfusion is needed (baby) (e.g. due to Rhesus isoimmunisation).

Risk factors (NHLBI, 2012)

- Incompatibility – the transfusion of incompatible blood causes an antigen:antibody reaction leading to the agglutination or clumping together of red blood cells. This is almost always caused by human error and on rare occasions can be fatal.
- Circulatory overload – due to rapid transfusion or too much fluid being transfused.
- Transmission of disease – a rare but serious complication of transfusion.
- Haemolysis with febrile reaction – due to incorrect blood being transfused following either an error in labelling a blood sample, collecting an incorrect unit of blood from the storage refrigerator or inadequate checking of the unit to be transfused.
- Allergic reaction or anaphylaxis – a rare but serious complication of transfusion.
- Hypothermia – this can impair haemostasis and oxygenation of the tissues.
- Thrombophlebitis – inflammation of the vein where a clot is loosely attached.

Management of a blood transfusion

Information from the UK Serious Hazards of Transfusion (SHOT) (Bolton-Maggs, 2016) initiative has shown that as many as 1 in 13000 units of blood component is transfused into the wrong patient. This may result in a fatal outcome. Therefore, the safe transfusion of a blood product is determined by the following:

- Right blood.
- Right patient.
- Right time.
- Right place.

Pretransfusion blood sampling (JPAC 4.7, 2017c)

- In-patients should wear an identity wristband containing: name, date of birth, hospital ID number.
- Sample tube(s) must not be prelabelled.
- Sampling and labelling should be done as one process by one person using the same identifying data as on the patient's wristband plus the date and time of the sampling and the name of the sample taker.
- Handwritten labels must be legible.

Authorisation/prescription for transfusion

(JPAC 4.5, 2017b)

All prescriptions must include:

- Patient's identifying data.
- Blood component that is required.
- The volume to be transfused.
- Rate of transfusion.
- Any special requirements.

Preparation for transfusion

- Informed, verbal consent of patient (JPAC 4.4, 2017a).
- Arrange for collection of the blood component by a person who has been trained and is competent to do so as local policy dictates.
- Ensure comfort and privacy of the woman and consider the baby's feeding needs if appropriate.
- Cannulate the woman and ensure patency of the vein.
- Prepare electronic device to administer the infusion at a specific rate if appropriate.
- Prepare documentation in readiness for the transfusion.

Administration of the transfusion

- Check the blood component on arrival in the ward area with a second midwife to ensure **right blood, right patient, right time, right place** (NPSA, 2006) (see Figures 43.1, 43.2 and 43.3).
- Record the woman's baseline heart rate, blood pressure, temperature and respiratory rate prior to transfusion (no more than 60 minutes prior to commencement of the transfusion).
- Prepare the transfusion using a blood administration set containing a screen filter. **Priming the 'giving' set with 0.9% sodium chloride is no longer recommended.**
- Check the blood component with a second midwife at the woman's bedside ensuring:
  - that the identity of the woman (verbally if possible), the laboratory-generated label attached to the component pack and the transfusion prescription are an exact match
  - that the identity of the woman against the unit of component is the same
  - that the blood group and Rhesus factor of the woman matches her blood result form and the unit to be transfused
  - that the unit is inspected for bubbles, discolouration, tampering and leakage
  - that the expiry date of the unit and that all details of the unit match those recorded on the labels and accompanying forms from the blood bank.
- Record in the woman's notes and on the observation chart the woman's heart rate, blood pressure, temperature and respiratory rate 15 minutes after the start of the transfusion.
- Observe the woman throughout the transfusion and refer any new local or systemic symptoms/reactions, for example, pain, changes in blood pressure, facial flushing, dyspnoea.
- Repeat the woman's heart rate, blood pressure and temperature within 60 minutes of completion of the transfusion.
- As an in-patient the woman should be observed for late reactions over the following 24 hours.

44 Artificial rupture of membranes

Figure 44.1 Amnihook.

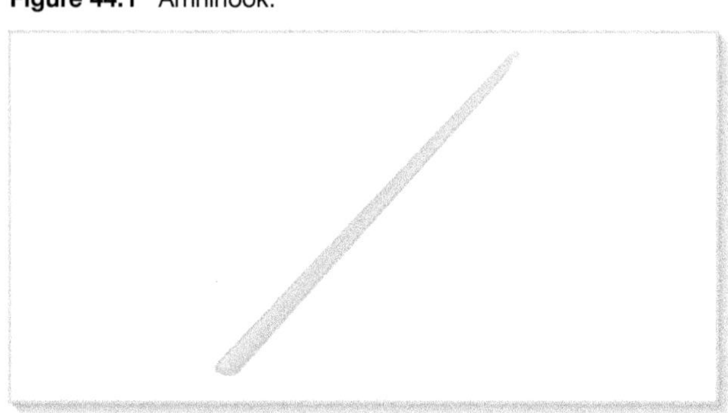

Box 44.1 Normal appearance of forewaters.

- Lie in front of/below the presenting part
- Bulge down against dilating internal os
- Tense during contractions
- 6-12 mm deep
- Clear
- Pale straw coloured
- pH 7-7.5
- Non-offensive smell

Box 44.2 Abnormal appearances of liquor.

- Pink or red coloured – can be a sign of bleeding or infection
- Pale green coloured – meconium stained from non-recent acute anoxia
- Dark green or black plus thick and tenacious – considered significant meconium staining associated with recent hypoxia/anoxic episode
- Any meconium lumps – considered significant meconium staining associated with recent hypoxia/anoxic episode

Box 44.3 Review notes prior to amniotomy.

Ensure no contraindications (and that theatre, obstetric and anaesthetic cover is available):

- No low-lying placenta on scan
- No polyhydramnios on scan
- No evidence of vasa praevia nor vellamentous insertion of cord
- Not preterm labour
- No vaginal infection nor HIV
- No directive forbidding ARM
- No maternal refusal to ARM
- Established labour or planned induction
- Normal fetal heart sounds

Box 44.4 Prior to amniotomy.

Gain maternal consent to perform abdominal palpation, vaginal examination (VE) and auscultation, to ensure:

- Established labour (unless planned induction/augmentation)
- Longitudinal lie
- Presenting part not high
- No compound presentation
- No malpresentation
- Membranes present
- No pulsation or cord felt
- Membranes not applied to face
- Normal fetal heart sounds

Box 44.5 Equipment list for amniotomy.

- Sterile vaginal examination pack (disposable sheet, gauze swabs, gallipot)
- Sterile gloves
- Apron
- Waterproof bed protector
- Water soluble sterile lubricant
- Amnihook
- Washing fluid
- Pinard stethoscope

Artificial rupture of membranes (ARM), also known as amniotomy, involves puncturing the membranes vaginally using an amnihook (a long handled, plastic hook, similar in appearance to a crochet hook – see Figure 44.1) (Smyth *et al.*, 2013). Routine amniotomy should not be practised (King & Pinger, 2014; NICE, 2014). Individualised management should determine the indications, benefits and risks, and ensure there are no contraindications. Evidence is then weighed against the benefits of maintaining intact forewaters (supports fetal rotation, prevents compression of the cord and presenting part [PP], averts cord prolapse, and protects against chorioamnionitis) (King & Pinger, 2014). Bulging membranes may also apply pressure on the cervix (first stage of labour) and introitus (second stage of labour) to aid effacement, dilatation and perineal stretching.

Indications

- Induction of labour – secondary to prostaglandin administration and alongside oxytocin administration as required (NICE, 2008).
- Augmentation of labour – controversial in the literature. King & Pinger (2014) found no evidence of amniotomy accelerating labour, but NICE (2014) supports benefits when there is delay in an established first stage of labour.
- Screening and diagnostic purposes – assessment of colour (evidence of meconium/blood – see Boxes 44.1 and 44.2), fetal blood sampling or fetal scalp electrode.
- To control descent and stabilisation of a high, unstable PP or where there is mild polyhydramnios. Reduces the risk of spontaneous rupture without obstetric management. Can allow slowing of fluid loss, descent, stability, and immediate identification of complications such as cord prolapse.
- Prior to birth and management of second twin.

Contraindications

- Lack of maternal consent.
- Placenta praevia, vasa praevia or vellamentous insertion of cord.
- Absence of labour – unless induction is planned.
- Normally progressing spontaneous labour – risks outweigh benefits (Smyth *et al.*, 2013).
- Known vaginal infection or HIV risk – unless prophylactic antibiotics balance the risk.
- Face presentation where the eyes or fontanelle are at risk of damage.
- High fetal head, malpresentation and/or unstable lie (when not under theatre conditions) – increases the risk of cord prolapse (NICE, 2008), compound presentation and abnormal lie or presentation.
- Use as a primary method of induction of labour – prostaglandins must be the primary method unless contraindicated (NICE, 2008).
- Preterm labour – intact membranes protect against compression and improve cervical pressure around the ill-fitting PP.
- Polyhydramnios – rapid reduction in uterine size may cause abruptio placenta and excessive gush of fluid may cause prolapsed cord (unless controlled ARM is possible).

Possible benefits

- Shortening of length of labour – NICE (2014) supports shortening of labour by approximately an hour when used for induction. Not effective at shortening when labour is normally progressing and spontaneous (King & Pinger, 2014). Oxytocin alongside ARM has greater support for augmenting labour.
- Combined with oxytocin may slightly reduce the likelihood of Caesarean after delay in normal progress of labour (Wei *et al.*, 2013).
- Stabilisation of an unstable lie.
- Descent and stabilisation of a high PP within the pelvis.

Potential risks and possible complications

- May increase pain and strength of contractions (NICE, 2014).
- Prolapsed umbilical cord (NICE, 2008).
- Infection – introduced to the vagina, uterus or fetus (Ray & Ray, 2014); chorioamnionitis (King & Pinger, 2014).
- Increased fetal heart decelerations (Smyth *et al.*, 2013; King & Pinger, 2014) – as a result of rapid descent, cord or PP compression, or maternal distress due to increased pain.
- Increased likelihood of Caesarean section (King & Pinger, 2014).
- Amniotic embolism – pathophysiology is unclear. One theory is that cervical lacerations or partially separating placentae allow amniotic fluid into the maternal circulation, causing anaphylactic or inflammatory reactions (Ito *et al.*, 2014; Kaur *et al.*, 2016). Both are potential risks of ARM. Consideration should be given to not performing the ARM at the height of a contraction to reduce these risks, cause less discomfort and enhance cooperation.

Management of ARM

- Ensure there are no contraindications (see Boxes 44.3 and 44.4).
- Gain informed consent and support bladder emptying in advance.
- Hand washing and aseptic non-touch procedure to be followed.
- Gather the equipment required (see Box 44.5).
- Perform abdominal examination to ensure there are no contraindications (see Box 44.4).
- Perform auscultation of fetal heart to confirm heart sounds are normal.
- Woman adopts semirecumbent position, knees bent, ankles together and, knees apart. Remove bed covers just prior to examination.
- Prepare sterile field and equipment.
- Vulval cleansing – swab from front to back and outer to inner layers with single use swabs. Maintain clean hand/dirty hand technique.
- Separate the vulva with the non-dominant hand. Enter vagina with lubricated index and second finger of dominant hand.
- Perform vaginal examination between contractions – confirm intact membranes and no contraindications (see Box 44.4).
- Non-dominant hand places Amnihook to face towards the underside of the fingers and slides it along their length, between the two fingers.
- When contraction is subsiding, rotate the Amnihook until it faces the softening but still slightly bulging membranes.
- Apply downward pressure to pierce the membranes and slightly extend the hole.
- Turn the Amnihook back to facing the underside of the fingers; slide it between the two fingers and back out of the introitus to remove it.
- Keep the two fingers in the vagina as the amniotic fluid flows away.
- Observe the colour and smell of the liquor for evidence of blood, meconium or signs of infection.
- Recheck for any evidence of cord prolapse and any other changes before removing fingers from vagina. Auscultate fetal heart.
- Make the woman comfortable, explain your findings and record all elements in the notes.

45 Oxytocic augmentation

Table 45.1 Bishop's score.

Score	Dilatation	Effacement	Station	Position	Consistency
0	Closed	0–30%	−3	Posterior	Firm
1	1–2 cm	40–50%	−2	Mid-position	Moderately firm
2	3–4 cm	60–70%	−1, 0	Anterior	Soft
3	5+	80+%	+1, +2		

Table 45.2 An example of an infusion regime.

Time (minutes after start)	Millilitres per hour	Units per minute
Start	6	2
30	12	4
60	18	6
90	24	8
120	36	12
150	48	16
180	60	20
210	72	24
240	84	28
270	96	32

Figure 45.1 Diagram of an infusion.

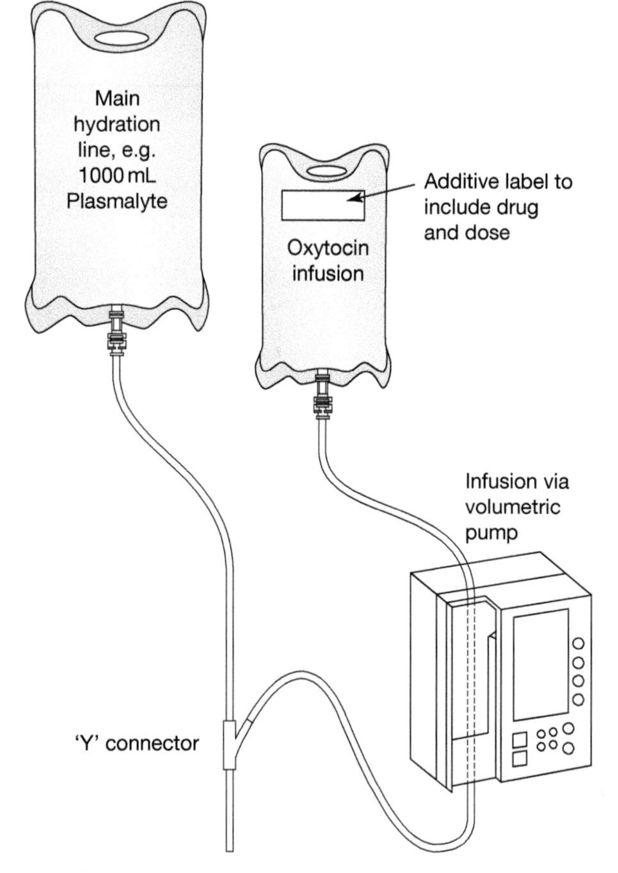

Slow progress in labour (labour dystocia) can be augmented by enhancing the efficiency of the contractions, by increasing their frequency, length and intensity. This is traditionally achieved by the administration of oxytocic therapy and/or amniotomy after the spontaneous onset of labour (WHO, 2014).

Physiology

Oxytocin, a naturally occurring hormone, is usually produced in increasing quantities by the posterior pituitary gland towards the end of pregnancy. This hormone causes the smooth muscle fibres contained in the myometrium of the uterus to contract, resulting in corresponding cervical dilatation.

Causes of delay

In the first stage of labour, causes of delay may include:
- Nulliparity.
- Inefficient uterine contractions.
- Malpresentation of the fetus.
- Malposition of the fetal head.
- Deflexed/extended attitude of the fetal head.
- Cephalo-pelvic disproportion (CPD).
- Full bowel.
- Full bladder.
- Maternal dehydration leading to ineffectual contractions.

Issues to take into consideration

Augmentation should be used with care and thus certain conditions should be considered – these may include:
- Previous uterine scarring.
- A woman experiencing eclampsia.
- The existence of any comorbidity such as cardiac disease.
- Favourability of the cervix according to the Bishop Score.
- Has an amniotomy been performed.
- Grandmultiparity.
- Fetal wellbeing should be assured before commencing an augmentation.

Should any of these situations exist, the woman's condition should be discussed with with an obstetric registrar/consultant.

Contraindications

The augmentation of labour should not be undertaken if there is:
- A lack of maternal consent.
- A confirmed malpresentation of the fetus such as breech, shoulder; or sub-optimal lie such as oblique or transverse.
- A known placenta or vasa praevia.
- A history of previous Caesarean section.
- A cord presentation or prolapse.
- Hypertonic contractions of the uterus.
- A pathological fetal heart rate.
- A known mechanical obstruction, such as, CPD.
- Persistent maternal pyrexia.
- Spontaneous labour.
- Known allergy or hypersensitivity to oxytocin.

Management

Consent

Augmentation of labour can only be undertaken following informed consent by the woman (GMC, 2008; NMC, 2015). It is imperative that language is used that both the woman and her birth partner(s) understand. Information to include that:
- The infusion will increase the frequency and strength of the contractions.
- The time interval until the birth of the fetus may be shortened.
- The mode of delivery or any other outcome cannot be guaranteed or altered.
- The fetus will be monitored before the start of the infusion and then constantly throughout the augmentation process.
- There may be possible adverse effects of the oxytocic infusion including:
  - maternal: nausea, vomiting, hypotension, tachycardia, hypertonic contractions (more than four contractions in 10 minutes lasting 2 minutes or more with <60–90 seconds between each contraction), increased risk of postpartum haemorrhage
  - fetal: bradycardia, fetal distress, emergency birth.

Procedure

- Perform and record baseline maternal observations to include: pulse, temperature, blood pressure, uterine activity palpated over 1 minute, abdominal palpation to determine the lie, presentation, position and station of the fetus. It is expected that the findings will show that the fetus has adopted a longitudinal lie with a cephalic presentation, a lateral or anterior position and that the fetal head is engaged.
- A cardiotocograph (CTG) recording is made for 20 minutes (or as local Trust protocol states) to establish fetal wellbeing prior to augmentation of labour. Continuous CTG monitoring will continue once augmentation is commenced.
- An examination *per vaginam* is performed and recorded to assess: cervical effacement, dilatation of the cervix, the state of the membranes and any liquor amnii in the case of ruptured membranes, the position and station of the fetal head (Bishops score, see Table 45.1).
- Intravenous cannulation is performed to secure access.
- The prescribed amount of oxytocin (e.g. Syntocinon) is added to 500 mL of 0.9% sodium chloride with an 'additive' label affixed to the bag, having been checked and recorded on the woman's prescription chart by two midwives.
- The fluid volume administered is recorded on a fluid balance chart as is urinary output.
- The intravenous administration set is connected to the bag of fluid to be infused and then to the intravenous cannula and run through, before being threaded through a volumetric pump. The infusion may be attached via a 'Y' connector to a main line infusion such as Plasmalyte (see Figure 45.1).
- The amount to be infused per minute is then set and the infusion is commenced once the right time, dose, person, route and drug have been checked with a second midwife.
- The rate of infusion is gradually increased as stated by Trust protocol (see Table 45.2) until approximately four contractions per 10 minutes is reached, at which point the rate of infusion is maintained.
- The augmentation should be recorded in the woman's notes and also on the partogram, together with the CTG findings and maternal observations of pulse, blood pressure and temperature.
- All deviations from 'the norm' will be referred to the obstetrician.

46 Third- and fourth-degree tears

Figure 46.1 Lines of third and fourth degree tears.

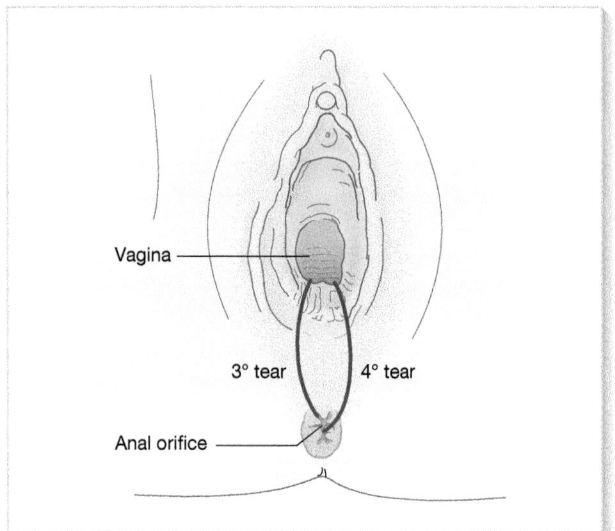

Figure 46.2 Muscle damage.

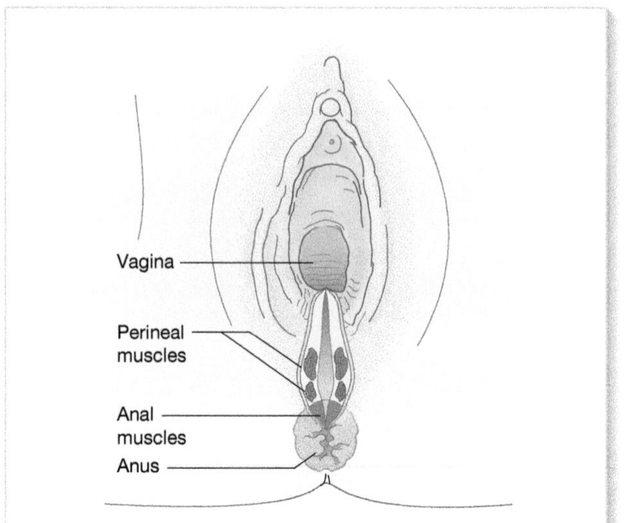

Box 46.1 OASI Care Bundle Project.

Readers are encouraged to follow the outcomes of the RCOG (2016) OASI Care Bundle Project. Their plan is to introduces interventions across 16 sites (in the UK) over the next 2.5 years. The intervention combines a campaign to raise awareness, multidisciplinary skills development and the following bundle:

- Communication with the woman to enable a slow controlled birth
- Performing an episiotomy when required
- Using the hands to enable perineal protection at the time of birth
- Thorough examination after birth to detect all tears

Box 46.2 Outcomes and complications. Source: Adapted from Priddis *et al.* (2014) and Fernando *et al.* (2015).

- 60–80% are asymptomatic at 12 months
- Prolonged pain
- Dyspareunia and sexual morbidity
- Wound dehiscence
- Sepsis
- Psychological morbidity
- Faecal incontinence
- Urinary problems
- Poor bonding with infant

A wide range of vulval, perineal, vaginal, anal, cervical and uterine trauma may occur during vaginal deliveries. This may result from a deliberate cut (episiotomy), a tear (laceration) or a combination of the two as an extended episiotomy. The degree of damage may include bruising, haematoma, first-, second-, third- and fourth-degree tears. This chapter will concentrate on third- and fourth-degree tears and their complications – obstetric anal sphincter injuries (OASI) (see Figure 46.1 and 46.2).

Classifications

These are all perineal tears, with the four degrees classified here to clarify the progressive stages involved. The classification used is that adopted by the Royal College of Obstetricians and Gynaecologists (RCOG) from Sultan (1999):

- **First-degree (1°)** – injuries to skin and/or vaginal mucosa.
- **Second-degree (2°)** – injuries involving perineal muscles but not involving the anal sphincter.
- **Third-degree (3°)** – injuries involving the anal sphincter complex:
  - Grade 3a: <50% of external anal sphincter (EAS) thickness torn
  - Grade 3b: >50% of EAS thickness torn
  - Grade 3c: both EAS and internal anal sphincter (IAS) torn.

  Note: Fernando *et al.* (2015) advocate classifying to the higher degree if there is any doubt.)
- **Fourth-degree (4°)** – injury to perineum involving the anal sphincter complex (EAS and IAS) and anorectal mucosa.

Incidence

The rate of reported OASIs between 2000 and 2012 tripled from 1.8 to 5.9% (Thiagamoorthy *et al.*, 2014). More recent evidence identified: an overall incidence across assisted and unassisted deliveries of 5.1% for primiparae and 1.8% for multiparae; unassisted deliveries have an incidence of 4.1% for primiparae and 1.5% for multiparae; and assisted deliveries are much higher at 7.8% for primiparae and 4.8% for multiparae (Carrol *et al.*, 2016). The tripling rate of reported OASIs between 2000 and 2012 from 1.8 to 5.9% (Thiagamoorthy *et al.*, 2014) alongside international and geographical variations (Birth Stats NSW, 2018; The Rotunda Hospital, 2014) raise significant concerns but this may be due to improved training and increased detection rather than poor standards of care (Thiagamoorthy *et al.*, 2014).

Predisposing factors (Melamed *et al.*, 2012; Gurol-Urganci *et al.*, 2013; Fernando *et al.*, 2015)

There are no risk factors which enable accurate prediction, but some individual or combined factors may make a third- or fourth-degree tear more likely:

- Episiotomy – as this may extend.
- Forceps delivery.
- Precipitate delivery.
- Persistent occipito-posterior positions.
- Vacuum extraction.
- Large for gestational age infants.
- Gestational age >40 weeks.
- Asian ethnicity.
- Nulliparity.
- Shoulder dystocia.
- Prolonged second stage of labour.

The Clinical Indicators Project (Carrol *et al.*, 2016) found there were clusters associated with types of delivery:

- Both assisted or unassisted deliveries – age group, deprivation, ethnicity, placenta praevia and abruption, abnormal fluid volume, birthweight, gestational age, pre-existing or gestational diabetes in pregnancy, pre-existing hypertension, pre-eclampsia.
- Unassisted only – age group, deprivation, ethnicity, birthweight, gestational age.
- Assisted – age group, deprivation, ethnicity, gestational age, pre-existing hypertension, pre-eclampsia, previous Caesarean section since 2000.

Prevention (Fernando *et al.*, 2015) (see also Box 46.1)

- Health education.
- Mediolateral episiotomies (when indicated) – 60 degrees away from midline.
- Perineal protection at crowning.
- Warm compression to perineum during second stage.
- Previous OASIs – counselling and discussion prelabour/delivery.
- Prophylactic episiotomy should not be performed – performed only if clinically indicated.
- Previous OASIs and symptomatic (or abnormal ultrasonography) – counsel regarding optional elective Caesarean birth.

Management (Fernando *et al.*, 2013; Fernando *et al.*, 2015)

- Explanation and consent for repair procedures.
- Management of haemostasis if required, including vaginal pack.
- Typically transfer to theatre for regional/general anaesthetic and good lighting; senior obstetrician if repair to be in the delivery room.
- Digital rectal examination – assess the severity before suturing.
- Repair by a trained clinician or by a trainee under supervision.
- Avoid 'figure of eight' sutures – haemostasis causes ischaemia.
- Rectal examination post-repair – ensure no sutures pass through the anorectal mucosa; remove any identified.
- Anorectal mucosa repaired by continuous or interrupted technique.
- Where IAS can be identified, repair this separately with interrupted or mattress sutures; do not overlap the IAS.
- Repair of a full thickness EAS tear by either an overlapping or an end-to end (approximation) method.
- For partial thickness (all 3a and some 3b) tears, an end-to-end technique should be used.
- Use 3-0 polyglactin for anorectal mucosa – less irritation and discomfort.
- Use 3-0 PDS or modern braided sutures such as 2-0 polyglactin for repair of the EAS and/or IAS muscle.
- Bury surgical knots beneath the superficial perineal muscles.
- Broad-spectrum antibiotics following repair.
- Postoperative laxatives – without added bulking agents.
- Cold pack, analgesics and anti-inflammatories for pain relief.
- Good nutrition and hygiene.
- 6–12 week follow-up of women including exercises/physiotherapy.
- Referral to a specialist gynaecologist or colorectal surgeon if incontinence present.
- Monitor for any complications (see Box 46.2).

47 Perineal suturing

Figure 47.1 Infiltration.

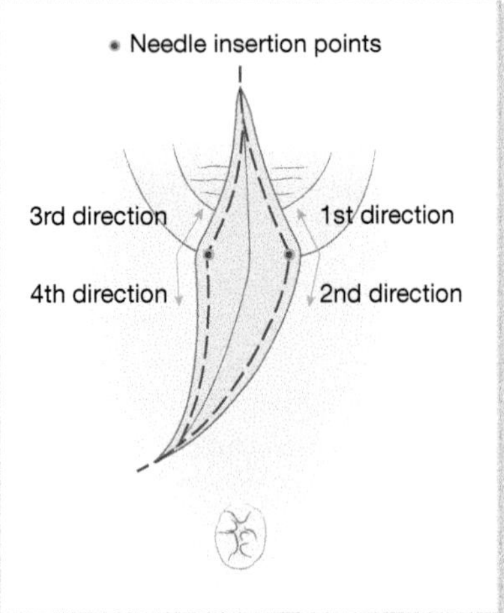

Figure 47.2 Needle guarded position.

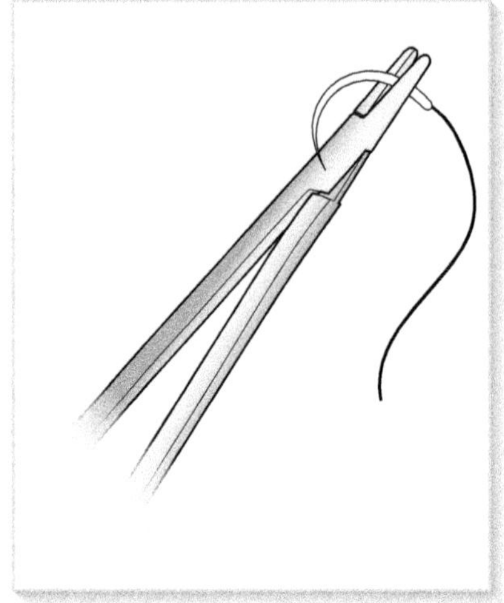

Figure 47.3 Square surgeon (anchor) knot.

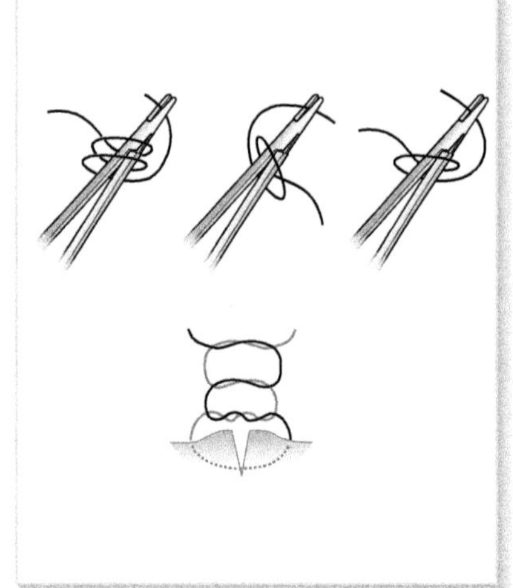

Figure 47.4 Suturing vaginal wall; ending in deep muscle layer.

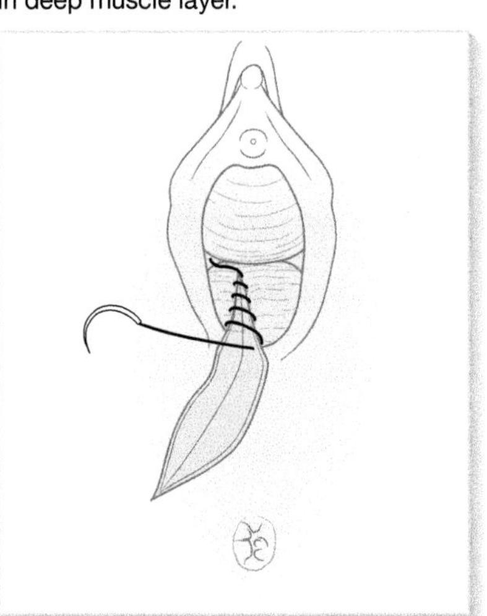

Figure 47.5 Deep muscle layer.

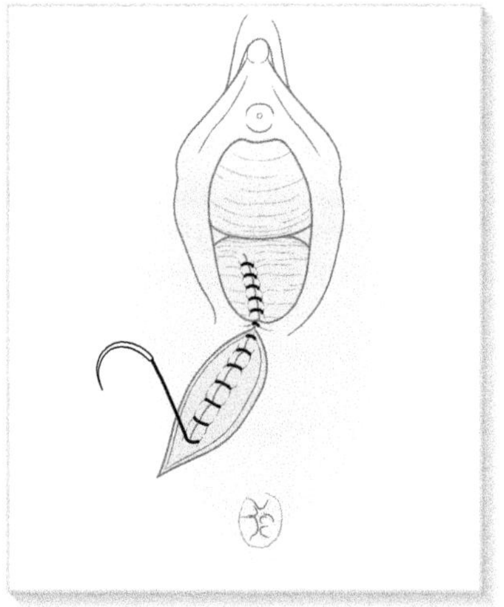

Figure 47.6 Skin layer.

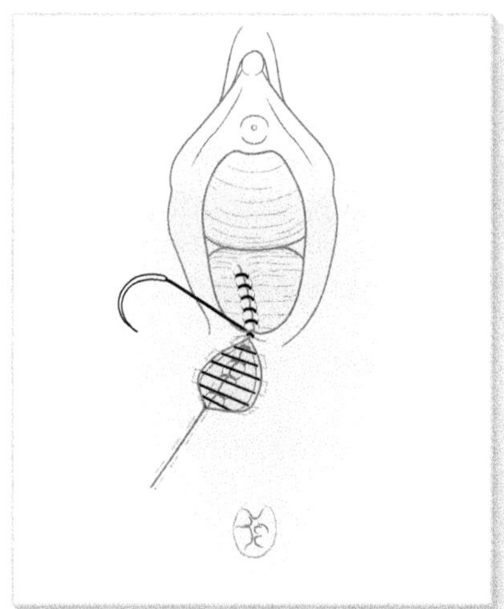

Figure 47.7 Aberdeen knot (AK) (within wound; leave loop left side as suture bites right side; make loop right side).

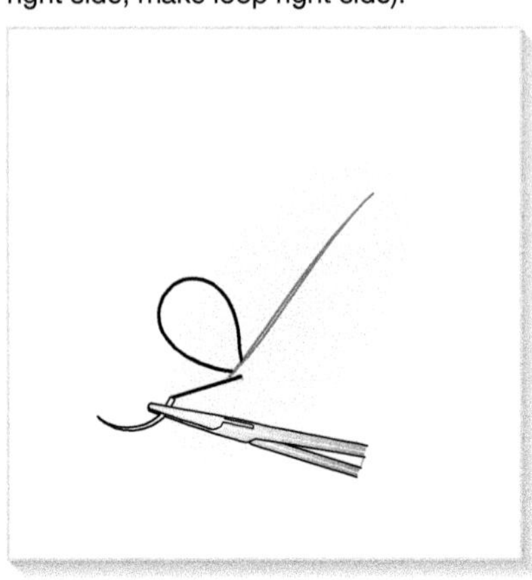

Figure 47.8 AK 2 (pull loop through other loop; tighten; repeat second time).

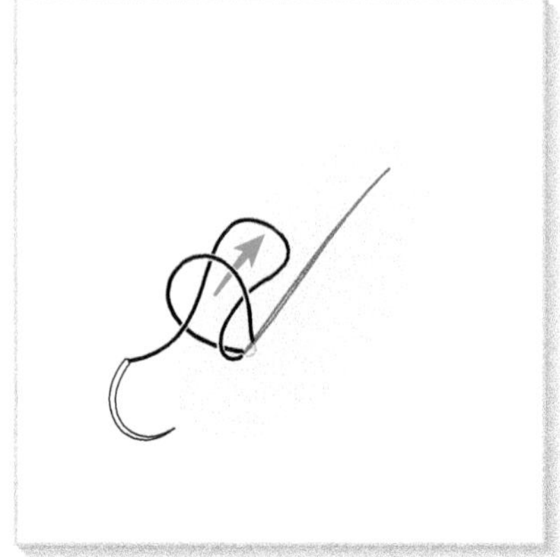

Figure 47.9 AK 3 (needle holder and all thread through loop; pull tight; cut both ends 0.5 cm long).

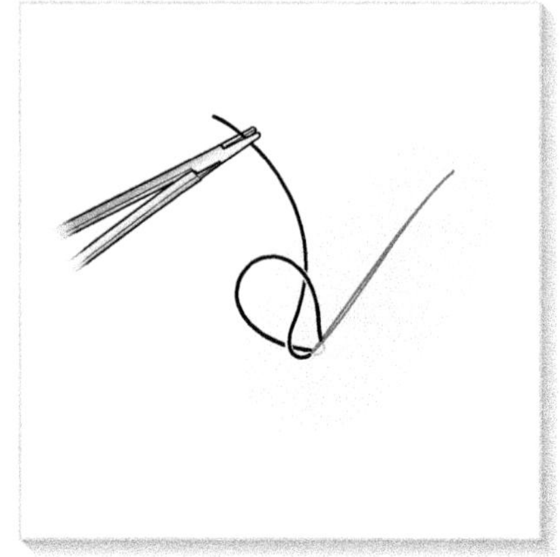

A wide range of trauma may occur during vaginal deliveries. The incidence of an intact perineum may be as low as 9.6% at a first delivery and 31.2% in subsequent deliveries (Smith *et al.*, 2013) which equates to approximately 350 000 women in the UK and millions more worldwide requiring perineal suturing (Dudley *et al.*, 2011). This chapter considers the repair of second degree tears/lacerations or episiotomies and the importance of applying best evidence.

Evidence gap

A number of surveys have identified that only around 6% of midwives follow best evidence in their suturing techniques (Bick *et al.*, 2012; Ismail *et al.*, 2013). Apart from failing to follow evidence throughout the three layers of suturing, these surveys showed that only 17% performed the necessary rectal examination (after suturing), more than 50% did not always suture second degree wounds, and only 22% felt confident about repairing wounds (typically senior midwives or those with >20 years' service (Bick *et al.*, 2012).

All practitioners have a duty to maintain their awareness of best evidence for discussions with the women they support and for application in practice. The current best evidence on perineal repair includes:

- Fast absorbable suture material should be used to reduce short- and long-term pain, wound dehiscence, and the need for suture removal (Kettle *et al.*, 2010; Kettle *et al.*, 2012).
- A continuous suturing technique for all layers reduces short-term pain (Kettle *et al.*, 2012).
- A continuous technique is quicker and requires less suture material making it more cost effective (Kindberg *et al.*, 2008).
- Non-sutured wounds result in a significantly higher proportion of open perineal wounds at 6 weeks. Evidence is limited about the advantages and disadvantages of leaving the muscle and skin unsutured – until evidence supports non-suturing second degree perineal wounds should be repaired (Elharmeel *et al.*, 2011).
- Rectal non-steroidal anti-inflammatory drugs should be offered routinely following repair of first and second degree trauma (if not contraindicated for the individual) (NICE, 2014).

Predisposing factors to perineal trauma

(Pergialiotis *et al.*, 2014)

- Nulliparity.
- Induction/augmentation of labour.
- Instrumental/operative vaginal deliveries.
- Longer duration of second stage.
- Heavier birthweight.
- Epidural anaesthesia.
- Hospital delivery.

Management of suturing (RCM, 2012; NICE, 2014)

- Gain informed consent and maintain ongoing explanation.
- Gather and prepare equipment (2.0 vicryl rapide, 36 mm taper cut suture, non-toothed dissecting forceps, needle holder, artery forceps, suture scissors, sterile towel, sponge forceps, gallipot of water based lubricant, bowl of sterile water, 20 mL syringe, green needle, 20 mL 1% lidocaine, tampon [not always required] and five X-ray detectable gauze swabs).
- Perform a swab, needle and equipment count.
- Position woman so that wound can be easily viewed with a good light source (lithotomy position is not always necessary).
- Use aseptic procedure throughout.
- Assess the degree of trauma and identify the wound apex – include a rectal assessment to exclude third or fourth degree tears if any muscle damage evident.
- Ensure adequate anaesthesia (spinal, epidural or local) – offer Entonox analgesia until anaesthesia achieved.
- If **local anaesthetic** required – check anaesthetic (substance, strength, dose and expiry date) with a second professional. Insert needle on left side, at introitus, below skin level; guide needle down along the line of the vagina to the apex, draw back to ensure needle is not in a blood vessel; inject 3-4 mL of anaesthesia gradually as needle is slowly withdrawn. As needle tip reaches the wound exit, reinsert but now along direction of perineal skin to extent of skin damage; then again draw back to ensure needle is not in a blood vessel; inject 3–4 mL of anaesthesia gradually as needle is slowly withdrawn. Repeat process on the right side of the wound. In addition, insert bolus doses into fourchette and distal ends of skin wound, then allow anaesthetic to work (see Figure 47.1).
- Remove suture from pack with needle holder gripping two-thirds from needle point; always turn needle into 'guarded' position (point resting on top of needle holder) using forceps when not suturing (see Figure 47.2).
- Assess if tampon required – lubricate and insert carefully; attach sponge forceps to X-ray detectable gauze tail.
- Insert anchor/square knot 5–10 mm above apex of vaginal wall, cutting short end of thread only (see Figure 47.3).
- Suture vaginal wall using three to four continuous non-interlocking sutures, 0.5 cm from wound edge and 1 cm apart. Use depth of round needle to reach trough of wound ending on the left side at hymenal remnants (see Figure 47.4).
- At hymenal remnants, suture is taken down into the deeper muscle layer. Close deep muscle layer using continuous sutures which reach from 0.5 cm below skin into full depth of laceration, aligning left and right side sutures to close dead space – may require two layers. End at anal end of skin wound (see Figure 47.5).
- Suture skin layer within subcutaneous tissue taking deep bites to avoid nerve endings. Align left and right edges (see Figure 47.6). Use non-toothed forceps to turn back skin edge and visualise subcutaneous tissue. End behind hymenal remnants using Aberdeen knot technique to finish (see Figures 47.7, 47.8 and 47.9).
- Remove tampon if used.
- Reassess wound for alignment – perform rectal examination to ensure no sutures can be felt; insert rectal analgesia if being used.
- Check swabs, needles and instruments are all present – dispose of these appropriately and then make the woman comfortable.
- Fully document procedure – time, anaesthetic, degree of damage repair required, sutures used, rectal examination performed, removal of tampon (if used) and swab, needle and instrument count.

Possible complications

- Infection.
- Wound dehiscence.
- Pain and inflammation – including dyspareunia.
- Haematoma.

48 Maternal sepsis

Figure 48.1 Maternal sepsis. Data from MBRRACE report (2014). *Saving lives, improving mothers' care* 2009 – 2012. Source: Knight *et al.*, (2014).

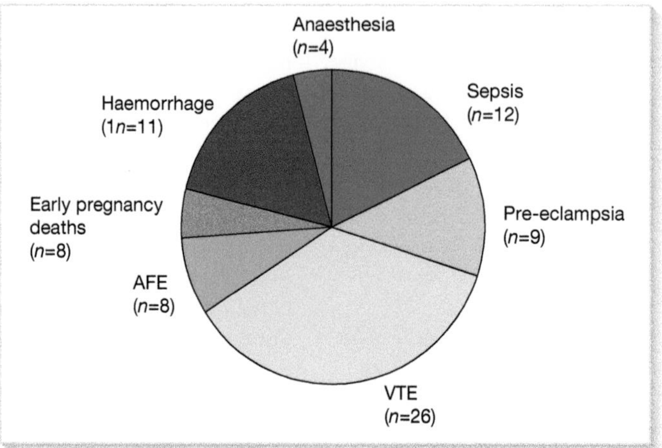

Figure 48.2 Sepsis 6 care bundle.

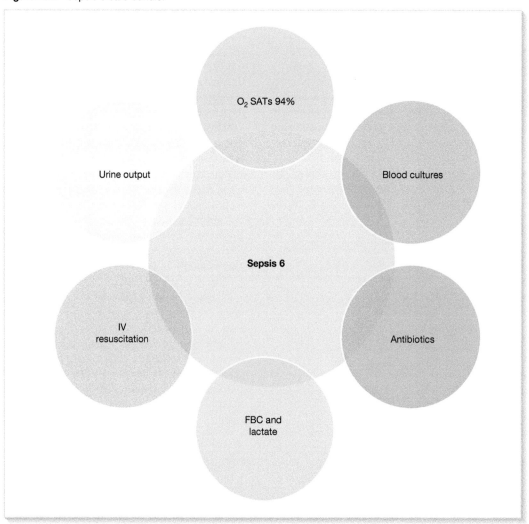

Sepsis 6

O_2 SATs 94%

Blood cultures

Antibiotics

FBC and lactate

IV resuscitation

Urine output

Maternal sepsis, may be defined as a condition in which a complex collection of symptoms results in a harmful response to infection, typified by organ dysfunction and failure, with tissue hypoperfusion resulting in lactic acidosis – a systemic inflammatory response (SIRS). Pregnant women have a greater predisposition to sepsis because physiological adaptations occur in pregnancy to enable the woman to accept foreign proteins from fetal antigens, thereby lowering her immunological response to infection.

Risk factors

Antenatal risk factors (Pasupathy *et al.*, 2012)

- Reduced/impaired maternal immunity.
- Anaemia.
- History of group B streptococcus infection.
- Maternal gestational diabetes mellitus.
- Prolonged spontaneous rupture of membranes.
- History of pelvic infection.
- Urinary tract infection.
- Chorioamnionitis.
- Vaginal discharge.
- Invasive procedure (e.g. amniotomy).
- Body mass index>35.

Specific postpartum risk factors

In addition to the previous list:

- Mastitis.
- Vaginal trauma.
- Caesarean section.
- Wound haematoma/infection.

Between 2009 and 2012 almost 25% of maternal deaths were caused by sepsis (Knight *et al.*, 2014) (see Figure 48.1). Sepsis remains a leading contributory factor in maternal death with causative organisms including (Morgan *et al.*, 2012):

- Group A *Streptococcus pyogenes* (GAS) infection.
- Influenza (H1N1).
- Pneumococcal disease (e.g. meningitis).
- *Staphylococcus aureus.*
- *Escherichia coli.*
- *Streptococcus pneumoniae.*
- Methicillin-resistant *Staphylococcus aureus* (MRSA).

Diagnosis

Collapse may occur without warning and thus women may appear to be well up to the point of collapse. Always include Red Flag Sepsis screening for SIRS: SIRS is confirmed if any two of the following are identified:

- Temperature above 38.3°C or below 36°C.
- Tachycardia >90 bpm.
- Tachypnoea >20 respirations per minute.

SIRS confirmed if any one of the following is identified:

- Systolic blood pressure <90 mmHg (or more than a fall of 40 mmHg from the baseline recording).
- Tachycardia >30 bpm.
- Hypoxia with oxygen saturations <91%.
- Tachypnoea >25 respirations per minute.
- Responds only to pain/voice or is unresponsive.

Other symptoms may include:

- Rash.
- Oliguria.
- Diarrhoea.
- Vomiting.
- Abdominal pain.
- Focus of infection (e.g. urinary tract, wound, chest).
- Subinvolution of the uterus ± offensive-smelling lochia.
- Productive cough.

It is essential that midwives and all medical staff are familiar with the signs and symptoms of the onset of sepsis. The onset may be insidious, but deterioration may be rapid.

Immediate management – prompt and rapid

Within 1 hour of diagnosis – The Sepsis 6 Care Bundle (see Figure 48.2)

- Take arterial blood gas and give high flow (10–15 l) facial oxygen via a reservoir mask to maintain oxygen saturation of 94%.
- Cannulate using two 16 G cannulae – one in each antecubital fossa.
- Take blood cultures.
- Take blood for: haemoglobin, group and save, coagulation screen, urea and electrolytes, glucose, liver function tests.
- Take blood for serum lactate levels.
- Commence broad-spectrum intravenous antibiotics (once all relevant swabs taken).
- Commence intravenous fluid resuscitation.
- Catheterise and monitor urine output hourly using urometer.

Actively identify source of the infection

- Take swabs:
  - wound
  - sputum
  - urine
  - stool
  - nose and throat
  - high/low vagina.
- Chest X-ray.

Immediate care as recommended by the Surviving Sepsis Campaign (Society of Critical Care Medicine, 2016)

- Early involvement of appropriate medical staff.
- Clear leadership is identified.
- Care for the woman in the high dependency area in delivery suite or high dependency/intensive care unit if a local facility is unavailable.
- Commence central venous pressure reading.
- Maintain close observation using a Modified Early Obstetric Warning Score (MEOWS) chart.
- Measure accurate fluid balance with hourly urine output measurements.

Source isolation nursing

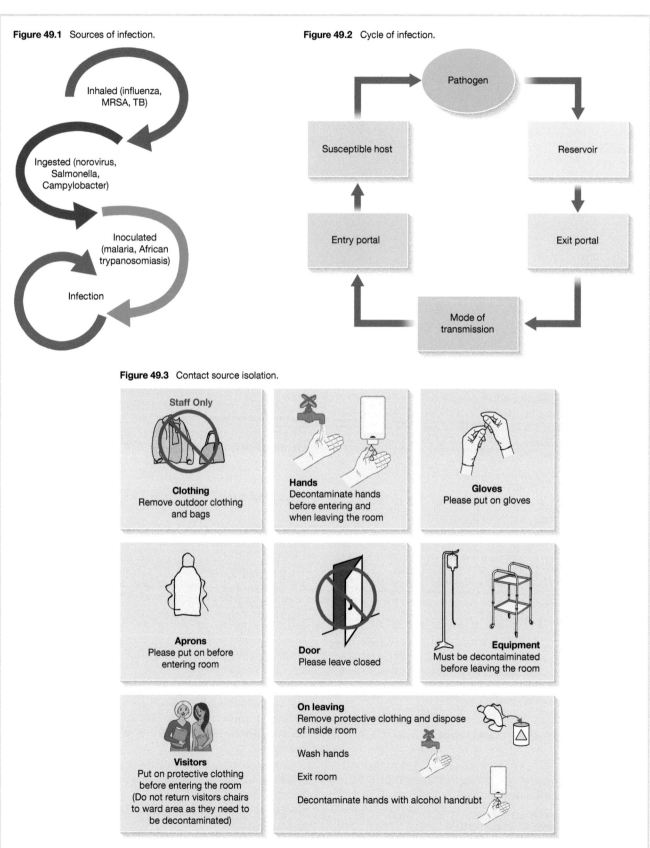

Figure 49.1 Sources of infection.

Inhaled (influenza, MRSA, TB)

Ingested (norovirus, Salmonella, Campylobacter)

Inoculated (malaria, African trypanosomiasis)

Infection

Figure 49.2 Cycle of infection.

Pathogen

Reservoir

Exit portal

Mode of transmission

Entry portal

Susceptible host

Figure 49.3 Contact source isolation.

Staff Only

Clothing
Remove outdoor clothing and bags

Hands
Decontaminate hands before entering and when leaving the room

Gloves
Please put on gloves

Aprons
Please put on before entering room

Door
Please leave closed

Equipment
Must be decontaiminated before leaving the room

Visitors
Put on protective clothing before entering the room (Do not return visitors chairs to ward area as they need to be decontaminated)

On leaving
Remove protective clothing and dispose of inside room

Wash hands

Exit room

Decontaminate hands with alcohol handrubt

Source isolation nursing can be defined as the separation of one patient from another in order to prevent the spread of infection to other patients, staff and members of the public. This was formerly known as 'barrier nursing' and aims to contain or isolate an infection from other women and babies cared for in the same locality. This means that the woman (and/or her baby) must be separated from other women and their babies – this may lead to increased levels of stress for the woman and a heavier workload for the staff caring for her.

Sources of infection and routes of transmission

These commonly include:

- Acute cases caused by **inhaling** droplets containing the bacterium or virus which the host has coughed or sneezed into the air – this includes organisms such as the H1N1 influenza virus, pulmonary tuberculosis, methicillin-resistant *Staphylococcus aureus* (MRSA).
- Infection caused by the **ingestion** of organisms such as *Clostridium difficile* or norovirus, leading to the colonisation of the alimentary tract and resulting in diarrhea and vomiting.
- Cases whereby the host has been **inoculated** with an organism such as malaria. These infections are rare in the UK but individual cases may appear in areas of particular significance, for example among groups of immigrating asylum seekers/refugees.

Therefore, the need for isolation is determined by the way the organism or disease is transmitted (see Figures 49.1 and 49.2).

General principles (Dougherty *et al.*, 2015)

- Isolate the woman to isolate the infection.
- Risk assessment will determine that isolation is necessary.
- Ensure that the woman understands the need for her to be isolated from other women as well as family and the general public.
- Consider the most appropriate environment in which the woman is to be nursed.
- If the woman has given birth to her baby, consider the need to separate them.

Precautions – a systematic approach

The approach to the management of a woman requiring source isolation should be systematic, taking into consideration all her possible needs when setting up the environment in which she will be nursed. Basic tenets apply (see Figures 49.3):

- Who is to care for the woman – a multidisciplinary approach.
- Where is the woman to be accommodated and how the room will be ventilated.
- What equipment will be necessary.
- How the woman's physical and mental health needs will be delivered.

Personnel

The approach to the care of the infected woman requires a multidisciplinary approach. The team is likely to include: midwives, obstetricians, microbiologists, physicians, the infection control team – each has their part to play. Ideally, one midwife should be allocated to the woman with responsibility for no-one else in the ward.

Accommodation and ventilation

The severity of the woman's condition may require her to be cared for in a high dependency or an intensive therapy unit with specially trained nurses and doctors, which may necessitate her removal from the maternity unit. However, the majority of women remain in isolation within the maternity unit:

- A side room with en suite facilities and preferably an ante-room between the main ward area and the woman's accommodation.
- A notice should be placed on the door alerting staff and members of the public. Relatives should be given instructions concerning isolation principles.
- Wherever possible, ventilation should be achieved by drawing air into the room from the nearby ward, but the air should be expelled via an external source (i.e. negative pressure).

Equipment

- Furniture should be kept to a minimum.
- All equipment should remain in the room for the duration of her stay (e.g. Pinard stethoscope and cardiotocograph machine/hand-held fetal heart monitor [where appropriate], sphygmomanometer, adult stethoscope, thermometer, 'sharps' boxes, etc.).
- Facilities for donning protective clothing before entering, such as gowns, gloves and goggles/face masks, should be available outside the room.

Physical and mental health needs of the isolated woman

- Physical needs: all routine physical and midwifery care should continue as for any other woman, ensuring that universal precautions are rigorously maintained at all times.
- Routine visits from the medical team(s) should be kept to a minimum and any visit should be the final port of call during the ward round.
- Any linen, equipment such as meal trays and rubbish for disposal must be suitably 'bagged' before leaving the room.
- Disposable protective clothing must be removed in the ante-room and placed in the bin prior to the carer rejoining the main ward area.
- Isolation can be a frightening time for the woman and her levels of anxiety and apprehension may increase. She may become bored, lonely and frustrated, with reduced social contact causing diminished communication and potential negative feelings such as the stigma associated with infection. Sensory deprivation in an environment lacking everyday stimuli such as conversation and the feeling of inferiority due to associations with being 'dirty' or 'contaminated', are the most common problems associated with isolation nursing. Where possible, distractions such as a radio, television, books and magazines may be provided together with repeated explanations concerning the isolation and consequent care. Compassion and care should be demonstrated without conveying any sense of fear or disgust related to the infection (Gammon, 1999).

50 Group B streptococcus

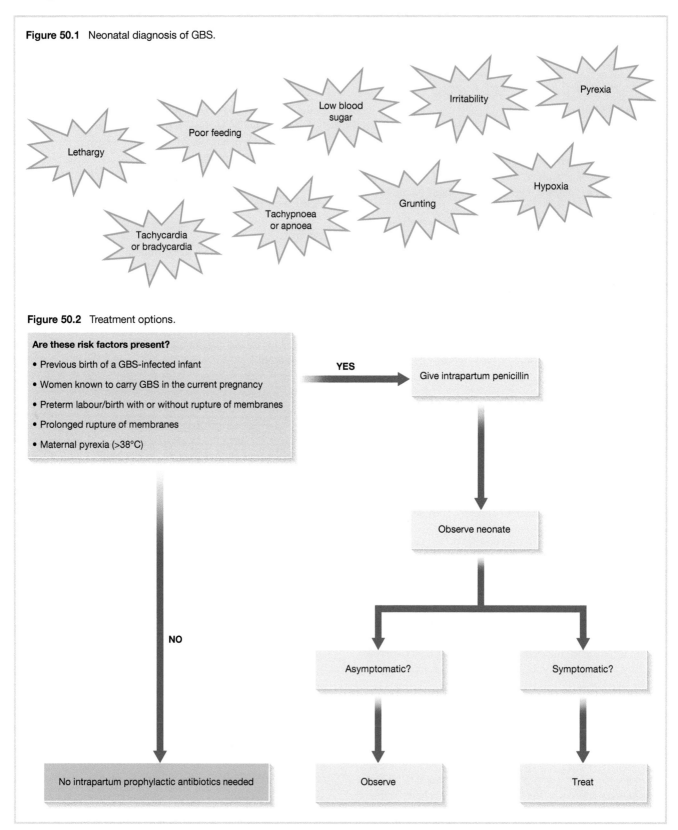

Figure 50.1 Neonatal diagnosis of GBS.

Figure 50.2 Treatment options.

Group B streptococcus (GBS) is a Gram-positive bacterium which can be found colonising the gastrointestinal and genital tracts of approximately 30–40% adults. Generally, these bacteria do not produce any symptoms in the host carrier, thriving as a commensal organism. However, up to 22% pregnant women may present with GBS in their vagina, increasing the risk of vertical transmission to the fetus during childbirth. GBS is recognised as the leading cause of severe, early-onset (between 0 and 7 days) infection in newborn infants.

Risk factors (NICE, 2016e)

Maternal factors increasing the risk of infection in the neonate

- Women who have given birth to a previously GBS infected infant.
- Women who are known to carry GBS in the current pregnancy.
- Preterm labour/birth with or without rupture of membranes.
- Prolonged rupture of membranes.
- Maternal pyrexia (>38°C).

Although the above are identified as risk factors, this does not suggest that immediate intrapartum antibiotic prophylaxis is required.

Maternal and fetal complications

Maternal:
- Preterm labour.
- Prolonged rupture of membranes.
- Maternal pyrexia (>38°C).
- Maternal infection (e.g. chorioamnionitis).

Fetal/neonatal:
- Late miscarriage.
- Stillbirth.
- Pneumonia.
- Sepsis.
- Meningitis.

Diagnosis – neonatal (Group B Strep Support, 2016) (see Figure 50.1)

- Lethargy.
- Reluctance to feed or intolerance of feed (e.g. vomiting).
- Low blood glucose.
- Irritability; seizure.
- Pyrexia >38°C or low body temperature <36°C.
- Tachycardia or bradycardia.
- Tachypnoea.
- Apnoea.
- ‘Grunting’; signs of respiratory distress.
- Hypoxia with central cyanosis and reduced oxygen saturation.

Management of maternal GBS infection

The management of potential infection caused by GBS falls into two areas (Hughes *et al.*, 2012):
- Prophylaxis – whether or not to offer prophylactic therapy.
- Treatment – when high risk situations are identified.

Prophylaxis – yes or no? (Hughes *et al.*, 2012)

- Screening for GBS. There is no evidence to support a national programme of routine, antenatal screening for all pregnant women (e.g. by taking a vaginal swab).
- If a woman has been diagnosed as GBS positive in a previous pregnancy, current evidence does not support either routine screening for GBS or the administration of prophylactic antibiotics.
- Incidental detection of GBS early in pregnancy does not warrant treatment with antibiotic therapy before the onset of labour.
- Women in preterm labour with intact membranes, with no known GBS colonisation, should not be offered intrapartum antibiotics.
- Women with preterm, prelabour rupture of membranes should not routinely be offered intrapartum antibiotic therapy.

Treatment (see Figure 50.2)

Maternal (NICE, 2016e)
- Women with a confirmed bacteriuria in pregnancy caused by GBS, should be offered treatment with antibiotics at the time of diagnosis as well as during the intrapartum period, as there is a higher risk of chorioamnionitis and subsequent neonatal disease.
- Intrapartum antibiotic therapy should be offered if GBS is detected on a vaginal swab.
- Spontaneous, prelabour rupture of membranes at >37 weeks gestation in a woman with known GBS colonisation should be offered immediate induction of labour and intrapartum antibiotic therapy.
- Maternal pyrexia >38°C – women should be offered a broad-spectrum antibiotic to reduce the risk of early-onset GBS disease in the neonate.
- If a woman has previously given birth to a baby affected by GBS disease, it is recommended that she is offered intrapartum antibiotics as there appears to be an increased risk of GBS disease to subsequent offspring.

Neonatal (Hughes *et al.*, 2012)

- Infants who are well but at risk of early-onset GBS disease should be observed for 12–24 hours after birth. Observations include heart rate, respiratory rate, temperature, quality of feeding and the general wellbeing of the infant.
- Before commencing antibiotic therapy, blood culture and sampling of cerebrospinal fluid should be undertaken.
- Infants demonstrating signs of early-onset GBS disease should be treated promptly with a narrow-spectrum antibiotic such as gentamicin, benzylpenicillin, etc.
- If an infant has a sibling previously treated for GBS disease, its condition should be assessed postpartum and observed for 24 hours. However, another option might be to obtain blood cultures and commence prophylactic antibiotics until the result of the blood culture analysis has been received.

51 Infection control

Figure 51.1 The stages of hand washing or gel application. Source: Campbell & Dolby (2018).

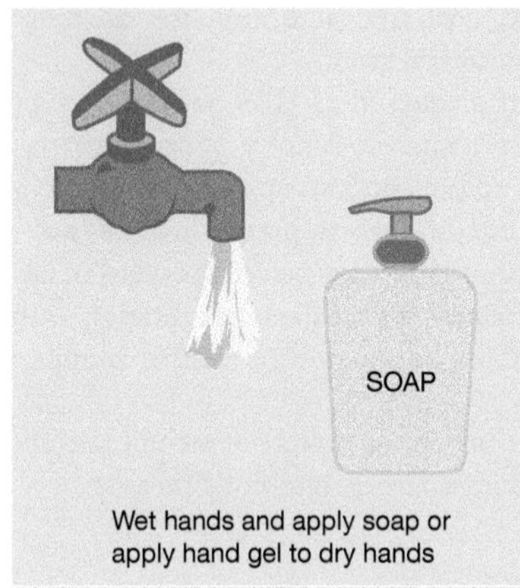

Wet hands and apply soap or apply hand gel to dry hands

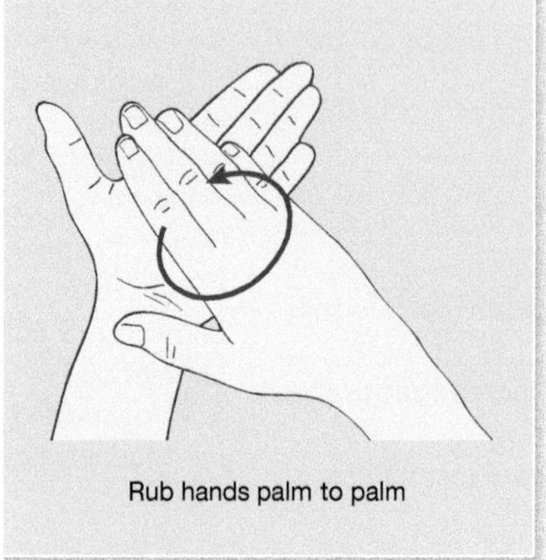

Rub hands palm to palm

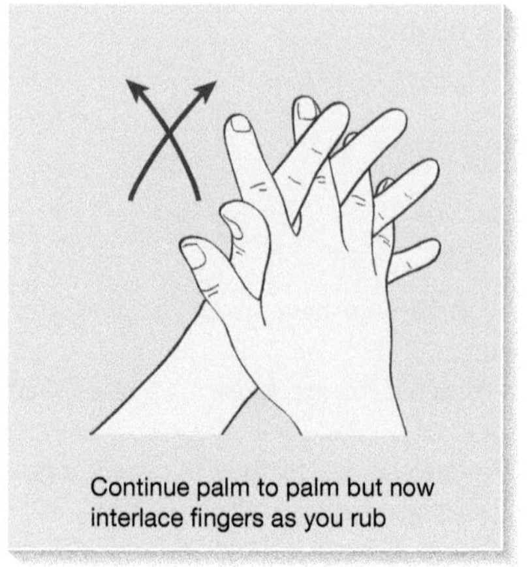

Continue palm to palm but now interlace fingers as you rub

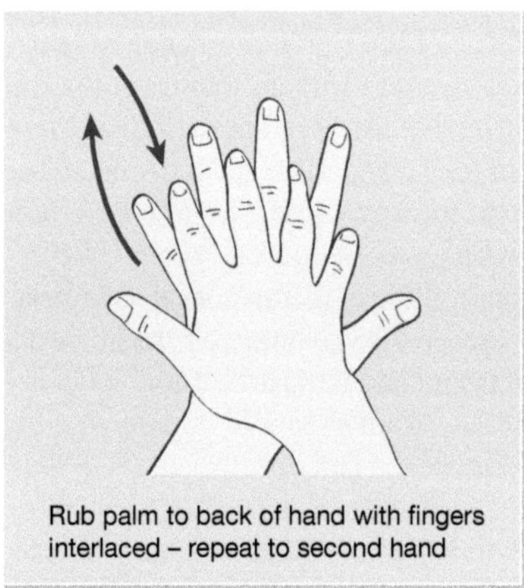

Rub palm to back of hand with fingers interlaced – repeat to second hand

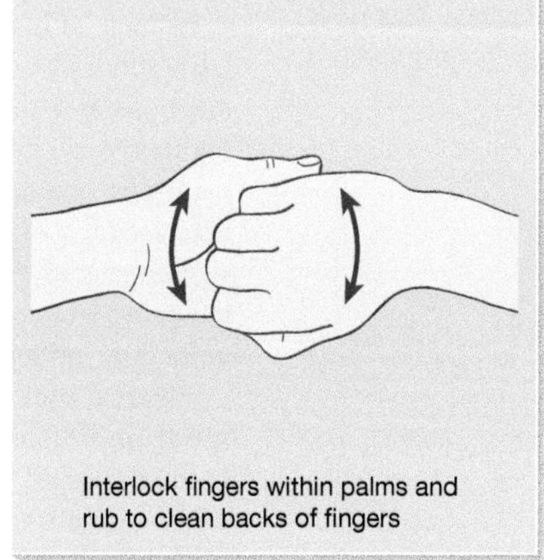

Interlock fingers within palms and rub to clean backs of fingers

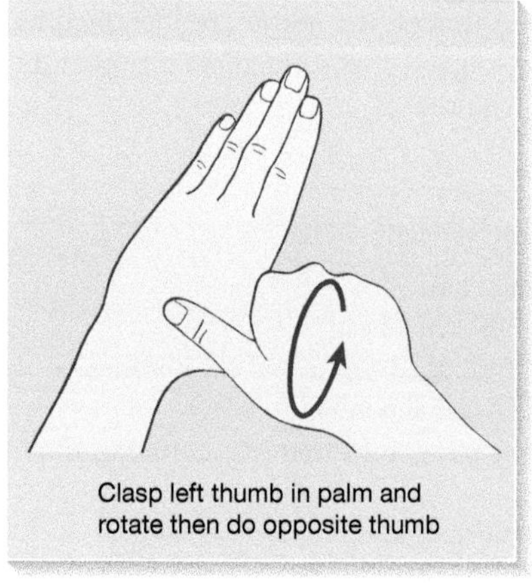

Clasp left thumb in palm and rotate then do opposite thumb

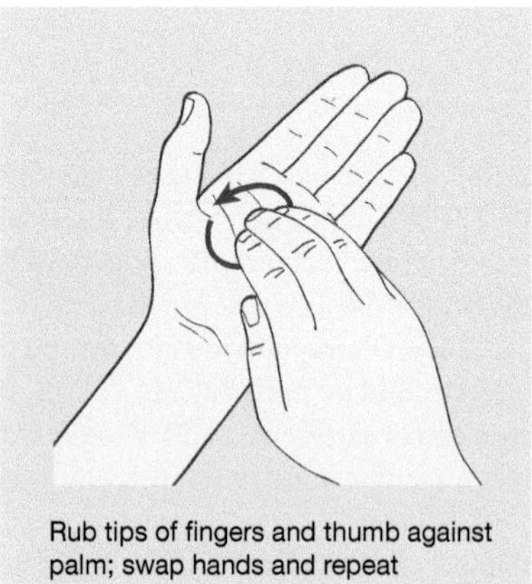

Rub tips of fingers and thumb against palm; swap hands and repeat

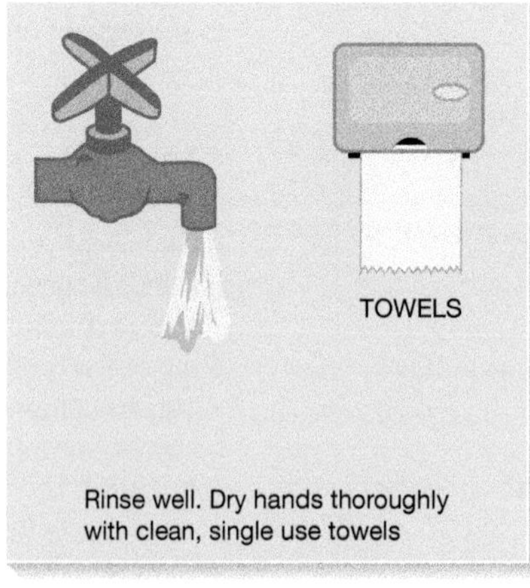

Rinse well. Dry hands thoroughly with clean, single use towels

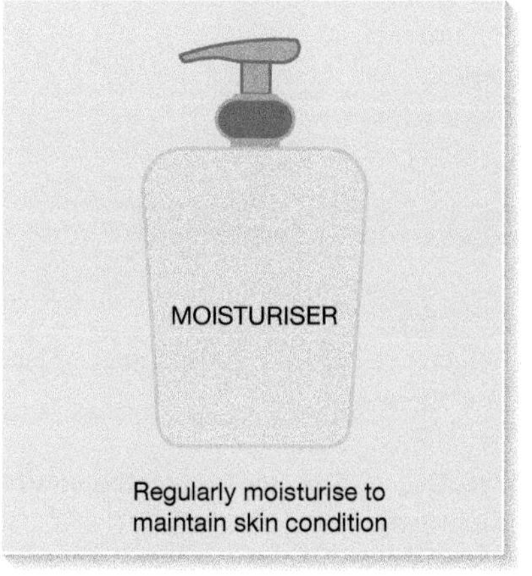

Regularly moisturise to maintain skin condition

This chapter considers the infection control responsibilities of all professionals involved in performing care. They have a duty to:

- Ensure that they do not introduce infection.
- Identify infection already present.
- Initiate appropriate treatment of any infection including senior review and antibiotic therapy.
- Control against spread of infection.
- Participate in the education of women and their families.
- Lead by example.

Infection risks

The risk of a health care-associated infection (HCAI) during a hospital stay is between 5 and 15% within developed countries, rising to as high as 19% in less developed countries. The risk increases further for higher risk women and those infants born prematurely or admitted to intensive care facilities (WHO, 2009). A number of factors increase infection risk:

- Increased levels of bacteria within hospital environments – airborne and carried by staff and equipment.
- Lowered resistance for newborns.
- Exposure as a fetus (e.g. via prolonged rupture of membranes).
- Increased maternal infection risk due to anaemia or operative delivery, for example.
- Close proximity within maternity wards increasing risk of spread.
- Sharing of equipment.
- Warm atmosphere allowing bacteria to multiply.
- High visitor numbers.
- Increased likelihood of body fluid exposure.

Infection prevention

Infection prevention is enhanced through an understanding of how infection may be transmitted during emergency procedures and the standard precautions which reduce this occurrence. The value of decontamination during hand hygiene was first appreciated by Ignaz Semmelweis in 1847. He was investigating considerably higher levels of puerperal fever in the clinic visited by medical students, compared with one which was run solely by midwives. His breakthrough came when a colleague was accidentally cut by a medical students' scalpel during a postmortem and died displaying the symptoms of puerperal fever. He realised that medical students were carrying infective body particles from the postmortem (despite hand washing). He escalated hand washing to include chlorinated lime, with an immediate 90% reduction in mortality rates. Sadly, his criticism of the hygiene of the medical profession and the lack of evidence for his theories lost him his career (and in time his mental health too). Louis Pasteur later provided evidence for all that Semmelweis had described and called it antisepsis, offering his own detailed theories concerning germs and disease.

Hand decontamination

Two categories of bacteria commonly exist on the hands – resident and transient (WHO, 2009). Transient bacteria are more likely to be responsible for cross-infection but are also more responsive to hand hygiene (WHO, 2009). The WHO (2009) Guidelines on Hand Hygiene in Health Care suggest that each mother and baby should be treated as a single patient zone and advocate five points at which hand hygiene is required. These are listed below with examples of how they should be applied during the physical examination:

1. **Before patient contact** – on entering the room.
2. **Before aseptic tasks.**
3. **After body fluid exposure risk.**
4. **After patient contact.**
5. **After contact with patient surroundings** – apply hand gel outside the door before moving on to a new task. In any situation of source isolation nursing or known infection risk, fully wash the hands.

The stages of hand washing or the application of alcohol gel are illustrated in Figure 51.1. A gel hand rub can only be used if the hands are clean. For some routine, non-invasive procedures (e.g. abdominal palpation, assessing vital signs) gloves are not normally required, but even this should be reconsidered on an individual basis for any additional potential risk (in which case a plastic apron should also be worn to protect clothing). For all emergency delivery management and aseptic procedures, gloves and plastic aprons should be worn. For all operative deliveries and some other theatre procedures, sterile gowns and masks are also worn to further enhance aseptic management.

Hand care

Hands should be examined daily for signs of broken skin, inflammation or torn cuticles (NICE, 2012b). Moisturising prevents drying and cracking from frequent hand washing and alcohol gel use. Nails must be short, smoothly filed and free from nail varnish, extensions or additions. A flat ring band does not prevent good hand hygiene but clothing below the elbow and all other jewellery (including watches) can both contaminate and interfere with washing and so should be removed (Hautemaniere *et al.*, 2010).

Signs of infection

Early identification enables appropriate management for the health of the woman and infant as well as prevention of spread. The reviewed history and risk factors will act as indicators and include:

- Drowsiness, lethargy and general malaise.
- Inflammation, redness or an area of localised pain or heat.
- Localised serous fluid or a purulent exudate.
- Vomiting and/or diarrhoea.
- Systemic temperature raised above 38°C, lower then 36°C or, being unstable.
- Increased or reduced respirations.
- An area of swelling and/or pain and tenderness.
- Bradycardia or tachycardia.
- Unusually blood-stained or purulent body fluid (e.g. urine or sputum).
- Increased and/or offensive lochia postpartum.

Additionally, the newborn may experience:

- Reduced responsiveness and/or lack of tone.
- Poor feeding.
- Jitteriness or seizures.
- Jaundice.
- Apnoea or shock.
- Respiratory distress.

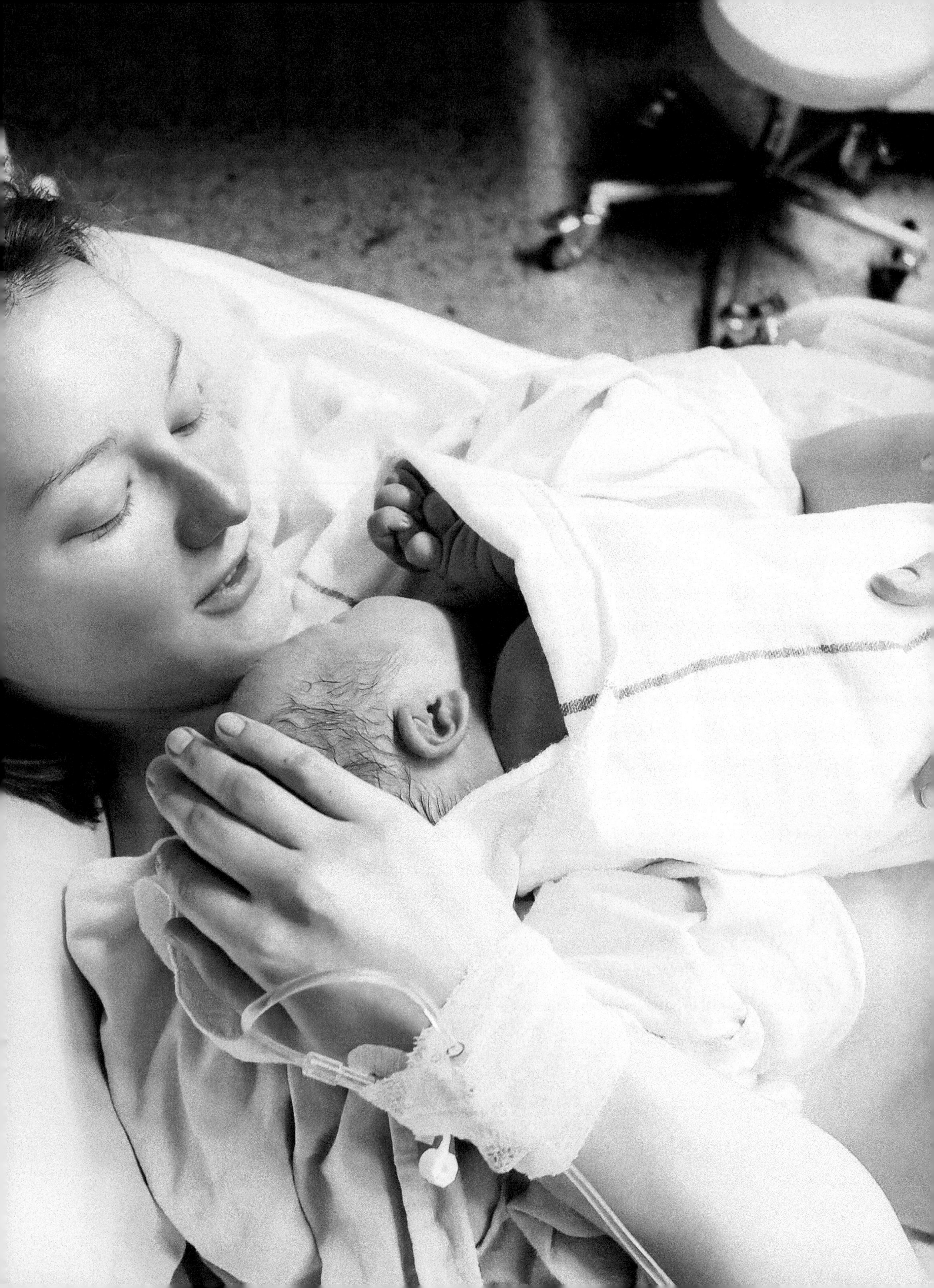

Self-assessment

Chapters

Section 19 Revision and self-assessment

Multiple choice questions 114

Multiple choice answers 120

Multiple choice questions

Chapter 3 Maternal resuscitation

1 **How many women died between 2011 and 2013 due to direct/indirect causes?**
A 147
B 200
C 214
D 260

2 **Which of the following can complicate the resuscitation of a pregnant woman?**
A Aortocaval compression/occlusion
B Relaxation of the cardiac sphincter
C Nasal and pharyngeal oedema
D All of the above

3 **During the initial assessment what is the rescuer looking, listening and feeling for?**
A Fetal movements
B Evidence of breathing
C Oedema of the glottis
D Oedema and movement of the lower extremities

4 **Approximately how much of the woman's total blood volume can be sequestered in the lower limbs during aortocaval compression?**
A 30%
B 20%
C 15%
D 10%

5 **How quickly should chest compressions be delivered?**
A 60–80 compressions per minute
B 80–100 compressions per minute
C 100–120 compressions per minute
D 120–140 compressions per minute

6 **To what depth should chest compressions be administered?**
A 4–5 cm
B 5–6 cm
C 6–7 cm
D No specified depth

7 **What is the ratio of chest compressions to rescue breaths?**
A 30 compressions to 2 breaths
B 15 compressions to 2 breaths
C 3 compressions to 1 breath
D 30 compressions to 1 breaths

8 **A perimortem Caesarean section should be performed within how many minutes of the decision to resuscitate?**
A 5 minutes
B 3 minutes
C 4 minutes
D 6 minutes

9 **Which of the following statements is true re: the use of an automated external defibrillator (AED)?**
A An AED can be used on a pregnant woman
B An AED can be used with caution when it is wet or raining
C An accidental shock cannot be administered
D All of the above

10 **When should efforts to resuscitate the woman cease?**
A When spontaneous respirations occur
B When spontaneous movement is seen
C When instructed by a senior member of staff
D Any of the above

Chapter 4 Neonatal resuscitation

1 **Which of the following might predispose a newborn infant to require support at birth?**
A Recent maternal sedation
B Precipitate delivery
C Obstetric emergency
D All of the above

2 **Which four elements are assessed regularly throughout the resuscitation?**
A Heart rate, respiratory effort, weight, blood glucose level
B Heart rate, respiratory effort, pupil reaction, Moro reflex
C Heart rate, respiratory effort, colour, tone
D Heart rate, respiratory effort, colour, reflexes

3 **Why is it important to dry the neonate?**
A To stimulate the baby to take a breath
B To dry the baby and prevent radiant heat loss
C To maintain the baby's temperature between 36.5°C and 37.5°C
D All of the above

4 **What position should the neonate's head be in to aid resuscitation?**
A Neutral position
B Extended position
C Flexed position
D Lateral position

5 **What is the purpose of the inflation breaths?**
A To remove the amniotic fluid in the alveoli in the lungs of the neonate and back-fill with air
B To maintain ventilation of the lungs
C To make the baby take a breath
D To open the airway

6 Approximately how much fluid may be present in the alveoli after birth in a term baby?

A 10–20 mL
B 30–50 mL
C 60–90 mL
D 100–150 mL

7 How frequently would you assess the baby's condition?

A Every 20 seconds
B Every 30 seconds
C Every 45 seconds
D Every 60 seconds

8 When is it appropriate to commence chest compressions?

A If the heart rate is below 60 beats per minute and you have seen the chest rise
B If the heart rate is below 60 beats per minute and you have not seen the chest rise
C If the heart rate is below 60 beats per minute, if you have seen the chest rise and if 30 seconds of ventilation breaths have been given
D If the chest has risen and if the heart rate is above 90 beats per minute

9 What is the acceptable preductal SpO_2 in a term baby at 3 minutes of age?

A 60%
B 70%
C 80%
D 90%

10 What drugs are likely to be used should the neonate require pharmacological support?

A Sodium bicarbonate 4.2% (1–2 mmol per kg); adrenaline 1 in 10 000 solution (10 mcg per kg); dextrose 10% (2.5 mL per kg)
B Sodium bicarbonate 4.2% (5 mmol per kg); adrenaline 1 in 10 000 solution (10 mcg per kg); dextrose 10% (2.5 mL per kg)
C Sodium bicarbonate 4.2% (1–2 mmol per kg); adrenaline 1 in 10 000 solution (5 mcg per kg); dextrose 10% (2.5 mL per kg)
D Sodium bicarbonate 4.2% (1–2 mmol per kg; adrenaline 1 in 10 000 solution (10 mcg per kg); dextrose 5% (2.5 mL per kg)

Chapter 5 Antepartum haemorrhage

1 Antepartum haemorrhage is defined as:

A Bleeding from the gastrointestinal tract after 24 weeks' gestation and before the birth of the baby
B Bleeding from the genital tract during the first trimester of pregnancy
C Bleeding from the genital tract after 24 weeks' gestation and before the birth of the baby
D A blood loss from the genital tract of an amount greater than 500 ml

2 Which is a predisposing factor for antepartum haemorrhage caused by placental abruption?

A Maternal cardiac conditions
B Raised body mass index (BMI)
C Pre-eclampsia
D Gestational diabetes mellitus

3 Which is a predisposing factor for antepartum haemorrhage caused by placenta praevia?

A Teenage pregnancy
B Primigravid woman
C Intrauterine growth retardation
D Multiple pregnancy

4 From the possible complications arising from an antepartum haemorrhage, which one is incorrect?

A Postpartum haemorrhage
B Disseminated intravascular coagulation
C Diabetes mellitus
D Renal failure

5 Which presenting factor is not an indicator of uterine rupture?

A Fetal heart rate abnormalities
B Constant lower abdominal pain
C Vaginal bleeding
D Cord prolapse

6 What other differential diagnoses might present with similar symptoms?

A Acute polyhydramnios
B Chorioamnionitis
C Trauma to the maternal abdomen
D All of the above

7 Which of the following is not part of the role of the midwife?

A Reassure the woman and her partner
B Undertake an examination *per vaginam* to ascertain the cause of the bleeding
C Make a rapid referral as the woman's condition can deteriorate quickly
D Ascertain as much detail as possible regarding the history of the blood loss

8 Placenta praevia may be considered when:

A There is a lack of vaginal bleeding
B The abdomen feels 'board-like' on palpation
C The presenting part of the fetus is palpated above the pelvis and/or the lie is unstable
D The placenta is located in the upper segment of the uterus on ultrasound scanning

9 How would a woman present when experiencing a placental abruption?

A Anxious and in pain
B Relaxed
C Flushed
D Bradycardic

10 A concealed antepartum haemorrhage may lead to:

A The uterus feeling hard on palpation
B Difficulty in palpation of the fetus
C Auscultation of the fetal heart becoming difficult or impossible
D All of the above

Chapters 6 and 7 Postpartum haemorrhage

1 **From the list below of the causes and predisposing factors for primary postpartum haemorrhage which one is incorrect?**
A Genital tract sepsis
B Uterine atony
C Genital tract trauma
D Preterm labour

2 **From the list below of the causes and predisposing factors for primary postpartum haemorrhage which one is correct?**
A White ethnicity
B Mismanagement of the third stage of labour
C Active management of the third stage of labour
D Maternal haemoglobinopathy

3 **The most common cause of postpartum haemorrhage is:**
A Uterine atony
B Trauma to the genital tract
C Retained fragments of the placenta, membranes or retroplacental clot
D Maternal clotting disorder

4 **Which pharmacological treatment is not used to manage uterine atony?**
A Syntocinon 5–10 IU given IM
B Syntocinon 40 IU in 500 mL 0.9% sodium chloride IV infusion
C Syntometrine 1 mL given IM
D Ergometrine 10 mL IM

5 **Which statement is correct in relation to strategies that can be used to manage postpartum haemorrhage?**
A Fluid replacement to counteract hypovolaemia
B Use uterine massage to 'rub up' a contraction
C Oxytocic therapy to counteract uterine atony
D All of the above

6 **Which of the following correctly define the '4 Ts' which are used to categorise the causes of postpartum haemorrhage?**
A Tone, Trauma, Tissue, Thrombin
B Tears, Tone, Toxaemia, Turgidity
C Thrombin. Tissue, Timing, Tone
D Transfusion, Thrombin, Trauma, Tone

7 **In the MBRRACE Report (2014), how many women died as a result of postpartum haemorrhage?**
A 11 women
B 12 women
C 13 women
D 14 women

8 **Which of the following antenatal risk factors for postpartum haemorrhage is incorrect?**
A Asian ethnicity
B Antepartum haemorrhage
C Previous spontaneous vaginal delivery
D Macrosomic baby

9 **In seeking to prevent postpartum haemorrhage, which of the following statements is correct?**
A Correct maternal anaemia antenatally
B Encourage staff training in the management of emergency postpartum haemorrhage
C Identify any risk factors
D All of the above

10 **When alerting the massive obstetric haemorrhage (MOH) team, who is not expected to respond immediately?**
A Senior midwife
B Delivery suite cleaner
C Anaesthetist
D Senior obstetrician

Chapters 8 and 9 Malpositions in labour

1 **An occipito-posterior position occurs when:**
A The denominator is the mentum
B The vertex is deeply flexed
C The sinciput is posterior
D None of the above

2 **An occipito-posterior position is the commonest cause of:**
A Postpartum haemorrhage
B Precipitate delivery
C Prolonged labour and instrumental delivery
D Third degree perineal tears

3 **One of the predisposing factors for an occipito-posterior can be:**
A Anthropoid pelvic shape
B Gestational diabetes
C Posterior placenta
D Macrocephaly

4 **On abdominal palpation of an occipito-posterior position:**
A The presenting part often engages earlier in pregnancy
B A depression may be felt below the umbilicus
C The fetal heart is auscultated at the fundus
D It is harder to feel fetal movements

5 **Occipito-posterior position may be indicated on vaginal examination when:**
A The presenting part is low in the pelvis
B The anterior fontanelle is identified anteriorly
C The posterior fontanelle is easily identified
D The presenting part is well flexed

6 **The engaging diameter in an occipito-posterior position is the:**
A Mento vertical
B Sub-occipito bregmatic
C Sub-mento bregmatic
D Occipito-frontal

7 **Which of the following accurately describes the attitude of the fetal head during a face presentation?**
A Complete extension
B Neutral
C Well flexed
D None of the above

8 **Which of the following is not a predisposing factor for face presentation?**
A Prematurity
B Fetal abnormality
C Pre-eclampsia
D Polyhydramnios

9 **A face presentation can be identified on vaginal examination when:**
A Fresh meconium is seen on the examining finger
B The three prominent features are felt in a straight line
C The sagittal suture can be easily palpated
D The three prominent features form a triangle

10 **What are the possible outcomes of a term brow presentation?**
A Obstructed labour
B Increased flexion to face presentation
C Both of the above
D Neither of the above

Chapter 10 Breech presentations

1 **What is the incidence of breech presentation at 28 weeks?**
A 5%
B 10%
C 15%
D 20%

2 **What is the incidence of breech presentation at term?**
A 1–2%
B 3–4%
C 5–6%
D 7–8%

3 **Which of the following is not a predisposing factor for breech presentation?**
A Uterine myoma
B Placenta accreta
C Fetal chromosomal disorders
D Uterine deformities

4 **Which of the following is the most common breech presentation?**
A Flexed/complete/full breech
B Frank/extended breech
C Footling breech
D Incomplete breech

5 **Which of the following is typically required to deliver flexed arms?**
A Løvset's manoeuvre
B Modified Mauriceau–Smellie–Veit manoeuvre
C Burns–Marshall manoeuvre
D Masterly inactivity

6 **Which of the following does not indicate a possible breech presentation?**
A A hard, round ballotable mass felt at the fundus
B Fresh meconium on a gloved hand after vaginal examination
C Landmarks identified on vaginal examination being in a straight line
D Increased Braxton Hicks contractions

7 **Which complication is not associated with breech presentation?**
A Cord prolapse
B Postpartum haemorrhage
C Cephalhaematoma
D Increased fetal morbidity

8 **What is the aim of the Mauriceau–Smellie–Veit manoeuvre?**
A To flex the head as it passes through the pelvis
B To avoid an episiotomy
C To enable a grip on the baby to prevent it pulling on the cord at delivery
D To prevent the use of forceps to deliver the head

9 **Which of the following manoeuvres must not be used to assist delivery of the breech-presenting infant?**
A Løvset's
B Rotating the fetal back to be posterior within the pelvis
C Modified Mauriceau–Smellie–Veit
D Rotating the fetal back to be anterior within the pelvis

10 **Which of the following is an absolute contraindication to external cephalic version?**
A Previous postpartum haemorrhage
B Macrosomia
C Twin pregnancy
D Gestational diabetes

Chapter 11 Cord presentation or prolapse

1 **What is the incidence of cord prolapse when the vertex is the lowest fetal pole?**
A 0.5%
B 1%
C 0.2%
D 2%

2 **What is the incidence of cord prolapse when the breech is the lowest fetal pole?**
A 1%
B 1.5%
C 2%
D 2.5%

3 **What is the incidence of cord prolapse with twin pregnancies?**
A 2%
B 4%
C 6%
D 8%

4 **Which of the following is not a predisposing factor for cord prolapse?**
A Low-lying placenta
B Oligohydramnios
C Premature labour
D High presenting part

5 **Which of the following is not specifically associated with cord prolapse?**
A Small fetus
B Premature labour
C Polyhydramnios
D Intact membranes

6 **How might cord prolapse be recognised?**
A Felt by the woman
B Visible at introitus
C Felt on vaginal examination
D All of the above

7 **Which complication is not associated with cord prolapse?**
A Fetal compromise
B Fetal morbidity
C Fetal pyrexia
D Fetal death

8 **If the cord is visible outside the vagina you should:**
A Replace it back inside the vagina
B Use it throughout the management to check for the fetal heart
C Not touch it in any circumstance
D Cover it in a sterile towel immediately

9 **How might you reduce pressure on a cord presentation/ prolapse?**
A Maternal knee–chest or exaggerated Sims positioning
B Firm digital pressure on the lowest fetal pole
C Fill the bladder with saline solution
D All of the above

10 **Which of the following is not routine management?**
A Maternal oxygen
B Episiotomy to expedite delivery
C Vaginal examination
D Preparation for Caesarean section unless delivery imminent or known fetal demise

Chapter 12 Twins

1 **In the UK in 2013 how many pregnancies were associated with twins?**
A 1:40
B 1:65
C 1:100
D 1:250

2 **Is an identical twin pregnancy the result of monozygotic or dizygotic conception?**
A Monozygotic only
B Dizygotic only
C Both
D Neither

3 **What is the rate of monozygotic to dizygotic twins in the UK?**
A 1:1
B 1:2
C 1:3
D 1:4

4 **How long can safely be left to await delivery of the second twin?**
A Up to 10 minutes
B Up to 20 minutes
C Up to 30 minutes
D Up to 40 minutes

5 **Which of the following is not a predisposing factor to non-identical twins?**
A Fertility care
B Body shape
C Race
D Social group

6 **Artificial rupture of membranes for twin 2 should only be considered if:**
A Presentation is uncomplicated
B The presenting part is below the ischial spines
C Regular contractions are present
D All of the above are confirmed

7 **In which twin pregnancies are two amnions and two chorions present?**
A Monozygotic only
B Dizygotic only
C Both
D Neither

8 **In how many twin pregnancies does a vertex–vertex presentation occur at term?**
A 5%
B 9%
C 40%
D 45%

9 **What should the obstetrician consider if a transverse lie of the second twin is identified after vaginal delivery of twin 1?**
A Caesarean section delivery is the only option now possible
B External cephalic version or internal podalic version should be considered
C An episiotomy is required to increase outlet diameters
D Wait for 15 minutes and then reassess if lie has become longitudinal as a result of contractions

10 **Which of the following is the least likely complication of vaginal twin delivery?**
A Postpartum haemorrhage
B Placental abruption
C Third-degree perineal tear
D Compound presentation

Chapter 13 Shoulder dystocia

1 **Shoulder dystocia occurs in what percentage of births?**
A Less than 1%
B 3%
C 5%
D 10%

2 **Which of the following are not predisposing risk factors for shoulder dystocia?**
A Previous shoulder dystocia, previous large baby, maternal obesity
B Tall stature, advanced maternal age, high parity
C Short stature, teenage mother, preterm labour
D Diabetes mellitus, previous gestational diabetes mellitus, postmaturity

3 **Which is not an indicating factor for shoulder dystocia?**
A Prolonged second stage of labour
B Slow advance of the presenting part in the second stage of labour
C Following a slow birth, the fetal head recoils against the maternal perineum
D Rapid restitution of the baby's head after delivery

4 **Which of the following is the correct expansion of the mnemonic 'HELPERR'?**
A Help (call for); Evaluate for episiotomy; Legs (McRoberts manoeuvre); fundal Pressure; Enter manoeuvres; Remove anterior arm; Roll the woman onto 'all fours'
B Help (call for); Evaluate for episiotomy; Legs (McRoberts manoeuvre); Pressure – suprapubic; Enter manoeuvres (internal rotation); Remove posterior arm; Roll the woman onto "all fours"
C Help (call for); Elevate head of the bed; Legs (McRoberts manoeuvre); Pressure – suprapubic; Enter manoeuvres (internal rotation); Remove anterior arm; Roll the woman onto 'all fours'
D Help (call for); Evaluate for episiotomy; abduct Legs; fundal Pressure; Elevate head of the bed; Roll the woman onto 'all fours'

5 **The McRoberts manoeuvre involves the following action:**
A Application of fundal pressure
B Positioning the woman's legs so that they are hyperflexed against her abdomen
C Positioning the woman's legs so that her legs are abducted to an angle of 45°
D Placing the woman's feet on the hips of midwives standing on her left and on her right

6 **In relation to the baby's shoulders, external suprapubic pressure over the baby's anterior scapula is intended to achieve what?**
A Increased flexion of the baby's head
B Movement of the shoulders into the antero-posterior pelvic diameter
C Reduction of the bisacromial diameter by adducting the baby's shoulders
D Reduction of the bisacromial diameter by abducting the baby's shoulders

7 **Which of the following are not possible complications of shoulder dystocia for the woman?**
A High blood pressure, pelvic fracture, subfertility
B Postpartum haemorrhage
C Recto-vaginal fistula, uterine rupture
D Genital tract infection, post-traumatic stress

8 **Which is the correct statement in relation to the possible complications of shoulder dystocia for the neonate?**
A Brachial plexus injury/palsy
B Fractured clavicle and/or humerus
C Hypoxia/asphyxia leading to neurological damage
D All of the above

9 **Which of the following statements is correct in relation to possible last resort methods for shoulder dystocia?**
A Deliberate clavicle fracture
B The Zavanelli manoeuvre
C Symphysiotomy
D All of the above

10 **Which of the following has no evidence to recommend its use in the prevention of shoulder dystocia?**
A Careful weight control of the obese woman
B Induction of labour at term can reduce the incidence of shoulder dystocia in women with gestational diabetes
C Compulsory elective Caesarean section
D 'Deliver through'

Chapters 22 and 23 Eclampsia and pre-eclampsia

1 **Which is not a sign of fulminating pre-eclampsia?**
A Continuing rise in blood pressure
B Increasing protein urea
C Oliguria
D Left, lower quadrant, abdominal pain

2 **What is the accepted regime for magnesium sulphate administration?**
A Immediate intravenous (IV) loading dosage, followed by 4–6 hourly IV doses
B Immediate IV loading dosage, followed by 4–6 hourly oral doses
C Immediate IV loading dosage, followed by 4–6 hourly intramuscular doses
D Immediate IV loading dosage, followed by a maintenance infusion

3 **Which of the following is not immediate care of an eclamptic woman?**
A Calling for help
B Initiating cardiac massage
C Protecting against injury
D Placing her in the left lateral position

4 **Which of the following correctly details the presentation of pre-eclampsia?**
A Headaches and visual disturbances
B Epigastric pain and tenderness
C Proteinurea, oedema and hypertension
D All of the above

5 **Which of the following is not a complication of eclampsia?**
A Stroke
B Infection
C Seizure
D HELLP syndrome

6 In the immediate management of an eclamptic seizure which of the following would be a priority?

A Calling for help
B Darkening the room
C Inserting an airway
D Ensuring the tongue is not bitten

7 Which of the following is not a complication of pre-eclampsia for the fetus?

A Macrosomia
B Growth retardation
C Premature birth
D Death

8 Which of the following best describes eclampsia?

A A chronic condition in pregnancy including glycosuria, oedema and a history of pre-eclampsia
B An acute condition in a woman with pre-existing epileptic seizures
C An acute, life-threatening condition in pregnancy including neurological symptoms and seizures
D An acute, non-life-threatening condition in pregnancy including neurological symptoms and seizures

9 Which of the following statements reflect the MBRRACE (2016) report around eclampsia deaths?

A At the lowest ever recorded rate
B Static at present
C At the highest ever recorded rate
D Not recorded in this report

10 Which of the following best describes the clonic stage of a convulsion?

A Dissociation with surroundings
B Generalised muscle spasm
C Alternating muscle spasm and relaxation
D Continuous seizures

Multiple choice answers

Chapter 3 Maternal resuscitation

1 **How many women died between 2011 and 2013 due to direct/indirect causes?**
The correct answer is C.

2 **Which of the following can complicate the resuscitation of a pregnant woman?**
The correct answer is D.

3 **During the initial assessment what is the rescuer looking, listening and feeling for?**
The correct ansswer is B.

4 **Approximately how much of the woman's total blood volume can be sequestered in the lower limbs during aortocaval compression?**
The correct answer is A.

5 **How quickly should chest compressions be delivered?**
The correct answer is C.

6 **To what depth should chest compressions be administered?**
The correct answer is B.

7 **What is the ratio of chest compressions to rescue breaths?**
The correct answer is A.

8 **A perimortem Caesarean section should be performed within how many minutes of the decision to resuscitate?**
The correct answer is A.

9 **Which of the following statements is true re: the use of an automated external defibrillator (AED)?**
The correct answer is D.

10 **When should efforts to resuscitate the woman cease?**
The correct answer is D.

Chapter 4 Neonatal resuscitation

1 **Which of the following might predispose a newborn infant to require support at birth?**
The correct answer is D.

2 **Which four elements are assessed regularly throughout the resuscitation?**
The correct answer is C.

3 **Why is it important to dry the neonate?**
The correct answer is D.

4 **What position should the neonate's head be in to aid resuscitation?**
The correct answer is A.

5 **What is the purpose of the inflation breaths?**
The correct answer is A.

6 **Approximately how much fluid may be present in the alveoli after birth in a term baby?**
The correct answer is D.

7 **How frequently would you assess the baby's condition?**
The correct answer is B.

8 **When is it appropriate to commence chest compressions?**
The correct answer is C.

9 **What is the acceptable preductal SpO_2 in a term baby at 3 minutes of age?**
The correct answer is B.

10 **What drugs are likely to be used should the neonate require pharmacological support?**
The correct answer is A.

Chapter 5 Antepartum haemorrhage

1 **Antepartum haemorrhage is defined as:**
The correct answer is C.

2 **Which is a predisposing factor for antepartum haemorrhage caused by placental abruption?**
The correct answer is C.

3 **Which is a predisposing factor for antepartum haemorrhage caused by placenta praevia?**
The correct answer is D.

4 **From the possible complications arising from an antepartum haemorrhage, which one is incorrect?**
The correct answer is C.

5 **Which presenting factor is not an indicator of uterine rupture?**
The correct answer is D.

6 **What other differential diagnoses might present with similar symptoms?**
The correct answer is D.

7 **Which of the following is not part of the role of the midwife?**
The correct answer is B.

8 **Placenta praevia may be considered when:**
The correct answer is C.

9 **How would a woman present when experiencing a placental abruption?**
The correct answer is A.

10 **A concealed antepartum haemorrhage may lead to:**
The correct answer is D.

Midwifery Emergencies at a Glance, First Edition. Denise (Dee) Campbell and Susan M. Carr. Published 2018 by John Wiley & Sons, Ltd.
Companion website: www.ataglanceseries.com/midwiferyemergencies

Chapters 6 and 7 Postpartum haemorrhage

1 **From the list below of the causes and predisposing factors for primary postpartum haemorrhage which one is incorrect?**
The correct answer is D.

2 **From the list below of the causes and predisposing factors for primary postpartum haemorrhage which one is correct?**
The correct answer is B.

3 **The most common cause of postpartum haemorrhage is:**
The correct answer is A.

4 **Which pharmacological treatment is not used to manage uterine atony?**
The correct answer is D.

5 **Which statement is correct in relation to strategies that can be used to manage postpartum haemorrhage?**
The correct answer is D.

6 **Which of the following correctly define the '4 Ts' which are used to categorise the causes of postpartum haemorrhage?**
The correct answer is A.

7 **In the 2014 MBRRACE Report, how many women died as a result of postpartum haemorrhage?**
The correct answer is D.

8 **Which of the following antenatal risk factors for postpartum haemorrhage is incorrect?**
The correct answer is C.

9 **In seeking to prevent postpartum haemorrhage, which of the following statements is correct?**
The correct answer is D.

10 **When alerting the massive obstetric haemorrhage (MOH) team, who is not expected to respond immediately?**
The correct answer is B.

Chapters 8 and 9 Malpositions in labour

1 **An occipito-posterior position occurs when:**
The correct answer is D.

2 **An occipito-posterior position is the commonest cause of:**
The correct answer is C.

3 **One of the predisposing factors for an occipito-posterior can be:**
The correct answer is A.

4 **On abdominal palpation of an occipito-posterior position:**
The correct answer is B.

5 **Occipito-posterior position may be indicated on vaginal examination when:**
The correct answer is B.

6 **The engaging diameter in an occipito-posterior position is the:**
The correct answer is D.

7 **Which of the following accurately describes the attitude of the fetal head during a face presentation?**
The correct answer is A.

8 **Which of the following is not a predisposing factor for face presentation?**
The correct answer is C.

9 **A face presentation can be identified on vaginal examination when:**
The correct answer is D.

10 **What are the possible outcomes of a term brow presentation?**
The correct answer is C.

Chapter 10 Breech presentations

1 **What is the incidence of breech presentation at 28 weeks?**
The correct answer is D

2 **What is the incidence of breech presentation at term?**
The correct answer is B

3 **Which of the following is not a predisposing factor for breech presentation?**
The correct answer is C.

4 **Which of the following is the most common breech presentation?**
The correct answer is B.

5 **Which of the following is typically required to deliver flexed arms?**
The correct answer is D.

6 **Which of the following does not indicate a possible breech presentation?**
The correct answer is D.

7 **Which complication is not associated with breech presentation?**
The correct answer is C.

8 **What is the aim of the Mauriceau–Smellie–Veit manoeuvre?**
The correct answer is A.

9 **Which of the following manoeuvres must not be used to assist delivery of the breech-presenting infant?**
The correct answer is B.

10 **Which of the following is an absolute contraindication to external cephalic version?**
The correct answer is C.

Chapter 11 Cord presentation or prolapse

1 **What is the incidence of cord prolapse when the vertex is the lowest fetal pole?**
The correct answer is A.

2 **What is the incidence of cord prolapse when the breech is the lowest fetal pole?**
The correct answer is C.

3 **What is the incidence of cord prolapse with twin pregnancies?**
The correct answer is B.

4 **Which of the following is not a predisposing factor for cord prolapse?**
The correct answer is B.

5 **Which of the following is not specifically associated with cord prolapse?**
The correct answer is D

6 **How might cord prolapse be recognised?**
The correct answer is D.

7 **Which complication is not associated with cord prolapse?**
The correct answer is C.

8 **If the cord is visible outside the vagina you should:**
The correct answer is A.

9 **How might you reduce pressure on a cord presentation/ prolapse?**
The correct answer is D

10 **Which of the following is not routine management?**
The correct answer is B.

Chapter 12 Twins

1 **In the UK in 2013 how many pregnancies were associated with twins?**
The correct answer is B.

2 **Is an identical twin pregnancy the result of monozygotic or dizygotic conception?**
The correct answer is A.

3 **What is the rate of monozygotic to dizygotic twins in the UK?**
The correct answer is C.

4 **How long can safely be left to await delivery of the second twin?**
The correct answer is C

5 **Which of the following is not a predisposing factor to non-identical twins?**
The correct answer is D.

6 **Artificial rupture of membranes for twin 2 should only be considered if:**
The correct answer is D.

7 **In which twin pregnancies are two amnions and two chorions present?**
The correct answer is C.

8 **In how many twin pregnancies does a vertex–vertex presentation occur at term?**
The correct answer is D.

9 **What should the obstetrician consider if a transverse lie of the second twin is identified after vaginal delivery of twin 1?**
The correct answer is C.

10 **Which of the following is the least likely complication of vaginal twin delivery?**
The correct answer is D.

Chapter 13 Shoulder dystocia

1 **Shoulder dystocia occurs in what percentage of births?**
The correct answer is A.

2 **Which of the following are not predisposing risk factors for shoulder dystocia?**
The correct answer is C.

3 **Which is not an indicating factor for shoulder dystocia?**
The correct answer is D.

4 **Which of the following is the correct expansion of the mnemonic 'HELPERR'?**
The correct answer is B.

5 **The McRoberts manoeuvre involves the following action:**
The correct answer is B.

6 **In relation to the baby's shoulders, external suprapubic pressure over the baby's anterior scapula is intended to achieve what?**
The correct answer is C.

7 **Which of the following are not possible complications of shoulder dystocia for the woman?**
The correct answer is A.

8 **Which is the correct statement in relation to the possible complications of shoulder dystocia for the neonate?**
The correct answer is D.

9 **Which of the following statements is correct in relation to possible last resort methods for shoulder dystocia?**
The correct answer is D.

10 **Which of the following has no evidence to recommend its use in the prevention of shoulder dystocia?**
The correct answer is C.

Chapters 22 and 23 Eclampsia and pre-eclampsia

1 **Which is not a sign of fulminating pre-eclampsia?**
The correct answer is D.

2 **What is the accepted regime for magnesium sulphate administration?**
The correct answer is D.

3 **Which of the following is not immediate care of an eclamptic woman?**
The correct answer is B.

4 **Which of the following correctly details the presentation of pre-eclampsia?**
The correct answer is D.

5 **Which of the following is not a complication of eclampsia?**
The correct answer is B.

6 **In the immediate management of an eclamptic seizure which of the following would be a priority?**
The correct answer is A.

7 **Which of the following is not a complication of pre-eclampsia for the fetus?**
The correct answer is A.

8 **Which of the following best describes eclampsia?**
The correct answer is C.

9 **Which of the following statements reflect the MBRRACE (2016) report around eclampsia deaths?**
The correct answer is A.

10 **Which of the following best describes the clonic stage of a convulsion?**
The correct answer is C.

References

Abdel-Aleem, H., Shaaban, O.M. & Abdel-Aleem, M.A. (2013) Cervical pessary for preventing preterm birth. *Cochrane Database of Systematic Reviews*, Issue 5. Art. No.: CD007873. doi: 10.1002/14651858.CD007873.pub3.

Alfirevic, Z., Stampalija, T., Roberts, D. & Jorgensen, A.L. (2012) Cervical stitch (cerclage) for preventing preterm birth in singleton pregnancy. *Cochrane Database of Systematic Reviews*, Issue 4. Art. No.: CD008991. doi: 10.1002/14651858.CD008991 .pub2.

American College of Obstetricians and Gynaecologists (2012) *Placenta Accreta*. Committee opinion No. 529. July. Reaffirmed 2015. ACOG Retrieved April 5, 2018 from http://www.acog.org/Resources-And-Publications/Committee-Opinions/Committee-on-Obstetric-Practice/Placenta-Accreta#3

American Psychiatric Association (APA) (2013) *Diagnostic and Statistical Manual of Mental Disorders (DSM-5)*, 5th edn. Washington DC: APA.

Amos, T., Stein, D.J. &; Ipser, J.C. (2014) Pharmacological interventions for preventing post-traumatic stress disorder (PTSD). *Cochrane Database of Systematic Reviews*, Issue 7. Art. No.: CD006239. doi: 10.1002/14651858.CD006239.pub2.

Andersen, L.B. *et al.* (2012) Risk factors for developing post-traumatic stress disorder following childbirth: a systematic review. *Acta Obstetrica et Gynecologica Scandinavica*, 91, 1261–1272. doi: http://dx.doi.org/10.1111/j.1600-0412.2012.01476.x.

Ayers, S. *et al.* (2016) The aetiology of post-traumatic stress following childbirth: a meta-analysis and theoretical framework. *Psychological Medicine*, 46, 1121–1134. doi: http://dx.doi .org/10.1017/S0033291715002706.

Bahl, R., Strachan, B.K. & Murphy, D.J. (2011) *Operative Vaginal Delivery. Green Top Guideline no 26*, 3rd edn. London: Royal College of Obstetricians and Gynaecologists.

Banfield, P. & Roberts, C. (2015) The early detection of maternal deterioration in pregnancy. *The Health Foundation. Inspiring Improvement.* Retrieved April 5, 2018 from http://patientsafety .health.org.uk/resources/early-detection-of-maternal-deterioration-pregnancy

Barr, J.A. & Beck, C.T. (2008) Infanticide secrets: qualitative study on postpartum depression. *Canadian Family Physician*, 54, 1716–1717.

Bastos, M.H. *et al.* (2015) Debriefing interventions for the prevention of psychological trauma in women following childbirth. *Cochrane Database of Systematic Reviews*, Issue 4. Art. No.: CD007194. doi: 10.1002/14651858.CD007194.pub2.

Berg, C.J. *et al.* (2010) Pregnancy related mortality in the United States, 1998–2005. *Obstet Gynaecol* 116, 1302–1309. doi: http://dx.doi.org/10.1097/AOG.0b013e3181fdfb11.

Bergink, V. *et al.* (2012) Prevention of postpartum psychosis and mania in women at high risk. *The American Journal of Psychiatry*, 169, 609–615. doi: 10.1176/appi.ajp.2012.11071047.

Bergink, V. *et al.* (2015) Treatment of psychosis and mania in the postpartum period. *The American Journal of Psychiatry*, 172, 115–123. doi: 10.1176/appi.ajp.2014.13121652.

Bick, D.E. *et al.* (2012) How good are we at implementing evidence to support the management of birth related perineal trauma? A UK wide survey of midwifery practice. *Bio Med Central. Pregnancy and Childbirth*, 12, 57. doi: http://doi.org/10.1186/1471-2393-12-57.

Birth Stats NSW (2018) Birth complications: perineal tears. Retrieved April 5, 2018 from http://www.healthstats.nsw.gov.au/Indicator/mab_pnspvbth_cat/mab_pnspvbth_cat_hos

Bisson, J.I. *et al.* (2013) Psychological therapies for chronic post-traumatic stress disorder (PTSD) in adults. *Cochrane Database of Systematic Reviews*. Issue 12. Art. No.: CD003388. doi: 10.1002/14651858.CD003388.pub4.

Bolton-Maggs, P. on behalf of the Serious Hazards of Transfusion (SHOT) Steering Group. (2016) *The 2015 Annual SHOT Report (2016)*. Manchester: SHOT.

British HIV Association (2014) British HIV Association guidelines for the management of HIV infection in pregnant women 2012 (2014 interim review). *HIV Medicine*, 15 (Supplement 4), 1–77. doi: 10.1111/hiv.12185.

Buchanan, S.L. *et al.* (2010) Planned early birth versus expectant management for women with preterm prelabour rupture of membranes prior to 37 weeks' gestation for improving pregnancy outcome. *Cochrane Database of Systematic Reviews*. Issue 3. doi: 10.1002/14651858.CD004735.pub3.

Buckley, S. (2004) Undisturbed birth – nature's hormonal blueprint for safety, ease and ecstasy. *MIDIRS*, 14, 203–209.

Campbell, D. (Dee) and Dolby, E. (2018) *Physical Examination of the Newborn at a Glance*. Chichester: John Wiley & Sons, Ltd.

Cantwell, R. *et al.* on behalf of the MBRRACE-UK mental health chapter writing group. (2015) Lessons on maternal mental health. In: Knight, M. *et al.* (eds) *Saving Lives, Improving Mothers' Care – Surveillance of maternal deaths in the UK 2011–13 and lessons learned to inform maternity care from the UK and Ireland Confidential Enquiries into Maternal Deaths and Morbidity 2009–13*. Oxford: National Perinatal Epidemiology Unit, pp. 22–41.

Carrol, F. *et al.* (2016) Patterns of maternity care in English NHS trusts 2013/2014. RCOG. Retrieved April 5, 2018 from https://www.rcog.org.uk/globalassets/documents/guidelines/research–audit/maternity-indicators-2013-14_report2.pdf

Chavan, R. & Latoo, M. (2013) Recent advances in the management of major obstetric haemorrhage. *British Journal of Medical Practitioners*, 6, a604.

Chongsomchai, C., Lumbiganon, P. & Laopaiboon, M. (2014) Prophylactic antibiotics for manual removal of retained placenta in vaginal birth. *Cochrane Database of Systematic Reviews*, Issue 10. Art. No.: CD004904. doi: 10.1002/14651858.CD004904.pub3.

Cloitre, M. *et al.* (2012) The ISTSS Expert Consensus Treatment Guidelines for Complex PTSD in Adults. Retrieved April 5, 2018 from http://www.istss.org/ISTSS_Main/media/Documents/ComplexPTSD.pdf

College of Operating Department Practitioners (CODP), Royal College of Midwives (RCM) & Association for Perioperative

Practice (AfPP) (2009) *Staffing of Obstetric Theatres – A Consensus Statement*. London: CODP. RCM. AfPP.

Cox, J.L., Holden, J.M. & Sagovsky, R. (1987) Detection of postnatal depression development of the 10-item Edinburgh Postnatal Depression Scale. *British Journal of Psychiatry*, 150, 782–786.

Crofts, J. *et al.* (2012) *Shoulder Dystocia. Green Top Guideline No. 42*. London: Royal College of Obstetricians and Gynaecologists.

Crowther, C.A. *et al.* (2015) Repeat doses of prenatal corticosteroids for women at risk of preterm birth for improving neonatal health outcomes. *Cochrane Database of Systematic Reviews*, Issue 6. doi: 10.1002/14651858.CD003935.pub4.

Cummings, K. *et al.* (2016) Timing of manual placenta removal to prevent postpartum hemorrhage: is it time to act? *Journal of Maternal-Fetal and Neonatal Medicine*, 29, 3930–3933. doi: 10.3109/14767058.2016.1154941.

Cunningham, F.G. *et al.* (2014) *Williams Obstetrics*, 24th edn. London: McGraw Hill Education.

Davey, M.A. *et al.* (2015) Risk-scoring systems for predicting preterm birth with the aim of reducing associated adverse outcomes. *Cochrane Database of Systematic Reviews*, Issue 10. Art. No.: CD004902. doi: 10.1002/14651858.CD004902.pub5.

Dawn, R., Hostetler, M. & Bosworth, D. (2000) Uterine inversion: a life-threatening obstetric emergency. *Journal of the American Board of Family Medicine*, 13, 120–123.

Dedhia, J. & Mushambi, M. (2007) Amniotic fluid embolism. *Continuing Education in Anaesthesia, Critical Care & Pain*, 7, 152–156.

Dekker, G. (2010) Hypertension. In: James, D.K. *et al.* (eds) *High Risk Pregnancy Management Options*, 4th edn. Philadelphia: Elsevier Saunders, pp. 997–1010.

Dougherty, L., Lister, S. & West-Oram, A. (2015) *The Royal Marsden Manual of Clinical Nursing Procedures*, 9th edn. Oxford: Wiley Blackwell.

Dudley, L.M., Kettle, C. & Ismail, K.M.K. (2011) Secondary suturing compared to non-suturing for broken down perineal wounds following childbirth. *Cochrane Database of Systematic Reviews*, Issue 2. Art. No.: CD008977. doi: 10.1002/14651858. CD008977.

Duffy, J.M. *et al.* (2015) Pharmacologic intervention for retained placenta: a systematic review and meta-analysis. *Obstetrics and Gynecology*, 125, 711–718. doi: 10.1097/ AOG.0000000000000697.

East, C.E. *et al.* & On behalf of The Flamingo Study Group. (2015a) Protocol for a randomised controlled trial of fetal scalp blood lactate measurement to reduce caesarean sections during labour: the Flamingo trial. [ACTRN12611000172909]. *BMC Pregnancy and Childbirth*, 15(285). doi: 10.1186/s12884-015-0709-7.

East, C.E. *et al.* (2015b) Intrapartum fetal scalp lactate sampling for fetal assessment in the presence of a non-reassuring fetal heart rate trace. *Cochrane Database of Systematic Reviews*, Issue 5. Art. No.: CD006174. doi: 10.1002/14651858.CD006174.pub3.

Eclampsia Trial Collaborative Group (1995) Which anticonvulsant for women with eclampsia? Evidence from the Collaborative Eclampsia Trial. *Lancet*, 345(8963), 1455–1463.

Elharmeel, S. *et al.* (2011) Surgical repair of spontaneous perineal tears that occur during childbirth versus no intervention. *Cochrane Database of Systematic Reviews*, Issue 8. doi: 10.1002/14651858.CD008534.pub2.

El Senoun, G.A., Dowswell, T. & Mousa, H.A. (2014) Planned home versus hospital care for preterm prelabour rupture of the membranes (PPROM) prior to 37 weeks' gestation. *Cochrane Database of Systematic Reviews. Cochrane Pregnancy and Childbirth Group*. doi: 10.1002/14651858.CD008053.pub3.

Erez, O., Mastrolia, S. & Thachil, J. (2015) Disseminated intravascular coagulation in pregnancy: insights in pathophysiology, diagnosis and management. *American Journal of Obstetrics and Gynaecology*, 213, 452–463.

Essali, A. *et al.* (2013) Preventative interventions for post natal psychosis (Review). *Cochrane* Database of Systematic Reviews. The *Cochrane* Collaboration. doi: 0.1002/14651858.CD009991.pub2.

Evensen, A. & Anderson, J. (2017). Postpartum haemorrhage. In Leeman, L., Quinlan, J., Dresang, L., & Gregory, D. (Eds.). *ALSO Provider Manual*. (Ch. J. pp1–16). Leawood: American Academy of Family Physicians.

Fernando, R.J. *et al.* (2013) Methods of repair for obstetric anal sphincter injury. *Cochrane Database of Systematic Reviews*, Issue 12. Art. No.: CD002866. doi: 10.1002/14651858.CD002866 .pub3.

Fernando, R.J. *et al.* (2015) *The management of Third- and Fourth-degree Perineal Tears. Green Top Guideline No. 29*. Retrieved April 5, 2018 from https://www.rcog.org.uk/en/guidelines-research-services/guidelines/gtg29/

Fitzpatrick, K.E. *et al.* (2012a) Uterine rupture by intended mode of delivery in the UK: a National Case-Control Study. *PLOS Medicine*, 9, e1001184. doi: 10.1371/journal. pmed.1001184.

Fitzpatrick, K.E. *et al.* (2012b) Incidence and risk factors for placenta accrete/increta/percreta in the UK: a National case-control study. *PLOS ONE*, 7, e52893.

Fitzpatrick, K.E. *et al.* (2014) The management and outcomes of placenta accreta, increta, and percreta in the UK: a population-based descriptive study. *British Journal of Obstetrics and Gynaecology*, 121, 62–71.

Frank, J., Baeseman, Z. & Leeman, L. (2017). Vaginal bleeding in late pregnancy. In Leeman, L., Quinlan, J., Dresang, L., & Gregory, D. (Eds.). *ALSO Provider Manual*. (Ch. C. pp1–14). Leawood: American Academy of Family Physicians.

Fung, A. (2015) Preterm labour including cervical insufficiency. In: Permezel, M., Walker, S. & Kyprianou, K. (eds) *Beischer & MacKay's Obstetrics, Gynaecology and the Newborn*, 4th edn. Chatswood: Elsevier, pp. 98–105.

Gammon, J. (1999) The psychological consequences of source isolation: a review of the literature. *Journal of Clinical Nursing*, 8, 13–21.

Gee, H. (2010) Dysfunctional labour. In: James, D.K. *et al.* (eds). *High Risk Pregnancy Management Options*, 4th edn. Philadelphia: Elsevier Saunders, pp. 1169–1184.

General Medical Council (2008) *Consent: Patients and Doctors Making Decisions Together*. London: General Medical Council.

Gentile, S. (2015) Managing antidepressant treatment in pregnancy and puerperium. Careful with that axe, Eugene. *Expert Opinion on Drug Safety*, 14, 1011–1014. doi: 10.1517/14740338.2015.1037273.

Getahun, B.S., Yeshi, M.M. & Roberts, D.J. (2012) Case records of the Massachusetts General Hospital: Case 34-2012: a 27-year-old woman in Ethiopia with severe pain, bleeding, and shock during labor. *New England Journal of Medicine*, 367, 1839–1845. doi: 10.1056/NEJMcpc1209508.

Gibson, J. *et al.* (2009) A systematic review of studies validating the Edinburgh Postnatal Depression Scale in antepartum and postpartum women. *Acta Psychiatrica Scandinavica*, 119, 350–364. doi: 10.1111/j.1600-0447.2009.01363.

Gobbo, B., Warren, J. & Hinshaw, K. (2017). Shoulder dystocia. In Leeman, L., Quinlan, J., Dresang, L., & Gregory, D. (Eds.). *ALSO Provider Manual*. (Ch. I. pp1–20). Leawood: American Academy of Family Physicians.

Grekin, R. & O'Hara, M.W. (2014) Prevalence and risk factors of postpartum posttraumatic stress disorder: a meta-analysis. *Clinical Psychology Review*, 34, 389–401. doi: 10.1016/j. cpr.2014.05.003.

Group B Strep Support (2016) *GBS infection in babies*. GBSS. Retrieved April 5, 2018 from http://gbss.org.uk/infection/

Guise, J-M. *et al.* (2010) Vaginal Birth After Cesarean: New Insights. Evidence Report/Technology Assessment No.191. (Prepared by the Oregon Health & Science University Evidence-based Practice Center under Contract No. 290-2007-10057-I). AHRQ Publication No. 10-E003. Rockville, MD: Agency for Healthcare Research and Quality.

Gupta, P., Sahu, R. & Huria, A. (2014) Acute uterine inversion: a simple modification of hydrostatic method of treatment. *Annals of Medical and Health Sciences Research*, 4, 264–267.

Gurol-Urganci, I. *et al.* (2013) Third- and fourth-degree perineal tears among primiparous women in England between 2000 and 2012: time trends and risk factors. *British Journal of Obstetrics and Gynaecology*, 120, 1516–1525.

Gutteridge, K. & Lazarus, R. (2008) Psychiatric disorders. In Robson, S.E. & Waugh, J. (eds) *Medical Disorders in Pregnancy. A Manual for Midwives*. Chichester: Blackwell Publishing, pp. 207–212.

Haas, D.M. *et al.* (2015) Ethanol for preventing preterm birth in threatened preterm labor. *Cochrane Database of Systematic Reviews*, Issue 11. Art. No.: CD011445. doi: 10.1002/14651858.CD011445.pub2.

Harper, L.M. *et al.* (2013) The risks and benefits of internal monitors in labouring patients. *American Journal of Obstetrics and Gynaecology*, 209(38), e1–e6.

Harris, J. (2008) How to … perform venepuncture. RCM. Retrieved April 5, 2018 from https://www.rcm.org.uk/news-views-and-analysis/analysis/how-to%E2%80%A6-perform-venepuncture

Harris, J. (2011). How to … perform a vaginal examination. *RCM*. Retrieved July, 5, 2017 from https://www.rcm.org.uk/news-views-and-analysis/analysis/how-to%E2%80%A6-perform-a-vaginal-examination.

Harty, E. (2017) Inserting peripheral intravenous cannulae – tips and tricks. *Update in Anaesthesia*. Retrieved April 5, 2018 from http://e-safe-anaesthesia.org/e_library/05/Peripheral_intravenous_cannulae_UPdate_2011.pdf

Haskett, R.F. (2010) Psychiatric illness. In: James, D.K. *et al.* (eds) *High Risk Pregnancy Management Options*, 4th edn. Philadelphia: Elsevier Saunders, pp. 997–1010.

Hautemaniere, A. *et al.* (2010) Factors determining poor practice in alcoholic hand gel rub technique in hospital workers. *Journal of Infection and Public Health*, 3, 25–34. doi: 10.1016/j/jiph.2009.09.005 PMID: 20701888.

Holmgren, C. *et al.* (2012) Uterine rupture with attempted vaginal birth after cesarean delivery. *Obstetrics and Gynecology*, 119, 725–731.

Hughes, R. *et al.* (2012) *The Prevention of Early-onset Neonatal Group B Streptococcal Disease. Green Top Guideline 36*, 2nd edn. London: Royal College of Obstetricians and Gynaecologists.

Impey, L.W.M. *et al.* on behalf of the Royal College of Obstetricians and Gynaecologists. (2017) Management of Breech Presentation. Green Top Guideline 20b. *British Journal of Obstetrics and Gynaecology*, 124, e151–e177. doi: 10.1111/1471-0528.14465.

Iribarren, J. *et al.* (2005) Post-traumatic stress disorder: evidence-based research for the third millennium. *Research Gate*, 2, 503–512. doi:10.1093/ecam/neh127.

Ismail, K.M.K. *et al.* (2013) Perineal Assessment and Repair Longitudinal Study (PEARLS): a matched-pair cluster randomized trial. *Bio Med Central, Medicine*, 11, 209. doi: http://doi.org/10.1186/1741-7015-11-209.

Israelsohn, N. (2015) Antepartum haemorrhage. In: Permezel, M., Walker, S. & Kyprianou, K. (eds) *Beischer & MacKay's Obstetrics, Gynaecology and the Newborn*, 4th edn. Chatswood: Elsevier, pp. 85–90.

Ito, F. *et al.* (2014) Incidence, diagnosis and pathophysiology of amniotic fluid embolism. *Journal of Obstetrics and Gynaecology*, 34, 580–584. doi: http://dx.doi.org/10.3109/01443615.2014.919996.

John, C.O., Orazulike, N. & Alegbeleye, J. (2015) An appraisal of retained placenta at the university of Port Harcourt teaching hospital: a five year review. *Niger J Med* 24, 99–102.

Johnson, R. & Taylor, W. (2016) *Skills for midwifery practice*, 4th edn. Edinburgh: Elsevier.

Johnston, T. & Grady, K. (2011) *Maternal Collapse in Pregnancy and the Puerperium. Green Top Guideline 56*. London: Royal College of Obstetricians and Gynaecologists.

Johnston, T.A. & Paterson-Brown, S. (2011) *Placenta Praevia, Placenta Praevia Accreta and Vasa Praevia: Diagnosis and Management. Green Top Guideline, No. 27*. London: Royal College of Obstetricians and Gynaecologists.

Joint United Kingdom (UK) Blood Transfusion and Tissue Transplantation Services Professional Advisory Committee (JPAC) (2017a) 4.4 Patient consent. Retrieved April 5, 2018 from https://www.transfusionguidelines.org/transfusion-handbook/4-safe-transfusion-right-blood-right-patient-right-time-and-right-place/4-4-patient-consent

Joint United Kingdom (UK) Blood Transfusion and Tissue Transplantation Services Professional Advisory Committee (JPAC) (2017b) 4.5 Authorising (or 'prescribing' the transfusion). Retrieved April 5, 2018 from http://www.transfusionguidelines.org/transfusion-handbook/4-safe-transfusion-right-blood-right-patient-right-time-and-right-place/4-5-authorising-or-prescribing-the-transfusion

Joint United Kingdom (UK) Blood Transfusion and Tissue Transplantation Services Professional Advisory Committee (JPAC) (2017c) 4.7 Pre-transfusion blood sampling. Retrieved April 5, 2018 from http://www.transfusionguidelines.org/transfusion-handbook/4-safe-transfusion-right-blood-right-patient-right-time-and-right-place/4-7-pre-transfusion-blood-sampling

Jones, I. *et al.* (2007) Bipolar affective puerperal psychosis: genome-wide significant evidence for linkage to chromosome 16. *American Journal of Psychiatry*, 164, 1099–1104. doi: 10.1176/appi.ajp.2008.08121899.

Kaur, K. *et al.* (2016) Amniotic fluid embolism. *Journal of Anaesthesiology Clinical Pharmacology*, 32, 153–159. doi: 10.4103/0970–9185.173356.

Kawakita, T. *et al.* (2016) Neonatal complications associated with use of fetal scalp electrode: a retrospective study. *British Journal of Obstetrics and Gynaecology*, 123, 1797–1803. doi: 10.1111/1471-0528.13817.

Kenyon, S., Boulvain, M. & Neilson, J.P. (2013) Antibiotics for preterm rupture of membranes. *Cochrane Database of Systematic Reviews*, Issue 12. Art. No.: CD001058. doi: 10.1002/14651858.CD001058.pub3.

Kettle, C., Dowswell, T. & Ismail, K. (2010) Absorbable suture materials for primary repair of episiotomy and second degree tears. *Cochrane Database of Systematic Reviews*, Issue 6. Art. No.: CD000006. doi: 10.1002/14651858.CD000006.pub2.

Kettle, C., Dowswell, T. & Ismail, K.M.K. (2012) Continuous and interrupted suturing techniques for repair of episiotomy or second-degree tears. *Cochrane Database of Systematic Reviews*, Issue 11. Art. No.: CD000947. doi: 10.1002/14651858.CD000947.pub3.

Kindberg, S. *et al.* (2008) Postpartum perineal repair performed by midwives: a randomised trial comparing two suture techniques leaving the skin unsutured. *British Journal of Gynaecology*, 115, 472–479. doi: 10.1111/j.1471-0528.2007.01637.x.

King, T. L. & Pinger, W. (2014) Evidence-based practice for intrapartum care: the pearls of midwifery. *Journal of Midwifery & Women's Health*, 59, 572–585. doi: 10.1111/jmwh.12261.

Knight, M. *et al.* (eds) (2014) On behalf of MBRRACE-UK. *Saving Lives, Improving Mothers' Care – Lessons Learned to Inform Future Maternity Care from the UK and Ireland Confidential Enquiries into Maternal Deaths and Morbidity 2009–12*. Oxford: National Perinatal Epidemiology Unit, University of Oxford.

Knight, M. *et al.* (eds) (2015) on behalf of MBRRACE-UK. *Saving Lives, Improving Mothers' Care – Surveillance of Maternal Deaths in the UK 2011–13 and Lessons Learned to Inform Maternity Care from the UK and Ireland Confidential Enquiries into Maternal Deaths and Morbidity 2009–13*. Oxford: National Perinatal Epidemiology Unit.

Lev-Wiesel, R., Daphna-Tekoah, S. & Hallak, M. (2009) Childhood sexual abuse as a predictor of birth-related post-traumatic stress and postpartum post-traumatic stress. *Child Abuse and Neglect*, 33, 877–887. doi: 10.1016/j.chiabu.2009.05.004.

Levi, M. (2015) Disseminated intravascular coagulation. *Medscape*. Retrieved April 5, 2018 from http://emedicine.medscape.com/article/199627-overview

Lewis, K.J.S., Foster, R.G. & Jones, I.R. (2016) Is sleep disruption a trigger for postpartum psychosis? *British Journal of Psychiatry*, 208, 409–411. doi: 10.1192/bjp.bp.115.166314.

Liddle, C. (2013) Postoperative care 1: principles of monitoring postoperative patients. *Nursing Times*, 109, 24–26.

Lissauer, T. & Fanaroff, A.A. (2011) *Neonatology at a Glance*, 2nd edn. Oxford: Wiley Blackwell.

Luettel, D., Beaumont, K. & Healey, F. (2007) *Recognising and Responding Appropriately to Early Signs of Deterioration of Hospitalised Patients*. London: National Patient Safety Agency.

Lupien, S.J. *et al.* (2011) Larger amygdala but no change in hippocampal volume in 10-year-old children exposed to maternal depressive symptomatology since birth. *Proceedings of the National Academy of Sciences*, 108, 14324.

Macdonald, S. & Johnson, G. (2017) *Mayes' Midwifery*, 15th edn. Edinburgh: Elsevier.

Mackeen, A.D. *et al.* (2014) Tocolytics for preterm premature rupture of membranes. *Cochrane Database of Systematic Reviews*, Issue 2. Art. No.: CD007062. doi: 10.1002/14651858.CD007062.pub3.

Mahendru, A.A. & Lees, C.C. (2011) Is intrapartum fetal blood sampling a gold standard diagnostic tool for fetal distress? *European Journal of Obstetrics and Gynecology and Reproductive Biology*, 152, 137–139. doi: http://dx.doi.org/10.1016/j.ejogrb.2010.12.044

Maher, M.A., Sayyed, T.M. & Elkhouly, N.I. (2017) Different routes and forms of uterotonics for treatment of retained placenta: a randomized clinical trial. *Journal of Maternal-Fetal and Neonatal Medicine*, 30, 2179–2184. doi: 10.1080/14767058.2016.1242124.

Martí-Carvajal, A.J. *et al.* (2009) Interventions for treating painful sickle cell crisis during pregnancy. *Cochrane Database of Systematic Reviews*, Issue 1. Art. No.: CD006786. doi: 10.1002/14651858.CD006786.pub2.

Martini, F., Nath, J. & Bartholomew, E. (2014) *Fundamentals of Anatomy and Physiology*, 10th edn. Harlow: Pearson Education Ltd.

Mavrides, E. *et al.* (2016) *Prevention and Management of Postpartum Haemorrhage. Green Top Guideline 52*. London: Royal College of Obstetricians and Gynaecologists.

Melamed, N. *et al.* (2012) Third- and fourth-degree perineal tears – incidence and risk factors. *Journal of Maternal-Fetal and Neonatal Medicine*, 26, 660–664. doi:10.3109/14767058.2012.746308.

Mercer, B.M. (2007) Is there a role for tocolytic therapy during conservative management of preterm premature rupture of the membranes? *Clinical Obstetrics and Gynecology*, 50, 487–496.

Moake, J. (2016) Disseminated intravascular coagulation. MSD Manual. Retrieved April 5, 2018 from http://www.msdmanuals.com/en-gb/professional/hematology-and-oncology/coagulation-disorders/disseminated-intravascular-coagulation-dic

Morgan, D., Hughes, R. & Kinsella, S. (2012) *Bacterial Sepsis in Pregnancy. Green Top Guideline 64b*. London: Royal College of Obstetricians and Gynaecologists.

Morrell, C.J. *et al.* (2016) A systematic review, evidence synthesis and meta-analysis of quantitative and qualitative studies evaluating the clinical effectiveness, the cost-effectiveness, safety and acceptability of interventions to prevent postnatal depression. *Health Technology Assessment*, 20, 1366–5278. doi: 10.3310/hta20370.

Murphy, N. and Cullinan, B. (2017) Maternal resuscitation and trauma. In: Leeman, L. *et al.* (eds). *ALSO Provider Manual*. Leawood: American Academy of Family Physicians, pp. 1–21.

Myatt, L. *et al.* (2012) On behalf of National Institute of Child Health and Human Development (NICHD) Maternal-Fetal Medicine Units (MFMU) Network. First-trimester prediction of preeclampsia in nulliparous women at low risk. *Obstetrics and Gynecology*, 119, 1234–1242. doi: 10.1097/AOG.0b013e3182571669.

Nahum, G.G. (2015) Uterine rupture in pregnancy. Medscape. Retrieved April 5, 2018 from http://reference.medscape.com/article/275854-overview

National Heart Lung and Blood Institute (NHLBI) (2012) What are the risks of a blood transfusion? Retrieved April 5, 2018 from https://www.nhlbi.nih.gov/health/health-topics/topics/bt/risks

National Institute for Health and Clinical Excellence (NICE) (2008) Induction of labour. Clinical Guideline CG 70. Retrieved April 5, 2018 from https://www.nice.org.uk/guidance/cg70/evidence/full-guideline-241871149

National Institute for Health and Care Excellence (NICE) (2010) Hypertension in pregnancy: diagnosis and management. Clinical Guideline CG 107. Retrieved April 5, 2018 from http://www.nice.org.uk/guidance/cg107

National Institute for Health and Care Excellence (NICE) (2011) Caesarean section. Clinical Guideline CG 132. Retrieved April 5, 2018 from nice.org.uk/guidance/cg132

National Institute for Health and Care Excellence (NICE) (2012a) NHS Evidence. Hypertension in pregnancy: Evidence Update 16 May 2012. A summary of selected new evidence relevant to NICE clinical guideline 107 'The management of hypertensive disorders during pregnancy' (2010). Retrieved April 5, 2018 from https://www.nice.org.uk/guidance/cg107/evidence/evidence-updates-pdf-134790445

National Institute for Health and Care Excellence (NICE) (2012b) Infection: prevention and control of healthcare associated infections in primary and community care. Clinical guideline CG 139. Retrieved April 5, 2018 from http://www.nice.org.uk/guidance/cg139

National Institute for Health and Care Excellence (NICE) (2013) *Induction of labour. Evidence update. Clinical Guideline CG 70*. London: Royal College of Obstetricians and Gynaecologists.

National Institute for Health and Care Excellence (NICE) (2014) Intrapartum care for healthy women and babies. Clinical Guideline CG 190. Retrieved April 5, 2018 from https://www.nice.org.uk/guidance/cg190/resources/intrapartum-care-for-healthy-women-and-babies-35109866447557

National Institute for Health and Care Excellence (NICE) (2015a) NICE Pathways. Intrapartum Care Overview. Retrieved April 5, 2018 from https://pathways.nice.org.uk/pathways/intrapartum-care

National Institute for Health and Care Excellence (NICE) (2015b) Preterm labour and birth. NICE Guideline NG 25. Retrieved April 5, 2018 from https://www.nice.org.uk/guidance/ng25

National Institute for Health and Care Excellence (NICE) (2016a) Diagnosing venous thromboembolism in primary, secondary and tertiary care. Retrieved April 5, 2018 from http://pathways.nice.org.uk/pathways/venous-thromboembolism

National Institute for Health and Care Excellence (NICE) (2016b) Treating venous thromboembolism. Retrieved April 5, 2018 from http://pathways.nice.org.uk/pathways/venous-thromboembolism

National Institute for Health and Care Excellence (NICE) (2016c) Preterm labour and birth. Quality standard QS135. Retrieved April 5, 2018 from https://www.nice.org.uk/guidance/qs135 8.1.16

National Institute for Health and Care Excellence (NICE) (2016d) Delay and complications in second stage labour. NICE Intrapartum care pathway. Retrieved April 5, 2018 from http://pathways.nice.org.uk/pathways/intrapartum-care

National Institute for Health and Care Excellence (NICE) (2016e) Recognising risk factors for infection during pregnancy, labour and birth. Pathway. Retrieved April 5, 2018 from http://pathways.nice.org.uk/pathways/antibiotics-for-early-onset-neonatal-infection

National Institute for Health and Care Excellence (NICE) (2017a) NICE Pathways. Care in 3rd stage of labour. Care overview. Retrieved April 5, 2018 from https://pathways.nice.org.uk/pathways/intrapartum-care/care-in-third-stage-of-labour

National Institute for Health and Care Excellence (NICE) (2017b) Interpretation of cardiotocograph traces. Clinical Guideline CG 190. Retrieved April 5, 2018 from https://www.nice.org.uk/guidance/cg190/resources/interpretation-of-cardiotocograph-traces-pdf-248732173

National Patient Safety Agency (NPSA) (2006) Right patient, right blood: advice for safer blood transfusions. NPSA. Retrieved April 5, 2018 from http://www.nrls.npsa.nhs.uk/resources/collections/right-patient-right-blood/

Neill, A. & Thornton, S. (2002) Secondary postpartum haemorrhage. *Journal of Obstetrics and Gynaecology*, 22, 119–122.

Neilson, J.P. (2015) Fetal electrocardiogram (ECG) for fetal monitoring during labour. *Cochrane Database of Systematic Reviews*, Issue 12. Art. No.: CD00011612. doi: 10.1002/14651858.CD000116.pub5.

Nelson-Piercy, C., MacCallum, P. & Mackillop, L. (2015) *Reducing the Risk of Venous Thrombo-Embolism During Pregnancy and the Puerperium. Green Top Guideline No. 37a.* London: Royal College of Obstetricians and Gynaecologists.

Nikpoor, P. & Bain, E. (2013) Analgesia for forceps delivery. *Cochrane Database of Systematic Reviews*, Issue 9. Art. No.: CD008878. doi: 10.1002/14651858.CD008878.pub2.

Nursing and Midwifery Council (NMC) (2007) *Standards for Medicine Management*. London: NMC.

Nursing and Midwifery Council (NMC) (2008) *Standards to Support Learning and Teaching in Practice*. London: NMC.

Nursing and Midwifery Council (NMC) (2009) *Standards for Pre-Registration Midwifery Education*. London: NMC.

Nursing and Midwifery Council (NMC) (2011) *Standards for Competence for Registered Midwives*. London: NMC.

Nursing and Midwifery Council (NMC) (2015) *The Code*. London: NMC.

Nursing and Midwifery Council (NMC) (2017) *Revalidation*. London: NMC.

O' Mahony, F., Hofmeyr, G.J. & Menon, V. (2010) Choice of instruments for assisted vaginal delivery. *Cochrane Database of Systematic Reviews*, Issue 11. Art. No.: CD005455. doi: 10.1002/14651858.CD005455.pub2.

Office for National Statistics. (ONS)(2016). Birth characteristics in England and Wales 2016. Statistical bulletin. ONS. Retrieved 23rd May 2018 from https://www.ons.gov.uk/peoplepopulationandcommunity/birthsdeathsandmarriages/livebirths/bulletins/birthcharacteristicsinenglandandwales/2016

Pasupathy, D. *et al.* (2012) *Bacterial Sepsis Following Pregnancy. Green Top Guideline 64a*. London: Royal College of Obstetricians and Gynaecologists.

Paterson-Brown, S. & Bamber, J. (2014) on behalf of the MBRRACE-UK haemorrhage chapter writing group. Prevention and treatment of haemorrhage. In Knight M *et al.* (eds) on behalf of MBRRACE-UK. *Saving Lives, Improving Mothers' Care – Lessons learned to inform future maternity care from the UK and Ireland Confidential Enquiries into Maternal Deaths and Morbidity 2009–12*. Oxford: National Perinatal Epidemiology Unit, University of Oxford, pp. 45–55.

Pergialiotis, V. *et al.* (2014) Risk factors for severe perineal lacerations during childbirth. *International Journal of Gynecology & Obstetrics*, 125, 6–14. doi: 10.1016/j.ijgo.2013.09.034.

Perkins, G., Colquhoun, M., Deakin, C., Handley, A., Smith, C. & Smyth, M. (2015). Resuscitation Council (UK) Guidelines. (2015). Adult basic life support and automated external defibrillation. *Resuscitation Council (UK)*. Retrieved November, 4, 2015 from https://www.resus.org.uk/resuscitation-guidelines/adult-basic-life-support-and-automated-external-defibrillation/

Permezel, M. (2015a) Caesarean section and trial of labour after caesarean. In: Permezel, M., Walker, S. & Kyprianou, K. (eds), *Beischer & MacKay's Obstetrics, Gynaecology and the Newborn*, 4th edn. Chatswood: Elsevier, pp. 267–275.

Permezel, M. (2015b) Hypertensive disorders of pregnancy eclampsia. In: Permezel, M., Walker, S. & Kyprianou, K. (eds), *Beischer & MacKay's Obstetrics, Gynaecology and the Newborn*, 4th edn. Chatswood: Elsevier, pp. 130–139.

Permezel, M. & Di Quinzio, M. (2015) The post dates pregnancy and rupture of the membranes before labour at term. In: Permezel, M., Walker, S. & Kyprianou, K. (eds), *Beischer & MacKay's Obstetrics, Gynaecology and the Newborn*, 4th edn. Chatswood: Elsevier, pp. 106–110.

Permezel, M. & Francis, J. (2015) Intrapartum Fetal Compromise. In: Permezel, M., Walker, S. & Kyprianou, K. (eds), *Beischer & MacKay's Obstetrics, Gynaecology and the Newborn*, 4th edn. Chatswood: Elsevier, pp. 277–284.

Permezel, M. & Paulsen, G. (2015) Instrumental delivery. In: Permezel, M., Walker, S. & Kyprianou, K. (eds), *Beischer & MacKay's Obstetrics, Gynaecology and the Newborn*, 4th edn. Chatswood: Elsevier, pp. 257–266.

Porreco, R.P. *et al.* (2009) The changing spectre of uterine rupture. *American Journal of Obstetrics Gynecology*, 200, 269. e1–4. doi: 10.1016/j.ajog.2008.09.874.

Priddis, H., Schmied, V. & Dahlen, H. (2014) Women's experiences following severe perineal trauma: a qualitative study. *Biomed Central (BMC) Women's Health*, 14, 32. doi: 10.1186/1472-6874-14-32.

Pusey, N. (2011) Women need scrub midwives. *Midwifery Matters, Summer* (129), 15.

Rather, H. *et al.* (2016) The art of performing a safe forceps delivery: a skill to revitalise. *Gynecology and Reproductive Biology*, 199, 49–54. doi: http://dx.doi.org/10.1016/j.ejogrb.2016.01.045.

Ray, A. & Ray, S. (2014) Antibiotic use before amniotomy (artificially rupturing the membranes) for reducing infections in mother and infant. *Cochrane Database of Systematic Reviews*. Art. No.: CD010626. doi: 10.1002/14651858.CD010626.pub2

Raynor, M., Marshall, J. & Jackson, K. (eds) (2012) *Midwifery Practice: Critical illness, Complications and Emergencies Case Book*. Maidenhead: Open University Press, Mc Graw-Hill Education.

Reichman, O. *et al.* (2008) Digital rotation from occipito-posterior to occipito-anterior decreases the need for cesarean section. *European Journal of Obstetrics and Gynecology and Reproductive Biology*, 171, 25–28. doi: 10.1016/j.ejogrb.2008.03.007.

Resuscitation Council (UK) Guidelines (2015) Adult basic life support and automated external defibrillation. Retrieved April 5, 2018 from https://www.resus.org.uk/resuscitation-guidelines/adult-basic-life-support-and-automated-external-defibrillation

Roberts, N.P. *et al.* (2010) Early psychological interventions to treat acute traumatic stress symptoms. *Cochrane Database of Systematic Reviews*. Issue 3. Art. No.: CD007944. doi: 10.1002/14651858.CD007944.pub2.

Roberts, N. P. *et al.* (2016) Psychological therapies for post-traumatic stress disorder and comorbid substance use disorder. *Cochrane Database of Systematic Reviews*. Art. No.: CD010204. doi: 10.1002/14651858.CD010204.pub2

Royal College of Midwives (2012) *Evidence Based Guidelines for Midwifery-Led Care in Labour. Suturing the Perineum*. Retrieved April 5, 2018 from https://www.rcm.org.uk/sites/default/files/Suturing%20the%20Perineum.pdf

Royal College of Obstetricians and Gynaecologists (RCOG) (2011) *Tocolysis for Women in Preterm Labour. Green Top Guideline 1B*. London: Royal College of Obstetrics and Gynaecology.

Royal College of Obstetricians and Gynaecologists (RCOG) (2014) *Perinatal Management of Pregnant Women at the Threshold of Infant Viability– the Obstetric Perspective (Scientific Impact Paper No. 41)*. London: Royal College of Obstetrics and Gynaecology.

Royal College of Obstetricians and Gynaecologists (RCOG) (2016) The OASI Care Bundle Project. Retrieved April 5, 2018 from https://www.rcog.org.uk/en/guidelines-research-services/audit-quality-improvement/third–and-fourth-degree-tears-project/

Saccone, G. & Berghella, V. (2015) Antibiotic prophylaxis for term or near-term premature rupture of membranes: metaanalysis of randomized trials. *American Journal of Obstetrics and Gynecology*, 212, 627. doi: 10.1016/j.ajog.2014.12.034.

Salim, R. *et al.* (2015) Precesarean prophylactic balloon catheters for suspected placenta accreta: a randomized controlled trial. *Obstetrics and Gynecology*, 126, 1022–1028.

Sangkomkamhang, U.S. *et al.* (2015) Antenatal lower genital tract infection screening and treatment programs for preventing preterm delivery. *Cochrane Database of Systematic Reviews*, Issue 2. Art. No.: CD006178. doi: 10.1002/14651858.CD006178.pub3.

Scales, K. (2008) A practical guide to venepuncture and blood sampling. *Nursing Standard*, 22, 29–36.

Shlamovitz, G. (2017) Intravenous cannulation. Medscape. Retrieved April 5, 2018 from http://emedicine.medscape.com/article/1998177-overview#a2

Sharma, V. & Burt, V.K. (2011) DSM-V: modifying the postpartum-onset specifier to include hypomania. *Archive of Women's Mental Health*, 14, 67–69. doi: 10.1007/s00737-010-0182-2.

Shinar, S. *et al.* (2016) Distribution of third-stage length and risk factors for its prolongation. *American Journal of Perinatology*, 33, 1023–1028. doi: 10.1055/s-0036-1572426.

Smith, L.A. *et al.* (2013) Incidence of and risk factors for perineal trauma: a prospective observational study. *Bio Med Central. Pregnancy and Childbirth*, 13, 59. doi: 10.1186/1471-2393-13-59.

Smyth, R.M.D., Markham, C. & Dowswell, T. (2013) Amniotomy for shortening spontaneous labour. *Cochrane Database of systematic Reviews*. Art. No.: CD006167. doi: 10.1002/14651858.CD006167.pub4

Society of Critical Care Medicine (2016) Bundles. Surviving Sepsis Campaign. Retrieved April 5, 2018 from http://www.survivingsepsis.org/Bundles/Pages/default.aspx

Song, J-M. & Chae, J-H. (2016) Update on Current Treatment Options for Posttraumatic Stress Disorder. ResearchGate. Retrieved April 5, 2018 from https://www.researchgate.net/publication/268441069_Update_on_Current_Treatment_Options_for_Posttraumatic_Stress_Disorder

Steiner, P. & Lushbaugh, C. (1941) Maternal pulmonary embolism by fluid as a cause of obstetric shock and unexpected deaths in obstetrics. *Journal of the American Medical Association*, 117, 1245–1254.

Stephenson, M., Shur, J., Black, J. (2013) *How to Perform Clinical Procedures*. Oxford: Wiley Blackwell.

Stone, A.B. (2008) Book reviews. The spectrum of psychotic disorders: neurobiology, etiology and pathogenesis. *Psychiatric Services*, 59, 118. doi: 10.1176/ps.2008.59.1.118.

Sultan, A.H. (1999) Editorial: obstetric perineal injury and anal incontinence. *Clinical Risk*, 5, 193–196.

Suwannachat, B., Lumbiganon, P. & Laopaiboon, M. (2012) Rapid versus stepwise negative pressure application for vacuum extraction assisted vaginal delivery. *Cochrane Database of Systematic Reviews*, Issue 8. Art. No.: CD006636. doi: 10.1002/14651858.CD006636.pub3.

Svigos, J.M., Dodd J.M. & Robinson, J.S. (2010) Prelabor rupture of the membranes. In: James, D.K. *et al.* (eds) *High Risk Pregnancy Management Options*, 4th edn. Philadelphia: Elsevier Saunders, pp 1091–1100.

The Rotunda Hospital (2014) The Rotunda Hospital Clinical Report 2014. Retrieved November, 11, 2016 from https://rotunda.ie/rotunda-pdfs/Clinical%20Reports/Rotunda%20Hospital%20Annual%20Clinical%20Report%202014.pdf

Thiagamoorthy, G. *et al.* (2014) National survey of perineal trauma and its subsequent management in the United Kingdom. *International Urogynecology*, 25, 1621–1627. doi: 10.1007/s00192-014-2406-x.

Thompson, A. & Greer, I. (2015) *Thrombo-Embolic Disease in Pregnancy and the Puerperium: Acute Management. Green Top Guideline No. 37b*. London: Royal College of Obstetricians and Gynaecologists.

Thomson, A. & Ramsay, J. (2011) *Antepartum Haemorrhage. Green Top Guideline No. 63*. London: Royal College of Obstetricians and Gynaecologists.

United Kingdom Teratology Information Services (UKTIS) (2011) Use of tobacco in pregnancy. Version 1. Summary. Retrieved April 5, 2018 from http://www.medicinesinpregnancy.org/bumps/monographs/USE-OF-TOBACCO-IN-PREGNANCY/

Urner, F., Zimmermann, R. & Krafft, A. (2014) Manual removal of the placenta after vaginal delivery: an unsolved problem. *Journal of Pregnancy*. doi: 10.1155/2014/274651

Walker, M.G. *et al.* (2013) Multidisciplinary management of invasive placenta praevia. *Journal of Obstetrics and Gynaecology Canada*, 35, 417.

Walsh, D. (2010) Labour rhythms. In: Walsh, D & Downe, S. (eds) *Essential Midwifery Practice: Intrapartum Care*. Oxford: Wiley Blackwell, pp. 63–80.

Webb, R. & Ayers, S. (2014) Cognitive biases in processing infant emotion by women with depression, anxiety and post-traumatic stress disorder in pregnancy or after birth: a systematic review. *Cognitive Emotion*, 29, 1278–1294. doi: 10.1080/02699931.2014.977849.

Wei, S. *et al.* (2013) Early amniotomy and early oxytocin for prevention of, or therapy for, delay in first stage spontaneous labour compared with routine care. *Cochrane Database Systematic Review*, Issue 7. Art. No.: CD006794. doi: 10.1002/14651858.CD006794.pub4.

Wesseloo, R. *et al.* (2016) Risk of postpartum relapse in bipolar disorder and postpartum psychosis: a systematic review and meta-analysis. *American Journal of Psychiatry*, 173, 117–127. doi: 10.1176/appi.ajp.2015.15010124.

Wojcieszek, A.M., Stock, O.M. & Flenady, V. (2014) Antibiotics for prelabour rupture of membranes at or near term. *Cochrane Database of Systematic Reviews, Cochrane Pregnancy and Childbirth Group*. doi: 10.1002/14651858.CD001807.pub2.

World Health Organization (WHO) (2009) Guidelines on hand hygiene in health care. Retrieved April 5, 2018 from http://apps.who.int/iris/bitstream/10665/44102/1/9789241597906_eng.pdf 7.7.16

World Health Organization (WHO) (2010) *International Statistical Classification of Diseases and Related Health Problems 10th Revision*. Retrieved April 5, 2018 from http://apps.who.int/classifications/icd10/browse/2010/en

World Health Organization (WHO) (2014) *Recommendations for Augmentation of Labour*. Geneva: WHO Press.

Wyllie, J., Ainsworth, S. and Tinnion, R. (2015) Resuscitation and support of transition of babies at birth. Resuscitation Council (UK). Retrieved April 5, 2018 from https://www.resus.org.uk/resuscitation-guidelines/resuscitation-and-support-of-transition-of-babies-at-birth/

Yonkers, K.A. *et al.* (2014) Pregnant women with posttraumatic stress disorder and risk of preterm birth. *Journal of American Medical Association Psychiatry*, 71, 897–904.

Yonkers, K.A., Vigod, S. & Ross, L.E. (2011) Diagnosis, pathophysiology and management of mood disorders in pregnancy and postpartum women. *Obstetrica Gynecologica*, 117, 961–977. doi: 10.1097/AOG.0b013e31821187a7.

Zhang, J., Troendle, J.F. & Yancey, M. (2002) Reassessing the labour curve. *American Journal of Obstetrics and Gynaecology*, 187, 824–828.

Index

Page numbers in *italic* refer to figures.
Page number in **bold** refer to tables and boxes.

Aberdeen knots, *102*
abruption of placenta, 14, 15
  twins, **28**
accelerations, fetal heart, **76**
accountability, 3
accreta syndromes, *36*, 37
acidosis (metabolic), fetus, 81
adherens/adherent placenta, 35, 36–37
adrenaline, neonatal resuscitation, **12**
agonal gasping, 11
airway
  maternal resuscitation, *8*, 9
  neonatal resuscitation, 11
alcohol hand rubs, 111
allergy, amniotic fluid embolism, 57
Amnihook, *96*, 97
amniotic fluid embolism, 56–57, 97
amniotomy *see* artificial rupture of membranes
anaesthesia
  Caesarean section, 69
  perineal repair, 103
anal sphincter, trauma, 100–101
anaphylactoid syndrome of pregnancy, 57
android pelvis, *20*, 21
antepartum haemorrhage, 14–15
anthropoid pelvis, *20*, 21
antibiotics
  group B *Streptococcus*, 109
  postpartum haemorrhage, 19
  prelabour rupture of membranes, 61
  uterine dystocia, 33
anticonvulsants
  labetalol, 53
  magnesium sulphate, **50**, **52**, 53, 62, 63
antidepressants, 47
aortocaval compression, 9
apnoea
  maternal, 8–9
  neonatal, 11
artificial rupture of membranes, **32**, 96–97
  twins, 29
augmentation of labour, 21, **32**, 33, 96–99, *see also* artificial rupture of membranes; oxytocin
auscultation, 79

back pain, occipito posterior positions, 21
bag-valve-mask systems, *11*
balloon catheters, internal iliac arteries, 37
basilic vein, 91
betamethasone, 62
bi-valve speculum, *86*
bicarbonate, neonatal resuscitation, **12**
bipolar disorder, 47, 49
Bishop's score, **98**
blood groups, *94*
blood loss assessment, 15
blood sampling
  fetus, 80–81
    equipment, 73
  maternal, 90–91
    for blood transfusion, 95
blood tests, for Caesarean section, 69
blood transfusion, 15, 17, 94–95
blues, 47
bradycardia, fetal, 77
breastfeeding
  lithium, 49
  oestrogen and antidepressants, 47
breathing
  maternal resuscitation, *8*, 9
  neonatal resuscitation, *10*, 11–13
breech presentations, 24–25
  Caesarean section, 69
  twins, *28*
brow presentation, 22–23

Caesarean section
  adherens/adherent placenta after, 37
  cord presentation, 27
  perimortem, 9
  preparation for, 69
  receiving baby, 72–73
  role of scrub midwife, 70–71
calcium gluconate, **50**
cannulation, intravenous, 92–93
carboprost, postpartum haemorrhage, *18*
cardiac arrest, maternal, 9
cardiotocography, **76**, 77, 79, 99
catheter insertion forms, *74*
catheterisation
  internal iliac arteries, 37
  urinary, *74*, 88–89
cephalo-pelvic disproportion, 33
cerclage, cervical, *62*, 63
cerebral hypoxia, 53
cervix
  cerclage, *62*, 63
  effacement, *84*
charts
  fluid balance, *74*
  maternal monitoring, 82–83
  SBAR, 73, 75, *82*
chest compressions
  maternal resuscitation, 8, 9
  neonatal resuscitation, *10*, *12*, 13
chronic hypertension in pregnancy, defined, 51
circulation, maternal resuscitation, 9
Clinical Indicators Project, on OASI, 101
clonic stage, seizures, 53
clothing, infection control, 111
coagulation disorders, 54–59
  postpartum haemorrhage, 19
communication, 4–5
consent, 5, 69, 99
continuing professional development, 3
contractions, 33
  hypertonic, 99
cord clamping, 13
cord presentation, 26–27
cord prolapse, 26–27
  prelabour rupture of membranes, 61
  twins, **28**, 29
corticosteroids
  hydrocortisone, 45
  prelabour rupture of membranes, 61
  preterm labour, 62, 63
Cusco speculum, *86*

D-dimer, 55
death *see* maternal mortality
debriefing, postnatal, 45
decelerations, fetal heart, *40*, 41, **76**, 77
deep transverse arrest, 33
deep vein thrombosis, 54–55
defibrillator, 9
dehiscence, uterine scars, 40–41
depression, *see also* bipolar disorder
  postnatal, 46–47
deteriorating woman, 82–83
dexamethasone, 62
dextrose, neonatal resuscitation, **12**
diazepam, 53
disseminated intravascular coagulation, 58–59
dizygotic twins, *28*, 29
drying neonate, 11
dystocia, 30–33
  instrumental vaginal delivery, 67
  manual removal of placenta, 35

early warning systems, *82*, 83
eclampsia, 51, 52–53
Edinburgh postnatal depression scale, **46**, 47
effacement, cervix, *84*
electrocardiotocography, 79
electronic fetal monitoring, 76–77
embolism, 54–59, *see also* thromboembolism
  amniotic fluid, 56–57, 97
emotional reactions to emergencies, 5
episiotomy
  breech presentations, 25
  face presentation, 23
  occipito posterior positions, 21
  twins, 29
ergometrine, postpartum haemorrhage, 17, *18*
escalation policy, deteriorating woman, 83
examination *per vaginam*, 84–87
exsanguination, second twin, **28**, 29
external cephalic version, 29, 69

face presentation, 22–23
failure to progress *see* augmentation of labour; uterine dystocia
fasting, for Caesarean section, 69
fetal blood sampling (see fetus)
fetus
  blood sampling, 73, 80–81
  fibronectin, 63
  hypoxia, *40*, 41, 61, 81
  monitoring, 76–81
  scalp electrodes, 78–79
  scalp stimulation, 77
  viability, 63
fibronectin, fetal, 63

Midwifery Emergencies at a Glance, First Edition. Denise (Dee) Campbell and Susan M. Carr. Published 2018 by John Wiley & Sons, Ltd.
Companion website: www.ataglanceseries.com/midwiferyemergencies

fluid balance charts, *74*
fluid therapy
antepartum haemorrhage, 15
neonatal resuscitation, **12**
postpartum haemorrhage, 17, *18*
pre-eclampsia, 51
focal placenta accreta, *36*, 37
forceps, *66*, 67
forewaters, **96**, 97
fourth-degree tears, 100–101
frank breech presentation, 24–25
fresh frozen plasma, for DIC, 59

gasping, agonal, 11
gel hand rubs, 111
gestational hypertension, definition, 51
gloves
infection control, 111
sterile, *70*
gowns, theatre staff, *70*, 71, 73
grand multiparity, retained placenta, 35
group B *Streptococcus*, 108–109

haemolysis, blood transfusion, 95
haemorrhage, **8**, 14–19, *see also* postpartum haemorrhage
antepartum, 14–15
hand hygiene, *110*
handovers, postoperative, 75
health care-associated infections, 111
heart rate
fetus, *40*, 41
neonatal resuscitation, *10*
HELLP syndrome, 51
HELPERR mnemonic, *30*, 31
Hemabate (carboprost), postpartum haemorrhage, *18*
heparin
for DIC, 59
for VTE, 55
HIV, fetal scalp electrodes and, 79
hydrocortisone, 45
hydrostatic replacement of uterus, 39
hypertension, definition, 51
hypertensive disorders, 50–53
hypertonic contractions, 99
hypoxia
cerebral (maternal), 53
fetus, *40*, 41, 61, 81
neonate, 11

identity bands
for baby, *72*, 73
for mother, 69
iliac arteries, balloon catheters, 37
immune response, amniotic fluid embolism, 57
incarcerated placenta, 35
indwelling catheters, *88*, 89
infections, 104–111
control, 110–111
fetal scalp electrodes and, 79
screening
group B *Streptococcus*, 109
preterm labour, 63
signs, 111
transmission, 107
urinary tract, 89
inflation breaths, 11, *12*
informed consent, 5, 69, 99
infusions, oxytocin, 98, 99
instrumental vaginal delivery, 66–67
instruments, surgical, *70*, 71
interlocked twins, **28**
intermittent catheterisation, 89
internal iliac arteries, balloon catheters, 37
intravenous cannulation, 92–93
inversion, uterus, 38–39
involution *see* subinvolution of uterus
isolation (source isolation nursing), 106–107

jaw thrust, *12*
jewellery, preparation for Caesarean section, 69

knee-chest position, *26*

labetalol, 53
labour
augmentation, 21, **32**, 33, 96–99, *see also* artificial rupture of membranes; oxytocin
dystocia, 32–33
instrumental vaginal delivery, 67
manual removal of placenta, 35
occipito posterior positions, 21
preterm, 62–63
instrumental vaginal delivery, 67
lactate, fetal blood, 81
liquor, **96**
lithium, 49
local anaesthesia, perineal repair, 103
lochia, observations, 75
long internal rotation, 21
Løvset manoeuvre, *24*, 25

magnesium sulphate, **50**, **52**, 53, 62, 63
major obstetric haemorrhage, 15
malpresentations, 20–27
manic depression (bipolar disorder), 47, 49
manual removal of placenta, 34–35
mask ventilation, 11, *12*
massive obstetric haemorrhage, 15
maternal monitoring, 82–89
maternal mortality, 9
amniotic fluid embolism, 57
mental health-related, *48*
postpartum haemorrhage, *40*, 41
maternal resuscitation, 8–9
blood transfusion, 15, 17
maternal sepsis, 104–105
MBRRACE report, 57, *104*
Mauriceau–Smellie–Veit manoeuvre, *24*, 25
MBRRACE report, maternal sepsis, 57, *104*
McDonald suture, *62*
McRoberts position, *30*, 31
meconium, 13, **96**
median cubital vein, 91
mento anterior face delivery, 22
mento vertical diameter, *22*, 23
MEOWS (Modified Early Obstetric Warning System), 83
metabolic acidosis, fetus, 81
misoprostol, postpartum haemorrhage, 17
Modified Early Obstetric Warning System, 83
monitoring
fetus, 76–81
maternal, 82–89
monozygotic twins, *28*, 29
mood disorders, 46–47
mortality, *see also* maternal mortality
infant, multiple pregnancy, 29
perinatal, vasa praevia, 27
multiple pregnancy, 29

National Early Warning System, 83
needle-stick injury, 90
needles, perineal repair, *102*
neonatal infection
group B *Streptococcus*, 108–109
signs, 111
neonatal resuscitation, 10–13
nifedipine, 62

OASI Care Bundle Project, **100**, 101
observations, postoperative, 75
obstetric anal sphincter injuries (OASI), 100–103
occipito posterior positions, 21
postpartum haemorrhage, 19
shoulder dystocia, 30–31
obstetric early warning charts, *82*
obstructed labour, 33

occipito posterior positions, 20–21
oestrogen, 47
oligohydramnios, 23
operating theatre
preparation and transfer to, 68–69
receiving the baby, 72–73
role of scrub midwife, 70–71
oxygen
antepartum haemorrhage, 15
maternal resuscitation, **8**
neonatal resuscitation, *10*, 13
oxytocin, *16*, 17, *18*, **32**, 97, 98–99, *see also* Syntocinon

pain
occipito posterior positions, 21
uterine rupture, 41
pelvis, shapes, *20*, 21
per vaginam examination, 84–87
perineal trauma, 100–103
occipito posterior positions, 21
postpartum haemorrhage, 19
pessary, cervical, *62*, 63
pH, fetal blood, 81
placenta
abruption, **14**, 15
twins, 28
adhered, 36–37
ischaemia, 51
manual removal, 34–35
succenturiate lobe, *26*, 27
placenta accreta, *36*, 37
placenta increta, *36*, 37
placenta percreta, *36*, 37
placenta praevia, **14**, 15
adherens/adherent placenta after, 37
platelet transfusions, 59
polyhydramnios, 23
positive end expiratory pressure, neonatal resuscitation, 11
post-ictal stage, eclampsia, 53
post-traumatic stress disorder, 44–45
postnatal debriefing, 45
postnatal depression, 46–47
postoperative care, 74–75
postoperative procedures, 71
postpartum haemorrhage
accreta syndromes, 37
manual removal of placenta, 35
maternal mortality, *40*, 41
primary, 16–17
secondary, 17, 18–19
postpartum psychosis, 48–49
pre-eclampsia, 50–51
pre-registration education, standards, *2*
prelabour rupture of membranes, 60–61
preoperative checklist, *68*
preoperative medication, 69
preterm babies, 61
breech presentations, 25
resuscitation, 13
preterm labour, 62–63
instrumental vaginal delivery, 67
primary postpartum haemorrhage, 16–17
professional standards, 2–3
progesterone, vaginal, 63
prolapse, uterus, 39
prolonged labour *see* uterine dystocia
prostaglandin analogues, postpartum haemorrhage, 17
puerperal psychosis, 48–49
pulmonary embolism, 54–55
pulse oximeters, 11

ranitidine, Caesarean section, 69
record keeping, 3
recovery rooms, 75
regional anaesthesia, Caesarean section, 69
respiratory arrest, magnesium sulphate, **50**

Resuscitaire, *72*, 73
resuscitation, 8–13
retained products of conception, 19
reverse Wood's screw, *30*
rotation, short internal, 21
Rubin manoeuvres, *30*
rupture, uterus, 40–41
rupture of membranes, *see also* artificial rupture of membranes
prelabour, 60–61

SBAR charts, 73, 75, *82*
scalp electrodes, fetal, 78–79
scalp stimulation, fetal, 77
scar dehiscence, uterus, 40–41
schistocytes, 59
screening for infections
group B *Streptococcus*, 109
preterm labour, 63
scrub midwives, 70–71
secondary postpartum haemorrhage, 17, 18–19
seizures, eclampsia, 53
selection of midwives, 3
self-assessment questions and answers, 113–122
semilunar valves, veins, 91
Semmelweis, Ignaz, 111
sepsis, maternal, 104–105
MBRRACE report, 57, *104*
Sepsis 6 Care Bundle, *104*, 105
Shirodkar suture, *62*
short internal rotation, 21
shoulder dystocia, 30–31
Sims speculum, *86*
SIRS (systemic inflammatory response), 105
skills, updates, 3
skin-to-skin contact, 73
sleep deprivation, 49
sodium bicarbonate, neonatal resuscitation, **12**
source isolation nursing, 106–107
speculum examination, 86–87
sphincter injuries, 100–103
square surgeon knot, *102*
standards, professional, 2–3
station, *84*
instrumental vaginal delivery, **66**
status eclampticus, 53
Streptococcus, group B, 108–109
sub-mento bregmatic diameter, *22*
sub-mento vertical diameter, *22*, 23
subinvolution of uterus, 19
succenturiate lobe, placenta, *26*, 27
suction, neonatal resuscitation, 13
suicide rates, *48*
suicide risk, 47
surgery, preparation for, 68–69
sutures, perineal trauma, 101, 102–103
Syntocinon, 6, 7
systemic inflammatory response (SIRS), 105

T-piece masks, *11*
teams
antepartum haemorrhage, 15
Caesarean section, 69
communication, 5
deteriorating woman, 83
postpartum haemorrhage, 17
source isolation nursing, 107
tears (perineal), 100–103
occipito posterior positions, 21
postpartum haemorrhage, 19
third-degree tears, 100–101
thromboembolism, venous, 54–55, 75
tocolytics, 62, 63
prelabour rupture of membranes, 61
tonic stage, seizures, 53
training, 3
tranexamic acid, 17
transient bacteria, 111
trauma, perineal, 100–103
twins, 28–29

ultrasound, retained products of conception, 19
umbilical cord, *see also* cord prolapse
breech presentations, 25
preterm labour, 63
twins, **28**, 29
urinary tract infections, 89
uterine dystocia, 32–33
instrumental vaginal delivery, 67
manual removal of placenta, 35
uterus
abnormalities, *32*
aorto-caval compression, 9
inversion, 38–39
rupture, 40–41
subinvolution, 19

vacuum extraction, 67
vagina, examination, 84–87
vasa praevia, 27
veins
anatomy, 91, 93
thromboembolism, 54–55, 75
velamentous insertion of cord, *26*
venepuncture, 90–91
ventilation, neonate, 11, *12*
ventilation (room), source isolation nursing, 107
version, external cephalic, 29, 69
viability, fetus, 63

washing (hand hygiene), *110*
Wood's screw, *30*

Notes